Practical Breastfeeding

AN ILLUSTRATED GUIDE FOR PARENTS

Caoimhe Whelan IBCLC, MSc (research)

Illustrated by Lauren Rebbeck

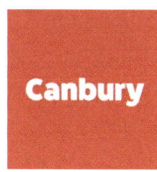

MEDICAL DISCLAIMER

The information in this book is the result of years of practice experience and research by the author. The information in this book, by necessity, is general in nature and not a substitute for an evaluation or treatment by a competent medical specialist. If you believe you need medical intervention, please see a medical professional as soon as possible. The information in this book is intended for parents in the United Kingdom and the Republic of Ireland.

First published by Canbury Press 2025
This edition published 2025

Publisher: Canbury Press (www.canburypress.com)
14 Beresford Rd, London, KT2 6LR, United Kingdom
EU Authorised Representative: Easy Access System Europe
- Mustamäe tee 50, 10621 Tallinn, Estonia, gpsr.requests@easproject.com
Printed and bound in Czechia by Finidr

Canbury Press
Kingston upon Thames, Surrey, United Kingdom
Canburypress.com

All rights reserved.

© Caoimhe Whelan and Lauren Rebbeck, 2025.

Caoimhe Whelan and Lauren Rebbeck have asserted their right to be identified as the authors and illustrators of this work in accordance with Section 77 of the Copyright, Designs and Patents Act 1988.

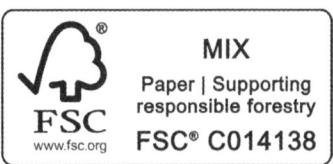

ISBN Paperback: 9781914487392
ISBN Ebook: 9781914487408

Design by Megan Sheer www.sheerbookdesign.com

I would like to dedicate this book to my mum
Mary Whelan (1944-2023)

Caoimhe

For Adam, my whole world
And for Quinn, my entire universe

Lauren

Contents

	Introduction	7
Chapter 1	Thinking About Breastfeeding	9
Chapter 2	Breasts, Colostrum, and Antenatal Hand Expression	37
Chapter 3	Birth and the Golden Hours	51
Chapter 4	The First Week	75
Chapter 5	Weeks Two and Three	103
Chapter 6	Life in the Fourth Trimester	121
Chapter 7	Using Social Media	135
Chapter 8	Sore Nipples and Tricky Nipples	143
Chapter 9	Mastitis, Blocked Ducts and Breast Pain	161
Chapter 10	Pumps and Pumping	173
Chapter 11	Postpartum Mental Health and Breastfeeding	189
Chapter 12	Breastfeeding and Sleep	207
Chapter 13	When Breastfeeding is Hard	225
Chapter 14	Low Milk Supply	245
Chapter 15	Drugs, Food and Alcohol	269
Chapter 16	Outside the Box Lactation	285
Chapter 17	Maternal Conditions/Illnesses and Breastfeeding	303
Chapter 18	Infant Conditions/Illnesses	311
Chapter 19	Breastfeeding Beyond the Fourth Trimester	323
Chapter 20	Stopping Breastfeeding	335
	Additional Resources	347
	Acknowledgements	350

Introduction

Hello and thanks for opening this book. I hope you and your baby have a positive experience of breastfeeding or providing your milk for your baby. As an International Board Certified Lactation Consultant (IBCLC) and the mother of three breastfed children, I know how rewarding breastfeeding can be. I also know it's not always easy. Unfortunately, social media can make new mothers feel worse by presenting a perfect image of motherhood and sometimes giving out unhelpful and incorrect advice.

I feel strongly that new parents should have access to good, clearly presented, evidence-based information. Which is why I wrote this book, because I couldn't find a modern, illustrated guide to breastfeeding. The topics covered have come up repeatedly during my work as an IBCLC supporting breastfeeding families.

While presenting my research findings into mothers' experiences of breastfeeding with low milk supply, I started working with Lauren Rebbeck, an illustrator (and a mum to toddler Quinn). Lauren's images blew me away: they were beautiful and conveyed sensitively and accurately what it is like to be a new mother, and the strong emotions that can be stirred up by feeding challenges.

Practical Breastfeeding is not intended to take the place of skilled peer and professional breastfeeding support. But hopefully it will give you some very useful information on breastfeeding and being a new mother, and some pointers on how to access specialist help.

It's been written so that you can either read it through or dip in and out of chapters when you need to know about a particular subject.

Best of luck with your breastfeeding journey! Please be kind to yourself as you navigate new parenthood. There will be times when it is joyful and times when it's really hard. Remember that breastfeeding looks different for everyone – it's not one-size-fits-all. Give yourself time and space to figure out what breastfeeding will look like for you, and expect that you will learn as you go.

Caoimhe Whelan

A note of terms and acronyms used:

COLOSTRUM:
This is the first milk that you start to make, usually around week 16 of your pregnancy. You make colostrum in small volumes for the first few days after your baby is born, until your milk volume increases with the onset of Lactogenesis II (often referred to as milk coming in).

LACTATION:
This is the word used to describe the physiological process of making milk.

LACTOGENESIS I:
This is the term used to describe the beginning of milk production which happens when your body starts to produce colostrum during pregnancy.

LACTOGENESIS II:
This is when your breasts start to produce larger volumes of milk, and it usually happens on around day three after you give birth.

FOURTH TRIMESTER:
There are three three-month long trimesters during your pregnancy. The fourth trimester describes the first three months of your baby's life after they are born.

SKIN-TO-SKIN CONTACT (SSC):
Skin-to-skin contact is simply holding your baby while they wear only a nappy and you have your top off, so that their skin is in contact with yours. You can read about SSC in Chapter 3.

LATCH:
This word describes how a baby attaches to your breast. They open wide, get a mouthful of breast tissue and remain attached so that they can breastfeed.

BREASTMILK:
This is the term I use in the book to describe the milk that your breasts make. Some people may prefer to use terms such as *mother's milk* or *human milk*.

BREASTFEEDING:
In the interests of clarity, I use this term in the book to refer to any kind of milk feeding your baby does at your breast. However, I acknowledge that some people may prefer to use other terms, for example, *chestfeeding*, *body feeding*, or simply *feeding*.

INTERNATIONAL BOARD-CERTIFIED LACTATION CONSULTANT (IBCLC):
An IBCLC is generally regarded as the gold standard qualification in breastfeeding and lactation support. IBCLCs must accrue 1000 hours of clinical lactation support and have relevant health and breastfeeding qualifications and education hours. For further information, see https://iblce.org/.

PUMPING:
This is the word used to describe removing milk from your breasts using a breast pump. Pumping is also sometimes described as *expressing*.

MOTHER/PARENT AND WOMAN/PERSON:
I use these terms interchangeably in the book. I am aware that not all lactating parents will identify as a *mother* or *woman* and I have endeavoured to use additive language as much as possible. This book aims to be inclusive and to support all parents, irrespective of gender identity or orientation.

CHAPTER 1

Thinking About Breastfeeding

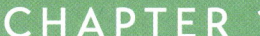

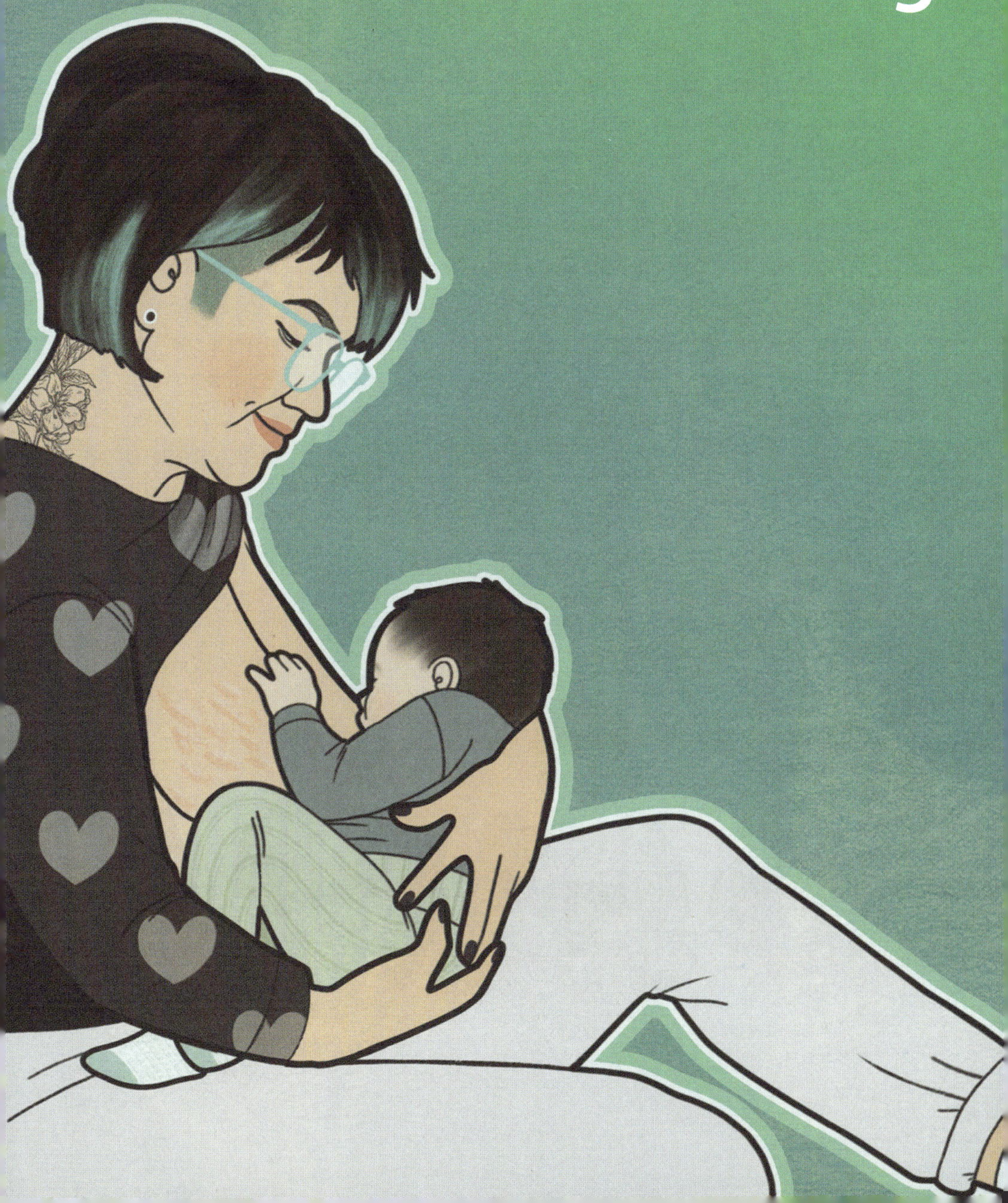

Introduction

Congratulations! If you are reading this chapter, you are probably pregnant or at the start of your parenting journey and thinking about either breastfeeding your baby or providing them with your milk. Breastfeeding is the optimal way to feed your baby as breast milk provides all the nutrients and immune protection they need. Breastfed babies are less likely to get respiratory and gut infections, need antibiotics or hospitalisation. They also have a lower risk of developing allergies, childhood cancers and type 1 diabetes. Breastfeeding is good for you too as it means you are less likely to develop type 2 diabetes, obesity, heart disease, osteoporosis, breast cancer and ovarian cancer. Breastfeeding also helps your body to recover after you give birth by shrinking your womb back to its normal size. The World Health Organisation recommends exclusively breastfeeding your baby for 6 months, and then continuing with other complementary foods for up to two years and beyond. This recommendation is based on the strong evidence that breastfeeding is the most healthy option for both mothers and babies. However, this does not mean that you *have to* breastfeed exclusively for six months to have a positive breastfeeding experience.

Some mothers choose to breastfeed for a shorter duration or to supplement with infant formula. And some mothers are unable to exclusively breastfeed. One of the messages I aim to convey in this book is that any amount of breastfeeding or breast milk that you provide for your baby is a good thing and should be celebrated.

Breastfeeding is free!

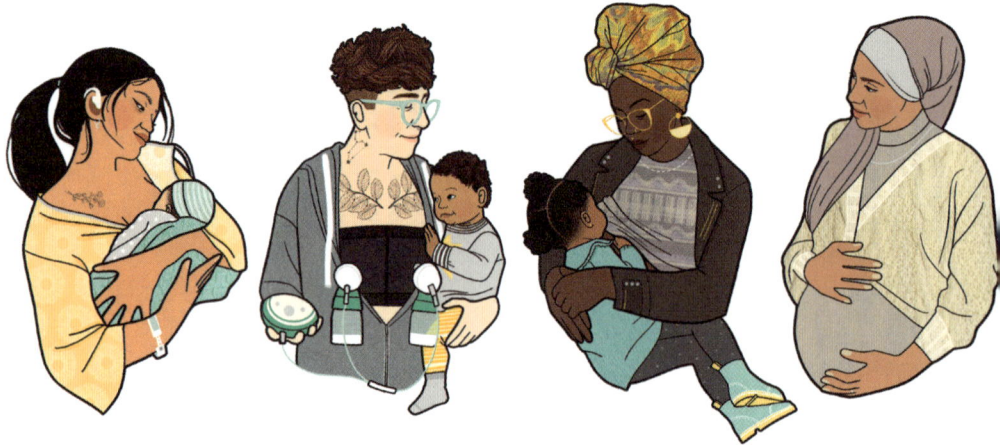

Breastfeeding is good for babies

- Provides all the nutrients babies need in the first 6 months
- Gives comfort to babies
- The antibodies in breastmilk help babies develop a strong immune system
- Lower risk of respiratory, ear and gut infections and of hospital admission
- Lower risk of asthma and allergies
- Lower risk of obesity, type 1 diabetes and sudden infant death syndrome (SIDS)
- Helps protect against some childhood cancers
- Less likely to need orthodontics
- Reduced likelihood of cardiovascular disease in adulthood
- Less likely to experience diarrhoea, constipation and vomiting
- Breastfeeding promotes cognitive development

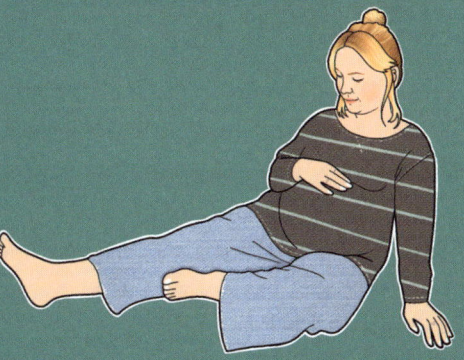

Breastfeeding is good for mothers

- Supports postpartum recovery – helps the womb contract to its normal size, and can aid weight loss
- Promotes the flow of feel good hormones oxytocin and prolactin and reduces the risk of postpartum depression
- Lower risk of obesity, breast and ovarian cancer, cardiovascular disease and osteoporosis
- Reduces the risk of type 2 diabetes, stroke and high blood pressure
- It's FREE!
- You don't have to wash, sterilise and prepare bottles
- Helps with bonding and attachment
- Breastmilk is always available, any time of the day or night
- Handy when you are out and about as you don't have to bring anything with you
- Breastfeeding can help some mothers heal from a traumatic birth experience
- Exclusive breastfeeding can be used as contraception – the Lactational Amenorrhea Method (LAM), See Chapter 6.

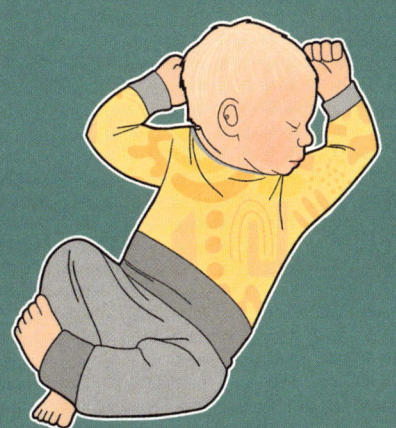

If you intend to exclusively breastfeed for six months — awesome! If you intend to just give your baby colostrum — yay! If you intend to breastfeed your baby for a month — fantastic! If you plan to exclusively pump milk for your baby — brilliant! Even breastfeeding for a short time can have health benefits for a mother and her infant. Perhaps you are not yet sure how you will feed your baby. That's OK too. But whatever hopes or goals you have for providing your baby with your milk, this book will provide you with information and guidance that will be helpful and practical.

Breastfeeding

Breastmilk is the only food that babies need in the first six months of life as it provides them with all they need to grow and develop optimally — energy, fat, vitamins and minerals, live cells that support their immune system, and constituents that play an important role in the development of the baby's endocrine system. It really is magic milk.

But breastfeeding is more than just food and protection against diseases. For many mothers and their babies, breastfeeding becomes a way to connect and communicate with each other. When a baby suckles at the breast, the hormone oxytocin is released, and contributes to feelings of attachment for both mother and baby. Breastfeeding encourages a mother to tune in to her baby and respond to cues, and as such it promotes two-way embodied communication. And for many mothers, breastfeeding is about motherhood self-identity — this often takes mothers by surprise. They may be quite shocked to discover that breastfeeding holds much more meaning for them than they had anticipated, and that breastfeeding is just as much about 'being' as it is about 'doing.'

Breastfeeding is an embodied practice. This means that you can hold feelings about it in your body, feelings that can be hard to understand. Breastfeeding is not simply a decision regarding a way of feeding, but an experience that involves your body, your baby's body, and emotions, feelings and instincts. Sometimes it can take time to start to feel at ease with your lactating body, to learn how it works and to let yourself be guided by it.

For babies, the experience of being at their mother's breast is about feeling safe. Babies are little mammals who are programmed to respond to instinct, and this

Breastfeeding helps to mitigate against the effects of climate change

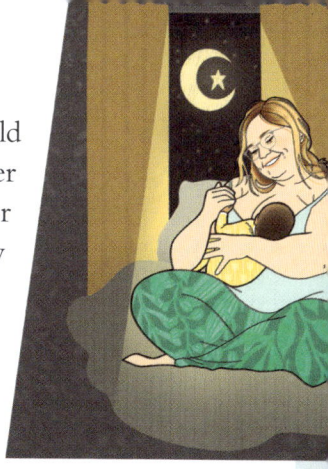

instinct tells them that if they are to survive in this world they need to stay close to the source of food. In other words, they don't like to be too far from the boobs for too long! Babies also experience physiologic stability when they feed at the breast: their mother's body keeps them warm and helps to stabilise their breathing and their heart rate. This kind of contact with the mother's body in the first few days of life can also help to reduce jaundice and raise blood glucose levels.

Suckling at the breast gives comfort to babies. There may be times when they feel alone or afraid, or there may be times when they feel some pain or discomfort, or some degree of discombobulation – especially towards the end of the day. And in these instances, being at the breast can help to soothe, calm and reassure them. There will be times when your baby is actively feeding at the breast – this is called *nutritive sucking*. And there will be times when your baby is suckling at the breast but not actively feeding – this is called *non-nutritive feeding*. The important thing is that they do enough nutritive feeding to get the milk they need.

Another amazing thing about breastfeeding is that it can help a baby get to sleep. Is it okay to let your baby fall asleep at the breast? Yes, absolutely! There are sleep-training and baby-care books that advise mothers not to get into the 'habit' of allowing their baby to fall asleep at the breast, but small babies are simply not designed to be able to self-soothe themselves to sleep. There are hormones in breastmilk that make babies sleepy, so it is normal to expect that they will fall asleep towards the end of a feed. Think of breastfeeding as a superpower that enables you to help your baby get to sleep, comfort them, calm them, boost their immune system, AND to supply the calories and nutrients they need to thrive.

> *Breastfeeding is a mother-to-child signaling system which programs the immune system, the endocrine system and the metabolism.*
>
> Professor Bodo Melnick, 2022

How Do You Feel about Breastfeeding or Lactating?

How do you *feel* about breastfeeding? One of the things I often hear from expectant parents, is the idea that infant feeding represents a straightforward choice, breast or formula – you pick one and that's that. If breastfeeding "doesn't work out," just formula feed. In general, little consideration is given to the mother's feelings about breastfeeding or feelings she may have if breastfeeding turns out to be more difficult than she anticipated. This may be due in part to the simplified way in which infant feeding is often presented to parents: breastfeed or formula feed. However, the reality is more complicated. Mothers who find breastfeeding more challenging than they expected are often shocked and confused by the strength of the feelings they have about it. A common refrain that I hear from mothers is: 'I said I would give it a go, and that I wouldn't beat myself up about it if it didn't work out.' And then in the days and weeks postpartum, they discover that they care more about making breastfeeding work than they thought they would. They struggle to understand why this is the case. I distinctly remember one mother saying to me 'I knew I would like breastfeeding, but I never expected that I would love it so much!.'

Breastfeeding is not simply an act of attaching a baby to a nipple. It involves not only a physical connection between the mother and her baby, but an emotional and psychological experience of being together and interacting with each other. For most mothers, the embodied aspects of breastfeeding are pleasurable – the feeling of their baby's body close to their body, the act of having breasts that can make nourishing milk, the two-way dance between them and their baby. But for some expectant parents, the prospect of lactating and/or putting their baby to their breast may make them feel uncomfortable or apprehensive. Or it might even trigger past traumas. Whatever feelings or ideas you have about breastfeeding or the act of lactation, this is a good time to explore what emotions or thoughts come up for you when

> I said I would give it a go, and that I wouldn't beat myself up about it if it didn't work out.

you think about what it may be like to have breasts that make milk or to have a baby feeding at your breast. If you discover that you have a deep desire to breastfeed and to *be* a breastfeeding mother, embrace and honour that. If you have ambivalent or uncomfortable feelings about breastfeeding or the idea of your breasts making milk, be accepting of those feelings while also considering where they may be coming from. There is no right way to feel about breastfeeding or lactation, particularly when we live in a society that gives us mixed messages about women's bodies, particularly their breasts.

> I knew I would like breastfeeding, but I never expected that I would love it so much!

Many expectant parents have not been breastfed themselves or may come from communities where formula feeding is the norm or the more socially acceptable way to feed a baby. Conversely, some parents will come from families or communities where breastfeeding is considered the normal way to feed a baby, and where there may even be a strong expectation that the mother will breastfeed. So, in addition to contemplating your own feelings about your body, motherhood and breastfeeding, it may be helpful to give some thought to how your expectations of feeding your baby may have been shaped by your family and community.

How Do Parents Learn About Breastfeeding?

Do women really need to *learn* how to breastfeed? Isn't it just instinctive? Well, yes, up to a point. We do have instincts to breastfeed that are triggered when we give birth and hold our babies. And babies are born with reflexes and instincts that help them find their mother's breast and latch on to the nipple when they are placed in skin-to-skin contact. But for breastfeeding behaviours to come naturally to us, it helps to have seen breastfeeding. We cannot assume that we will all just automatically know how to breastfeed. You may have heard the story about a gorilla born in captivity in an Ohio zoo some years ago. When she gave birth to her first baby she did not know how to breastfeed, and the baby subsequently died. When the gorilla became pregnant a second time, breastfeeding mothers from a local La Leche League group volunteered to sit beside the gorilla's enclosure and breastfeed their babies in order for her to learn how to do it. Initially, she ignored them, but as her due date became closer, the gorilla became more interested in observing the mothers. When her baby was born, mothers came again and breastfed their babies in front of her, showing her what to do. She watched, copied their behaviours, and held her baby close until it latched. So, breastfeeding is both an instinctive *and* a learned behaviour.

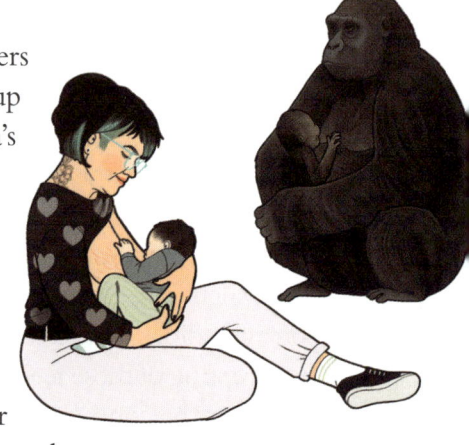

In the past, people would have learned about breastfeeding and lactation by seeing women in their families and communities feeding their babies. They would have seen how they held their babies and how babies latch at the breast. And they would have gained some understanding of how frequently babies feed and how much time they spend at their mother's breast. Simply by being around breastfeeding, people would have subconsciously learned about newborn infant behaviour. Mothers in previous generations probably also would have had women in their families to help them with breastfeeding difficulties. This is not something that many mothers can take for granted today. Life has changed dramatically in the last 150 years. Today, living separately to extended family, and in bigger urban communities where we may not even know our neighbours, is the norm for most people.

Another big change over the last few generations is the way in which formula feeding has become normalised, particularly in the United Kingdom and Ireland. In the early part of the 20th Century, infant formula came to represent wealth, modernity and freedom from the 'shackles of motherhood.' I sometimes see new mothers in my practice who have never really seen breastfeeding up close – they could be the first of their family or friend group to breastfeed, and they may only have been exposed to bottle feeding in schoolbooks, through the media or in films and television programmes. So, for them, breastfeeding has to be learned.

When we consider how we learn, we probably think in terms of reading books, doing research, attending courses, and memorising data.

This is probably how we did it at school. But this kind of learning cannot always be applied successfully to breastfeeding and lactation. Why? Because breastfeeding is an activity that is controlled by the more creative and emotional right side of the brain. Left-brained activities are more concerned with quantifiable data, numbers, hard facts, logic and analytical thinking, breastfeeding requires you to use your instinct and intuition, your feelings and embodied sensations to learn. It relies to a large extent on learning through experience and by being with other breastfeeding mothers. This is hard for a lot of new parents, because they want to be prepared, have some certainty around the postnatal period, and know that they will *succeed* at breastfeeding by mastering the facts. There is of course some left-brained learning involved in breastfeeding – I would encourage expectant parents to read as much as they can about breastfeeding and attend an antenatal breastfeeding class. But it's also important to be prepared to do the real learning after their baby is born. Remember that it is not just a case of you knowing what to do - babies are born with skills and instincts to breastfeed – so allow yourself to learn from your baby. And allow yourself to learn as you go.

Another factor to consider is all the variables that affect breastfeeding and lactation in the early days, that you may not be able to control for – for example, the nature of your baby's birth or the gestation at which your baby is born. The American politician Donald Rumsfeld (not talking about breastfeeding) put it like this:

> *There are known knowns – there are things we know we know, We also know there are known unknowns – that is to say, we know there are some things we do not know. But there are also unknown unknowns, the ones we don't know we don't know.*

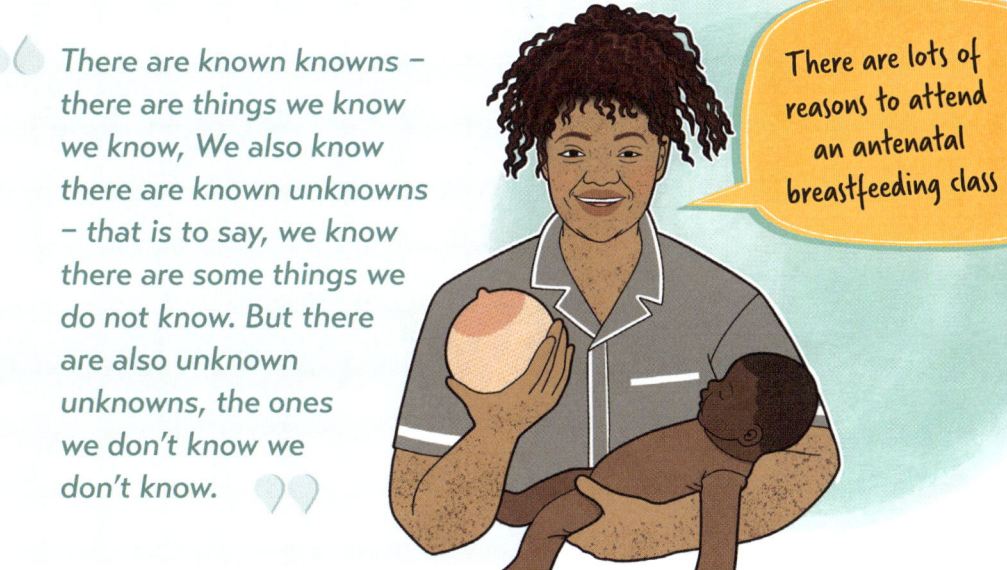

There are lots of reasons to attend an antenatal breastfeeding class

REASONS TO ATTEND AN ANTENATAL BREASTFEEDING CLASS

KNOWLEDGE IS POWER – doing a class can help you understand what to expect, how to overcome common challenges, and to set out some goals for breastfeeding.

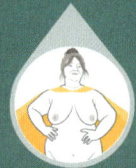
CONFIDENCE IS KEY – Breastfeeding is a new skill you will learn when your baby arrives. But having learned the basics at a class will help you feel more confident about navigating the early days postpartum.

MAKE CONNECTIONS – Attending a breastfeeding or birth preparation class can give you an opportunity to meet other expectant parents who are also planning to breastfeed. You can find your village.

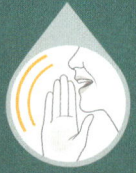
MYTH BUSTING – myths about breastfeeding and lactation abound, and you probably will have absorbed some of them, eg, 'Nipples need to be toughened up before you start breastfeeding' or 'You shouldn't drink coffee if you're breastfeeding.' Neither statement is true. Doing a class will dispel some of these myths and give you solid evidence-based information.

A CHANCE TO ASK QUESTIONS – whatever it is you've always wanted to know about breastfeeding or lactation, a class is a good opportunity to ask questions and receive reliable answers.

So, be prepared to encounter lots of unknowns. Allow yourself to be a beginner, to sometimes flounder, to make mistakes and to wing it. Try to cultivate an attitude of kindness and compassion to yourself as a beginner parent and a beginner breastfeeder. What kind of a learner are you? Are you more left or right-brained? Are there aspects of learning about parenting and breastfeeding that you anticipate will be challenging?

While you are pregnant, attending a hospital-run or private antenatal breastfeeding class is a good place to start with breastfeeding education.

Becoming a Mother

Rebecca Walker, writer and feminist, wondered how she would survive the transition to motherhood, asking:

> *Will I lose myself – my body, my mind,*
> *my options – and be left trapped,*
> *resentful, and irretrievably overwhelmed?*

These are valid fears. Becoming a mother can feel scary. For most women, it is probably the biggest and most life-changing experience they will ever undergo. No other life event has so many diverse and profound experiences – the pain and intensity of giving birth, the experience of falling in love with one's baby, a rollercoaster of emotions, vulnerability, role change and the responsibility of feeding a baby and keeping them safe. Motherhood is sometimes likened to stepping into a new country, starting a new chapter in your life, or being thrown into a different universe. But whatever way you like to think about it, becoming a mother is a journey that will take you to new and unfamiliar places, and that will present you with lots of unanticipated challenges. Motherhood can feel overwhelming, and it can push you to your limits and cause you to question who you think you are.

Motherhood can be a wonderful experience. The transition to becoming a mother is felt by many women as sublime (at least some of the time), and as one that brings with it opportunities for personal growth and a deepening of innate wisdom that we can apply to many facets of our lives. Toni Morrison described motherhood as '...the most liberating thing that ever happened to me....I could only be me – whatever that was – but somebody actually needed me to be that.'

When I was a teenager – in 1980s Ireland – motherhood didn't feature on our school curriculum. As students we were prepared for a trajectory that would see us leave school, enter higher-level education, join the workforce alongside our male colleagues and be successful career women. We would have it all, or at least we were led to believe we would. There was no discussion of the possibility that many of us would one day become mothers, and the potential challenges that motherhood might bring. Nobody told us that we might someday struggle to juggle motherhood with working outside the home, or that we might struggle to find affordable childcare. Nobody mentioned the possibility that we might choose to take an extended period off work to care for our children. The overarching impression that I came away with was that doing well academically and having a career equated to success, while being 'just a mother' equated to the worst-case scenario, and something to be avoided at all costs. As a result, I believe, we ended up being completely unprepared for practical, emotional and existential challenges that being and becoming mothers would present.

We don't talk enough about what it is like to become a mother in a world that to a large extent does not adequately support new mothers and parents. Challenges faced by mothers around the globe include economic pressures, lack of paid maternity leave, lack of connection with family and community (often due to migration), isolation, racism, lack of access to free or affordable healthcare services, lack of affordable childcare and lack of breastfeeding support. United Nations data shows that women are doing more than ever unpaid work at home, and that despite the gains made by the feminist movement, women still earn less, save less, hold less secure jobs, and are more likely to be employed in the informal sector. Modern society tends to undervalue motherhood and breastfeeding, perhaps because caring for a baby does not directly contribute to the economy.

Now may be a good time to reflect on your feelings about becoming a mother and how society may have shaped that view. Is there anything about becoming a mother that makes you feel anxious? Do you have some fixed ideas about the 'type' of mother you will be? How do you feel about your own mother, and how she mothered you? Did you plan your pregnancy or did you become pregnant by accident? Do you have a partner or will you be parenting solo? Did you have an arduous IVF journey to become pregnant? If you are a member of the LGBTQI+ community, has exposure to heteronormative representations of parenting been difficult for you? All of these things can shape how you feel about yourself as a mother or parent, and what kind of experience you will have after the birth of your baby. All feelings are valid. Sit with them, see what comes up for you. Consider seeking out support from like-minded people and/or doing some one-to-one counselling if fear or negative feelings about motherhood are overshadowing your pregnancy.

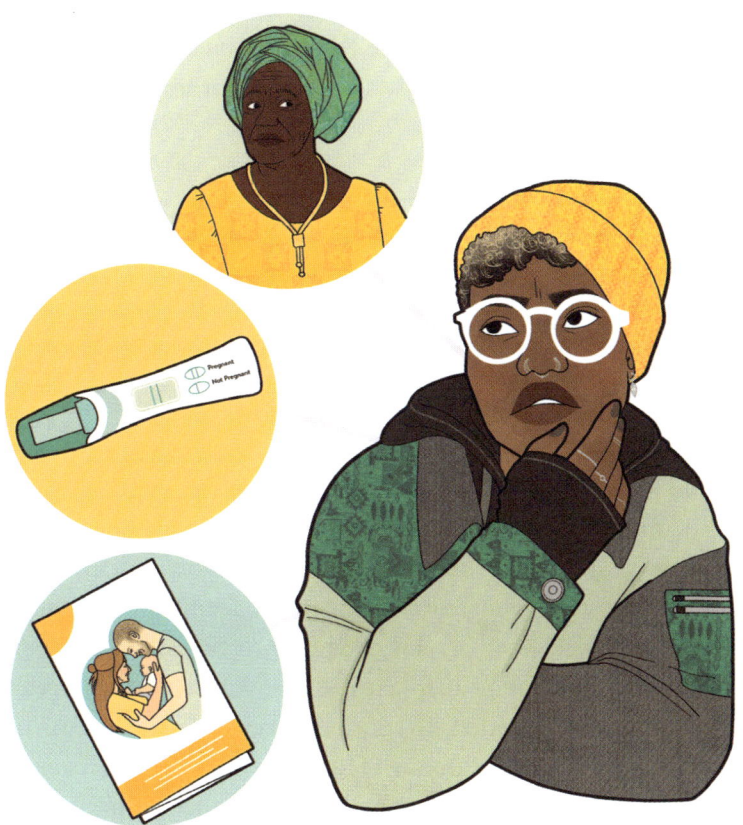

> *With the birth of a child, or acceptance of a child into her life, a woman, now a mother, arrives to a new country called 'motherhood', where she has to understand and find her existential bearings, learn a new culture and language, learn how to be 'at home' in this new unfamiliar 'being-in-the-world' as a mother*
>
> Victoria Garland

The last few years have seen a slew of honest and realistic memoirs about motherhood, which portray how challenging the first few months can be. A couple that I particularly like are *Milk* by the Irish writer Alice Kinsella and *Don't Forget to Scream* by British journalist Marianne Levy. They both capture the joy of becoming a mother, but also the vulnerability and loneliness of new motherhood.

Creating a Feeding Preferences Plan

Many expectant parents create a birth plan, also referred to as a *birth preferences* document, in the lead up to having their baby. This is a means of communicating with hospital staff how you would like to be supported during labour and birth and your preferences for interventions and pain relief. The hospital staff who support you while you are in labour and giving birth may not have met you beforehand. So, giving them a succinct document outlining your preferences can help them to provide you with individualised care. Likewise, you could give hospital staff some kind of *feeding preferences* plan. A feeding preferences plan can be one sentence, such as: 'I would like to breastfeed my baby and would appreciate as much help as possible.' Or a feeding preferences plan could be more detailed, if you have particular concerns that you would like staff to know about. Here are some more examples of sentences you could include in a feeding preference plan:

- 'I would like for my baby's first feed to be colostrum.'

- 'I would like to have at least an hour of uninterrupted skin-to-skin after I have my baby.'

- 'I had difficulty breastfeeding my first baby. I hope to have a more positive experience this time so I would be grateful for some extra support establishing breastfeeding baby #2.'

- 'I intend to exclusively express breastmilk for my baby.'

- 'It is important to me that my baby is not supplemented with infant formula.'

- 'I have large breasts and I feel anxious about breastfeeding. I think I will need some extra help with positioning.'

- 'I have flat nipples. I used nipple shields for the first couple of months when I breastfeed my first baby. I intend to use them again this time.'

- 'I have some concerns about my ability to make a full milk supply. I would like to get some lactation support to optimise milk production.'

- 'I would like to avoid having midwives touch my breasts. I would prefer verbal guidance with latching. Thank you.'

- 'I am autistic. I feel apprehensive about establishing breastfeeding and being able to interpret my baby's feeding cues. I would like to have some clear, simple guidance in the first few days to help me feel more confident about breastfeeding.'

- 'I have sensory issues. I am worried that breastfeeding may cause me sensory challenges.'

If you decide you would like to have a feeding preferences plan in your hospital file, discuss it with your obstetrician or midwife during an antenatal visit. Generally, parents find that having a feeding preferences plan is very helpful, both for them and for the staff who support them. Having one usually makes for a better breastfeeding or lactation experience.

How Babies Prepare to Breastfeed

Babies spend nine months in utero growing and developing skills, senses, reflexes and instincts that will enable them to find the breast, latch and feed when they are placed in skin-to-skin contact with their mother shortly after birth. This is something that is often overlooked in antenatal breastfeeding preparation. The emphasis is usually on what the mother or parent must do to establish breastfeeding, rather than on the fact that babies are born knowing how to breastfeed. Their breast-seeking and breastfeeding behaviours are *innate*. The job of the parent is to help their baby put their skills and instincts into action by placing them on the mother's chest after birth, offering gentle encouragement, and help when they need it. It is as if babies' brains have a little microchip that contains all of the instructions on how to breastfeed. These behaviours are triggered by the gentle pressure along the front of the baby's body when they are placed prone on their mother's body.

Babies learn in the womb how to swallow and how to suck, and how to coordinate these two skills. Swallowing has been observed in foetuses from around 12.5 weeks and sucking from week 26. Sometimes ultrasound images will capture a baby sucking their thumb. Babies also develop reflexes and senses that enable breast-seeking behaviours when they are in skin-to-skin contact with their mother. For example, newborn babies have a heightened sense of smell which enables them to smell their mother's colostrum. This encourages them to move towards the breast when they are in skin-to-skin contact. Newborn babies have limited vision, but it does enable them to see their mother's areola (the circular area of pigmented skin around the nipple). This is why the areolas usually darken during pregnancy, to act as a visual cue for babies seeking the breast.

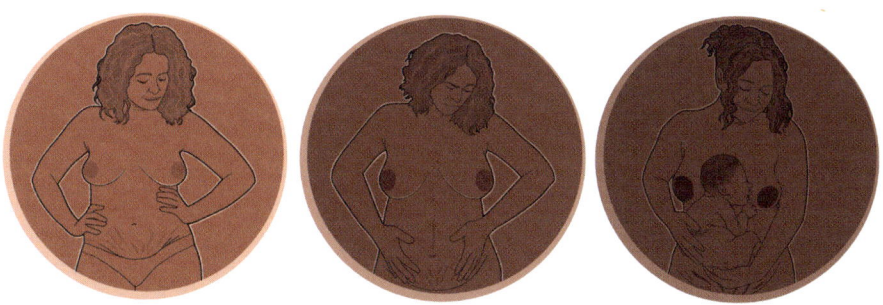

Considering all the skills and innate behaviours that babies are born with, it may be helpful to start thinking about breastfeeding not simply as a skill that YOU must learn, but as something that you and your baby will get the hang of together.

Breastfeeding Support

Generations ago, most mothers would have lived within extended families and smaller communities, and would have had women around them to help them establish breastfeeding and adapt to life in the *fourth trimester* – this is the term often given to a baby's first three months during which they adapt to being in the womb to being in the world. Now, however, the norm for many people is to live apart from extended family. As a result, many new mothers will not have people around who can help with breastfeeding and all that goes with having a new baby. Even mothers with family living close by may find that they have no lived experience of breastfeeding. Whatever level of experience or knowledge your partner and your extended family have about breastfeeding, now is the time to let them know that you intend to breastfeed and that having their support is important to you.

> *Without support, parenting an infant can be hell. Shared, it has moments of heaven.*
>
> (Julie Philips, 2022)

Breastfeeding is an emotive topic, especially for women who have had difficult breastfeeding experiences themselves or who harbour some feelings of failure around not having breastfed. There are also the women who never really got a chance to breastfeed due to lack of support. They may feel some sense of grief about that. So, be aware that if there are people close to you who do not seem particularly supportive of your choice to breastfeed, it is about them, not you. Stand your ground, but also see if you can understand where they may be coming from and why they dislike breastfeeding. Could you begin a conversation with people in your family who seem resistant to the idea of breastfeeding, to discover where that resistance is coming from? It may be that they know someone who had a difficult experience, or that they have been influenced by some of the myths about breastfeeding. Having a conversation can sometimes help people debrief and give you both space to express yourselves and gain a better understanding of where you are both coming from.

In addition to partner and family support, it is a good idea at this stage to consider what kind of breastfeeding support groups are available to you.

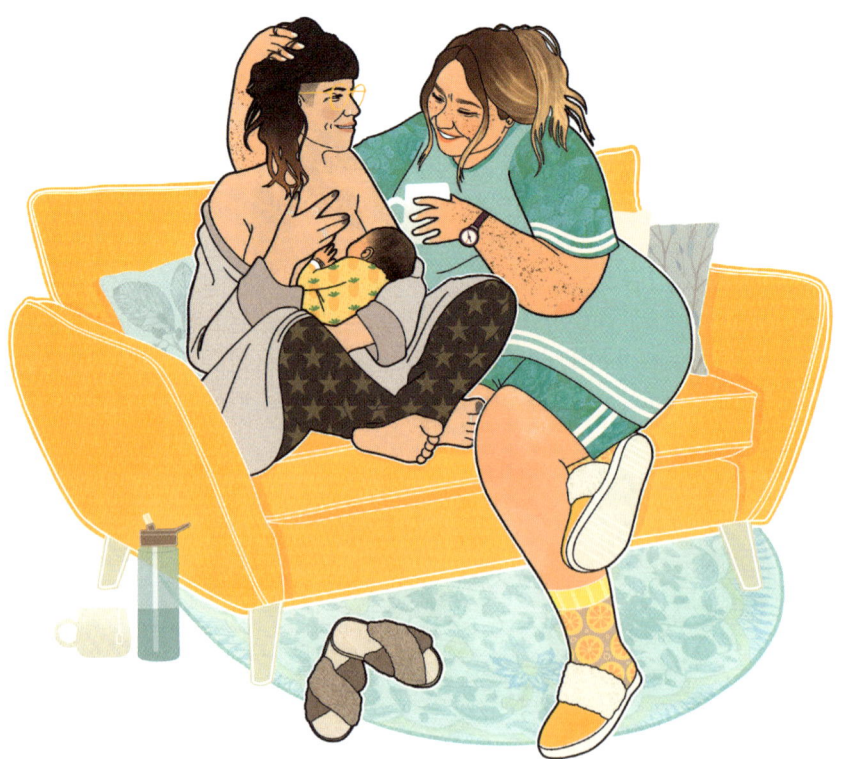

BREASTFEEDING SUPPORT GROUPS – These groups provide social support to breastfeeding mothers, help them have a positive experience of being a breastfeeding mother, and provide evidence-based information that can help them with common breastfeeding challenges. You don't have to have a breastfeeding problem to attend a group. In fact, most women who attend breastfeeding support groups are not experiencing significant problems. They attend to connect with other breastfeeding mothers and feel part of a *village*. Consider attending a group before your baby arrives. Being in a shared space with mothers breastfeeding their babies can help you feel more confident about getting off to a good start with breastfeeding yourself.

Social Media Breastfeeding Support and Information – Increasing numbers of mothers are looking to social media platforms like Instagram and Facebook for breastfeeding support and information. There are some excellent closed support groups on Facebook and accounts on Instagram that post practical and evidence-based information. However, bear in mind that anyone can post anything on social media, so for all the good information there are equal amounts of misinformation and unhelpful advice. If you are following breastfeeding and lactation accounts on Instagram, check the credentials of the person behind the account – are they qualified to give breastfeeding and lactation advice? If you like their content, keep following. If not, unfollow.

If you are a **Black or Black Mixed-Heritage Breastfeeding mother** or parent you may wish to contact a group or organisation that exists to support the Black pregnancy and maternal experience, for example The Motherhood Group https://themotherhoodgroup.org or https://dopeblackmums.co.uk. Similarly, if you are a member of any kind of minority group or feel that you don't fit in with mainstream support groups, you could try to find a group specific to your needs. There is evidence that people benefit from connecting with like-minded others who understand them. Social media has made it so much easier to find people like you. You may be solo-parenting, or identify as queer or non-binary, or perhaps you are breastfeeding a child with cancer, or breastfeeding with low milk supply. Sometimes finding a group or village that meets your needs can take a bit of time, but there will always be someone like you, somewhere, who is willing to connect.

What Do You Need to Buy?

Be prepared to be marketed to. As an expectant parent, you are the target market for a plethora of companies who want to sell you baby and feeding-related products, from breast massagers and pumps, to vibrating baby rockers and hi-tech electronic sleep monitoring devices. You are probably already noticing ads for these kinds of products on social media and the internet, because these companies probably know you are pregnant. They know that doing parenthood 'right' is important to you, and that you are going to want the 'best' for your baby. These companies will endeavour to capitalise on this by convincing you that their products will make parenting easier, result in more sleep and keep your baby safer. In her memoir on motherhood, the British journalist Marianne Levy captured the reality of how companies exploit the vulnerability of new parents in their marketing:

> The internet had offered us video monitors, and even sensory pads that beeped if the baby stopped breathing, or stood up. There seemed no particular method of distinguishing between the two. Their manufacturers knew what we were all afraid of: that while we slept, the baby would die. Why else were their products called names like Safe Sleep or Angelcare?

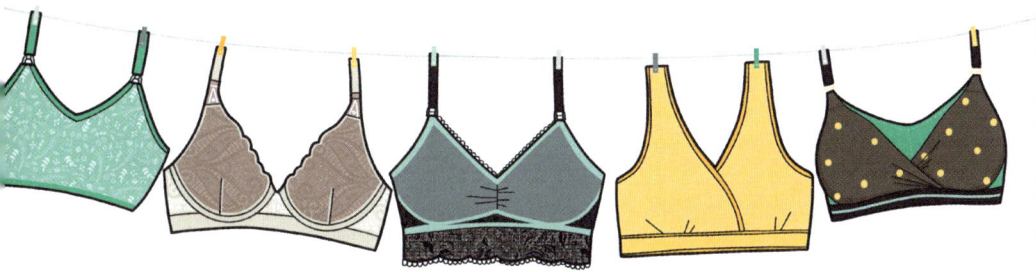

At a very basic level, babies need to be fed, clothed and cuddled. They do not need fancy stuff or expensive devices. The only products that I recommend parents buy in advance of their baby arriving are a couple of comfortable nursing bras and a box nursing pads (which you may or may not need – not every mother's breasts leak). You may need to buy larger bras earlier in your pregnancy due to breast growth that happens in the first trimester. But wait until around week 37 of your pregnancy to get nursing bras. A general rule is to go up a cup size and add two to the back size, so for example, if you are normally a 36C, you may need at least a 38D nursing bra. The main things to look for in a bra are comfort and support – remember, your breasts will be heavier when you are lactating, so your nursing bra will have a little more work to do to support that weight. Not wearing a bra at all is also an option, particularly if you have small breasts.

Nursing tops available now come in a variety of lovely styles and price ranges. But you don't absolutely have to have custom-designed nursing tops if you are breastfeeding. Instead, you can layer two tops – wear a stretchy vest top underneath a looser top. When you breastfeed, pull the outer top up and the vest top down, and hey presto, a DIY nursing top!

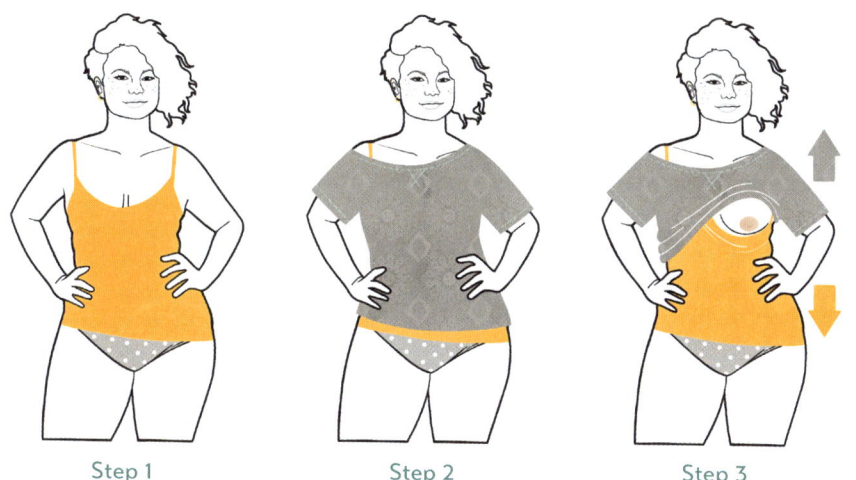

Step 1   Step 2   Step 3

Anything else breastfeeding-related that you may need after your baby is born can either be purchased in the hospital shop or a pharmacy, or ordered online for next-day delivery. Parents often ask me about breast pumps – should they get one, what type should they get, how much should they spend. My answer: it depends on why you will be pumping, how often you will be using your pump and for how long. I generally suggest parents wait until their baby is born and then see. Just by the way – not all breastfeeding mothers choose to or need to pump. If it's a case that you need to pump for a preterm or sick baby, or a baby that is unable to latch, the lactation team in your maternity hospital will probably provide you with access to a multiuser pump. On discharge, you will then be advised to rent a multiuser pump (sometimes referred to as a *hospital-grade pump*) that is designed for heavy-duty usage – a pump like this is much more efficient and durable than the type of commercially available pump you would buy for occasional use. Read more about pumping in Chapter 10.

Is buying a nipple cream essential? NO! Many women believe they must buy an expensive lanolin-based nipple cream if they are going to breastfeed. However, most mothers will not need any kind of cream for their nipples. In any case, there is no evidence that lanolin-based creams are more effective for sore or cracked nipples than breastmilk. If you do run into difficulties and find that your nipples are sore or cracked, get some skilled support from a lactation professional and follow their advice on nipple care (more about sore nipples in Chapter 8).

P.S. If you are having twins, do get yourself a good twin feeding cushion, and join the *Breastfeeding Twins and Triplets* Group on Facebook (more about breastfeeding twins in Chapter 16). There is no need to buy a feeding cushion if you are having a singleton.

Possible Challenges to Breastfeeding

Most women can breastfeed without experiencing significant challenges. However, there are certain situations where mothers or lactating parents will require extra breastfeeding help and support, and benefit from anticipatory guidance during pregnancy. If you have any concerns about your ability to breastfeed or make milk, seek out one-to-one support from an IBCLC (International Board-Certified Lactation Consultant) during your pregnancy or speak to your care providers, especially if you tick any of the following boxes:

- Concerns that your breasts look different (e.g. One breast is noticeably bigger than the other or tubular shape)
- Irregular periods or lack of breast growth during puberty
- Breast surgery
- Underlying hormonal issues such as polycystic breast growth (PCOS)
- Significant medical issues that have required medication
- No/minimal breast changes during pregnancy
- History of breast cancer, or other cancer
- History of eating disorders
- Infertility
- Difficulty breastfeeding a previous baby
- Inverted or very flat nipples
- Your mother or sisters were unable to breastfeed

Having one of the above conditions does not mean you can't breastfeed, but you may face certain challenges and need extra help. Putting a plan in place with the help of an IBCLC can maximise your chances of getting off to a good start and getting as close to reaching your breastfeeding or lactation goals as possible.

How You May Feel After You Have Your Baby

During pregnancy there is usually a lot of focus on what you need to learn and what you need to buy in advance of your baby arriving, with far less emphasis on how you may *feel* postpartum. Consequently, most new parents are often very surprised at the big emotions they experience. The postnatal period is a vulnerable time for most new mothers and birthing parents. They must contend with broken sleep, the demands of caring for a new baby, and learning to breastfeed. Some mothers may also experience physical and emotional pain following a difficult or traumatic birth. You may experience these feelings after your baby is born:

- Vulnerability
- Low Mood
- Anxiety
- Fear
- Loneliness
- Exhaustion
- Overwhelm
- Shock
- Confusion

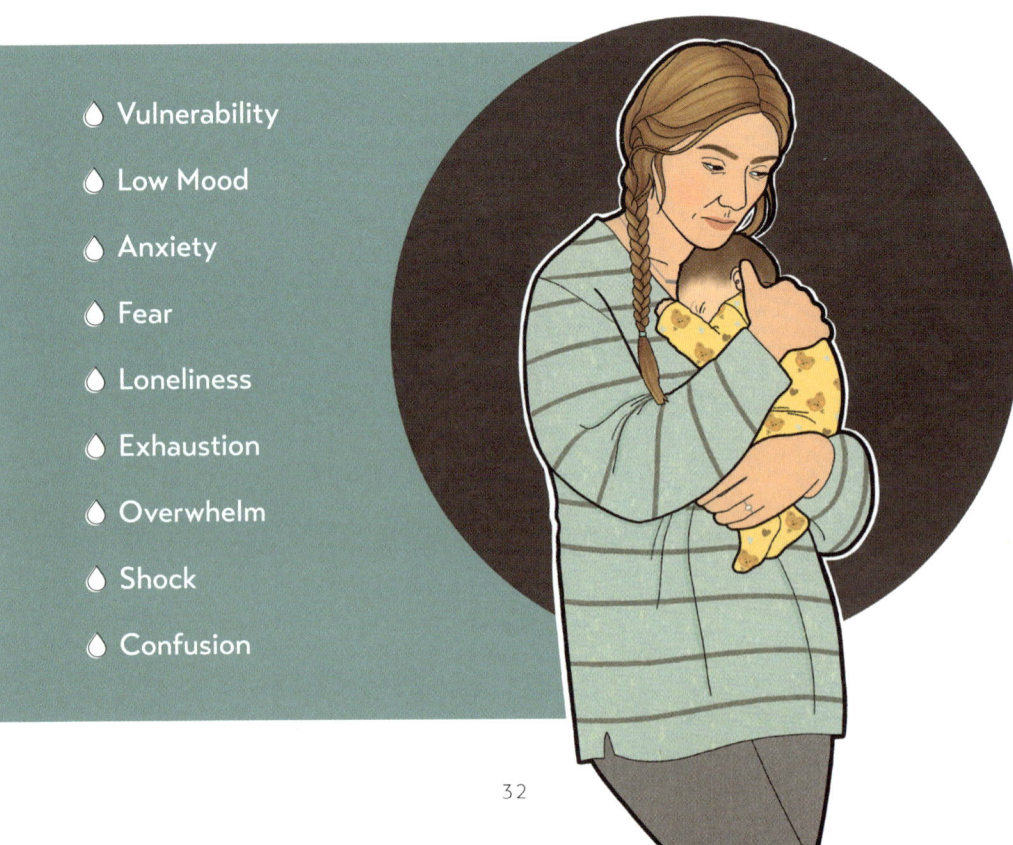

These feelings can co-exist alongside feelings of joy and immense love for your baby, happiness, and excitement for the motherhood journey that is ahead of you. Your heart opens up when you have a baby. This allows you to love and let your new little person take up their place in your heart. But the flipside is that opening up your heart can make you vulnerable. Some parents even find that this vulnerability can bring up past traumas (more about this in Chapter 11 on Mental Health). The important thing is to understand that experiencing a tsunami of emotions in the postpartum period is normal. You are not alone in having these feelings.

The key to surviving the postnatal period is support –

Support from a partner and/or family, friends, healthcare professionals, breastfeeding supporters, and community. Remember, at no stage are you on your own as you transition into motherhood, and that you are not meant to be able to do it all on your own! It may be a good idea now to start thinking about who will help you when your baby arrives. If you do not have family close by, are there friends who can help? Or could you consider postnatal doula support? A doula is a non-medical professional who can provide support during labour or after you have had your baby. Having realistic expectations of yourself in the postpartum period and an awareness of how emotionally vulnerable you may be, will help you navigate this time. After the birth of her son, the poet Alice Notley said 'He is born and I am undone – feel as if I will/never be, was never born.' This sense of being undone is very common among new mothers, but from this place of being undone emerges a new sense of self, a new place in the world, a new beginning, big wisdom and personal growth, and the opportunity for self-discovery.

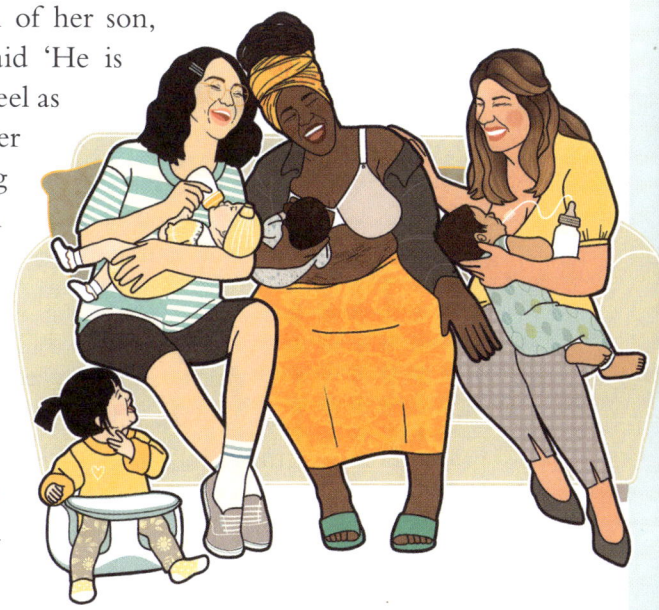

Parenting Your Way

There is no blueprint for how YOU will parent YOUR BABY. You can read all the books in the world on how to do it 'right' but ultimately you have to learn as you go, get to know your baby, figure out who you are as a parent, and determine what is going to work for you and your family.

You do not instantly become an expert in parenting the moment your baby is born (if only!). The process of becoming a parent is one of 'experiential learning.' Every day will bring something new. So, try to start cultivating a gentle attitude with yourself now that allows you space and time to make mistakes and to learn from them. Think in terms of *figuring it out* rather than *doing it right*.

> *My early motherhood asked more of me emotionally than any experience ever has, sometimes insisting on my capacity for bliss and tenderness, sometimes leaving me despairing at my limitations.*
>
> Julie Phillips, 2022

There are always new challenges when you are a parent. At times you will feel like you're being pushed out of your comfort zone, times when you feel grief for the life you had before you became a parent, times when you will feel overwhelmed and like you're failing, and there will be times when you do not enjoy parenting. There will also be times when you feel content and feel like you are a competent parent. There may be times when you experience strong feelings of bliss and gratitude that you are a parent. But at no point do you reach a stage where you think you have perfected the art of parenting. It is an ongoing journey of learning, growing, being humble, feeling vulnerable and raw, making mistakes, and being compassionate with yourself. Your journey with your family will be unique.

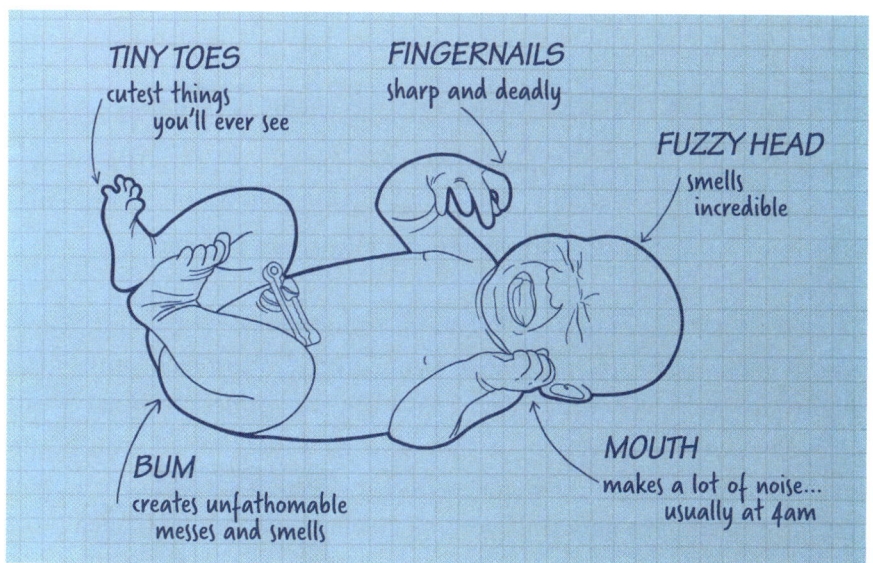

When I was pregnant with my first baby I watched a TV documentary about different parenting styles. One of the couples was very regimented in their approach to caring for their baby – everything was scheduled – and at the time this made total sense to me. Why would you do it any other way? There was another couple that leaned more towards attachment parenting – the baby slept in their bed and life revolved around the baby's needs. This seemed pretty insane to me. I did not understand why anyone would 'allow' their lives to be dominated by their baby. I decided I would opt for the more sensible, parent-led approach and bought a baby-care book, replete with daily feeding and sleeping schedules. That book was chucked into the recycling bin about three weeks after I gave birth. My baby was not on board with strict scheduling, and I discovered that neither was I! I ended up becoming a very different parent to the one I had imagined I would be.

FAQS:

Should I start pumping milk early on so my partner can help me with feeding? There are lots of ways that partners can help out. In the early weeks postpartum it may be easier for you to just focus on establishing breastfeeding without adding pumping into the mix. Even if your partner does give your baby a bottle of pumped milk, it does not necessarily make life easier for you as you still have to set aside time to pump and clean the pump parts.

I have breast implants. Can I breastfeed? Yes, you can! But talking to an IBCLC before your baby arrives would be a good idea as there are some challenges that breast augmentation can present.

I have very small breasts – will I make enough milk? Yes, you probably will. Most breasts, irrespective of size, can make sufficient milk for a mother to exclusively breastfeed. However, sometimes a tubular breast shape or asymmetry can be a sign of a condition called Insufficient Glandular Tissue (IGT) – a lack of milk-making tissue. This condition can affect milk production. If you are concerned about IGT, speak to a lactation consultant.

I am a member of the Traveller community – can I breastfeed? Most Traveller women can breastfeed. However, there are high rates of Galactosemia in the Traveller community, Galactosemia is a condition which means that babies are unable to tolerate breastmilk, so they have to be given a special lactose-free infant formula. As a result, Traveller babies can only start breastfeeding once they receive a negative Beutler test. A Beutler test is a test for galactosemia that is routinely done on Traveller babies. A small drop of blood is taken from the baby's foot before their first feed and sent to a laboratory for testing. Beutler test results can take anywhere between 12 hours and 3 days. Talk to your care team in the hospital about feeding your baby and protecting your milk supply while you wait for test results.

Do I need to toughen up my nipples with a nailbrush before I breastfeed? No, definitely not! Nipples are quite elastic and can become more protractile with breastfeeding. Also, nipples have more melanin, and this makes them more resistant to abrasion. So be nice to your nips.

I just don't want to breastfeed my baby. Can I express milk instead? Yes. Some mothers choose to exclusively pump milk for their babies instead of feeding them directly at the breast. Make sure your care providers know that this is how you intend to feed your baby and consider seeing a lactation consultant before your baby arrives.

CHAPTER 2

Breasts, Colostrum, and Antenatal Hand Expression

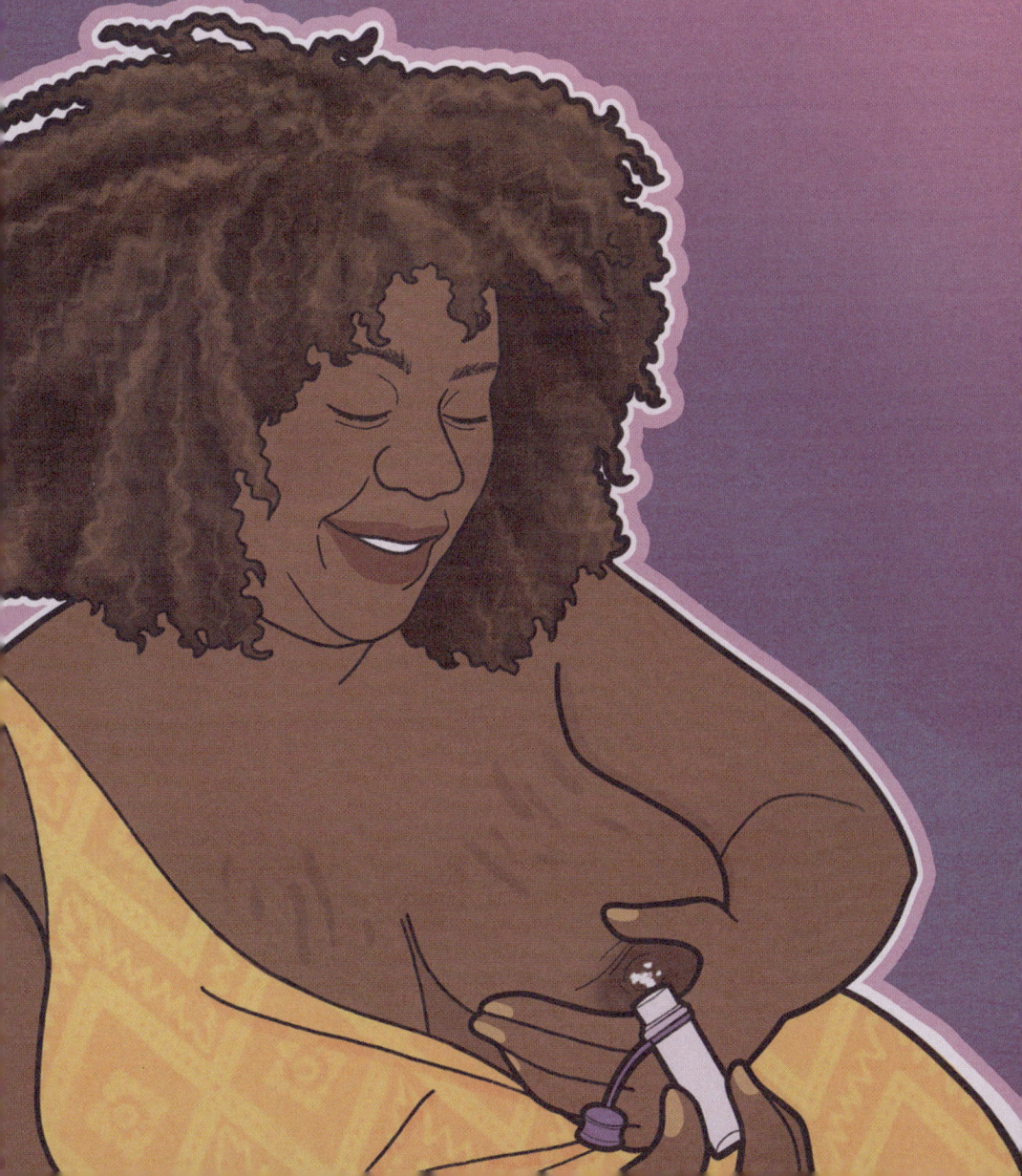

Breast Growth and Development

Breast development starts in the womb, continues during childhood in proportion to the rest of the body, and then speeds up in puberty with the with the onset of hormonal changes and menstruation. The main hormone involved in breast growth at this stage is oestrogen. With each menstrual cycle, more mammary *glandular,* or milk-making, tissue is laid down. Fatty tissue also grows in the breasts during puberty. As the breasts grow, the basic anatomy that ensures future milk production develops.

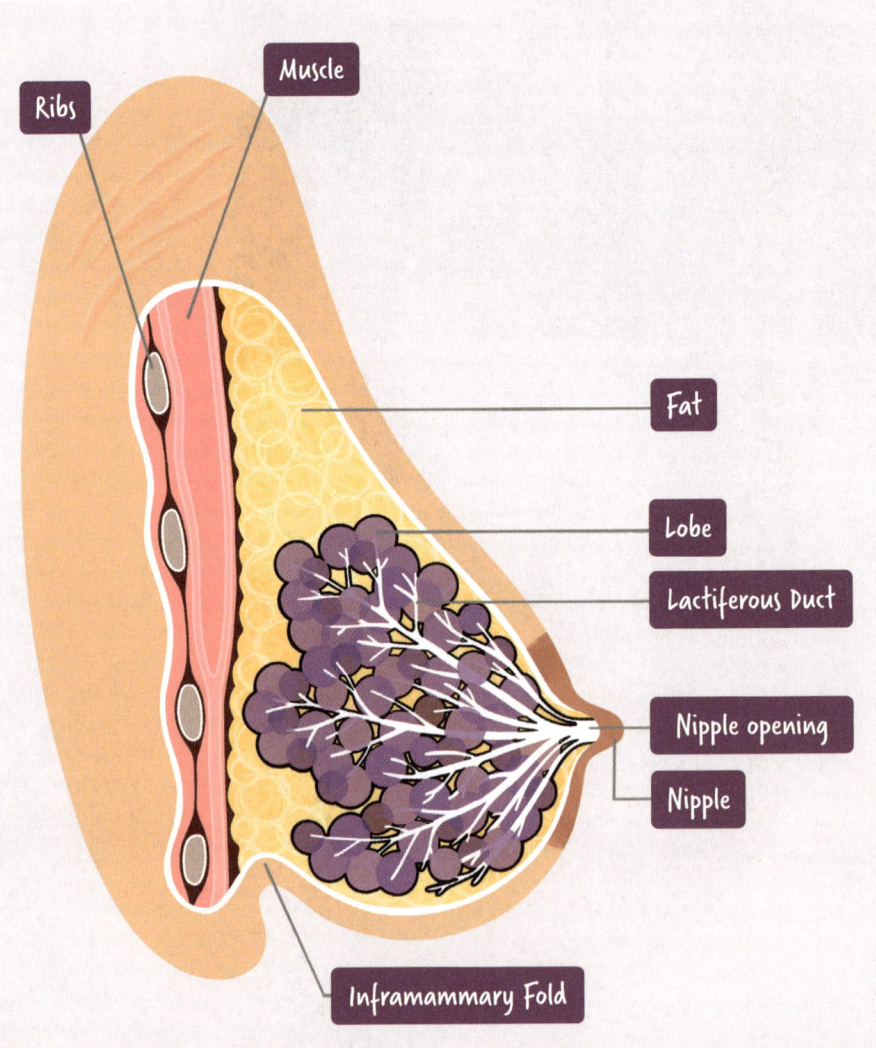

During the first trimester of pregnancy, rapid branching of the ducts and lobules occurs (aka *mammogenesis*) and this usually results in an increase in breast size. There is also an increase in the number of epithelial cells in the breasts. Epithelial cells are found on surfaces throughout the body, for example, they form the outer layer of your skin and they line your digestive tract. Epithelial cells perform different functions, depending on where they are located in the body. During the next stage of breast growth (*Lactogenesis I*), epithelial cells in the breasts develop into cells that can make milk - *lactocytes*. The first type of milk that these lactocytes secrete is called *colostrum*, and this can happen from around week 16 of pregnancy.

Breast Changes During Pregnancy

During pregnancy, your body starts to prepare to make plenty of milk once your baby is born. One of the first changes that women often notice is an increase in sensitivity of the breasts – sometimes this is the first obvious physical indication that they are pregnant. This sensitivity can happen during the first few weeks of pregnancy and is caused by increasing levels of the hormone progesterone (the hormone that helps to sustain your pregnancy). Other hormonal changes that take place during this first trimester spur breast growth, which is normally experienced at around 10 weeks. The cells that produce milk proliferate, milk ducts sprout, the blood supply to the breasts increases and new capillaries grow around the lobules (bunches of ducts). The upshot of all of this is that you may need to invest in a bigger bra by the end of the first trimester. Not everyone notices obvious breast changes in the first trimester.

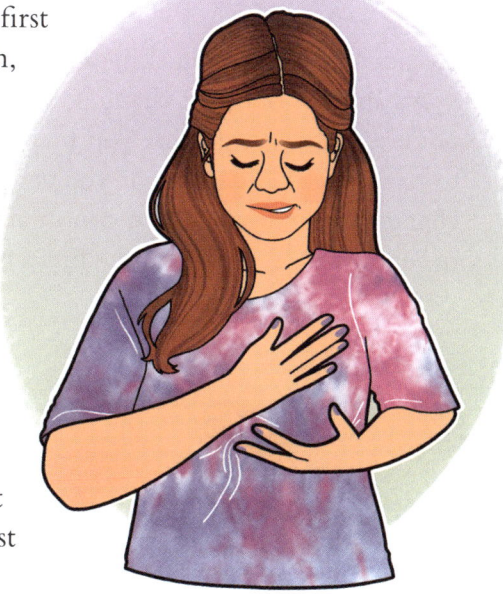

A few weeks into the second trimester a process called lactogenesis I starts. This is the beginning of milk production. The first milk your breasts make, *colostrum,* is produced in very small amounts. Colostrum is thick and yellow in colour. Some women find that their breasts leak small amounts of colostrum during pregnancy —this is normal. It is also normal for no leaking to occur. Another change that some women notice during pregnancy is the appearance of little bumps called Montgomery tubercles, around the areolas. These Montgomery tubercles secrete an anti-bacterial oil which helps to protect and lubricate the nipples and areolas.

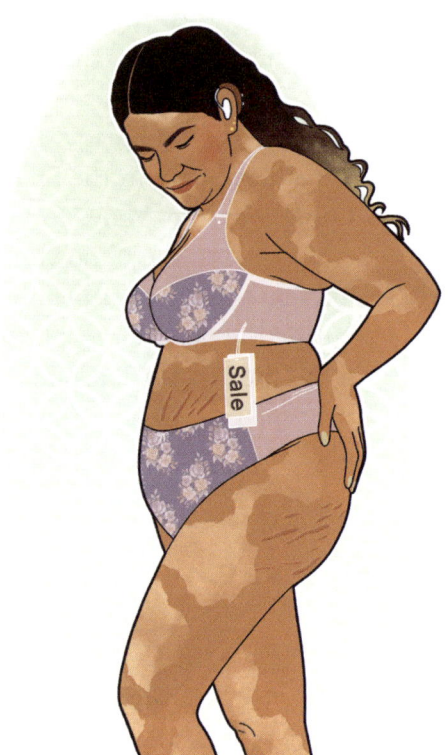

Other changes that you may notice during your pregnancy are a darkening of the nipples and areolas (the darker skin around your nipple) and more noticeable veining of your breasts, which is caused by an increase in blood supply to the area. The darkening of the nipple and areola makes them easier for your baby to see once they are born and placed in skin-to-skin contact with you.

An absence of breast changes during pregnancy can sometimes (but not always) be a sign that you may struggle to produce enough milk to exclusively breastfeed. If you are concerned about a lack of breast changes, talk to a lactation consultant who can help you make a plan to support you with breastfeeding once your baby is born.

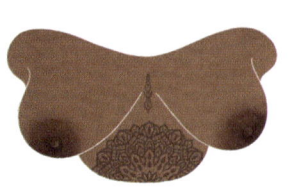 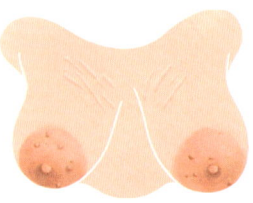 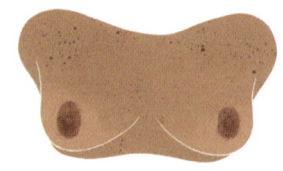

How Breasts Make Milk

Your breasts produce small volumes of *colostrum*, the first breastmilk, from around week 16 of your pregnancy, and during the first few days after you give birth (babies need only small volumes of colostrum during this time). Two to three days after birth, the volume of milk your breasts produce increases significantly — this is called *lactogenesis II*, or more commonly referred to as *'milk coming in.'* During pregnancy, the hormone progesterone inhibits the production of large volumes of milk. Once you have delivered your baby and the placenta, the progesterone levels drop. When this happens, levels of prolactin (the main hormone involved in milk production) rise and your breasts can start producing bigger volumes of milk. Lactogenesis II is usually noticeable — breasts increase in size, feel full and heavy, and veining becomes more obvious. Your breasts may also feel warm to touch. Once your milk is in, it is important to keep it flowing either by feeding your baby frequently (every 2 — 3 hours, or even more frequently) or by pumping (if your baby is not latching or feeding effectively at the breast). The volume of milk your breasts produce will continue to increase over the next few weeks to meet your baby's needs.

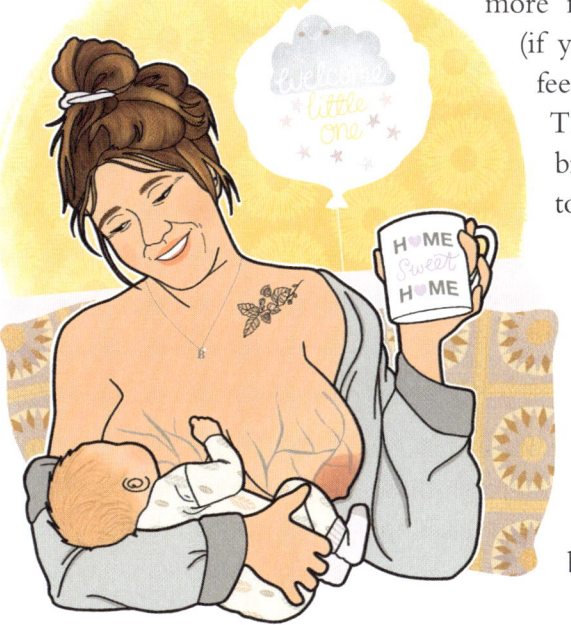

The more your baby feeds, the more milk your body will make. This is why it is important to keep your baby close and allow them easy access to your breasts.

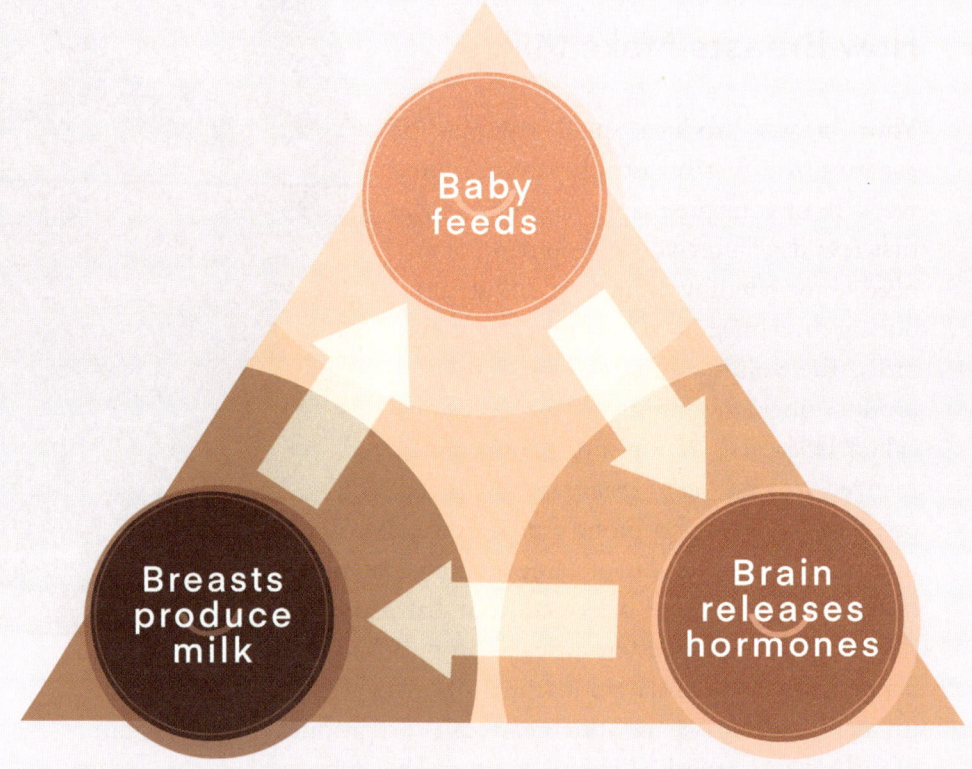

How does demand and supply work?

1. Your baby latches to your breast and starts to suckle. This sends a signal to the brain to release hormones prolactin and oxytocin. Prolactin is involved in milk production.

2. Oxytocin causes milk to start flowing. This release of milk is called a letdown, or milk ejection reflex, and is often experienced as a tingly sensation in the breasts although some women don't feel anything when their milk starts to letdown.

3. Once the letdown happens, your baby starts to get milk and is encouraged to keep drinking and suckling at the breast. Milk continues to flow.

4. As your baby continues to feed and remove milk from the breast, a signal is sent to the brain to start making more milk. This ensures that the milk that is being removed is constantly being replaced.

Think of the process as a continuum. Your baby feeds, your breasts produce milk, your baby feeds, your breasts produce milk — and on it goes. It is important that your baby feeds often. Leaving your breasts full for a long time can slow down milk production and put you at risk of engorgement and/or blocked ducts (more about this in Chapter 9).

Feedback Inhibitor of Lactation (FIL) is an active whey protein in your milk that inhibits milk production. When your breasts are full, FIL levels are high and milk production slows down. But when milk is removed from your breasts and they become soft, FIL levels drop and milk production increases.

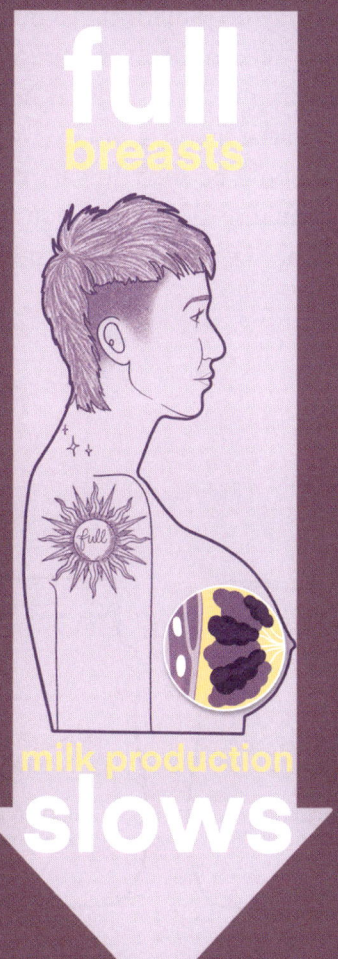

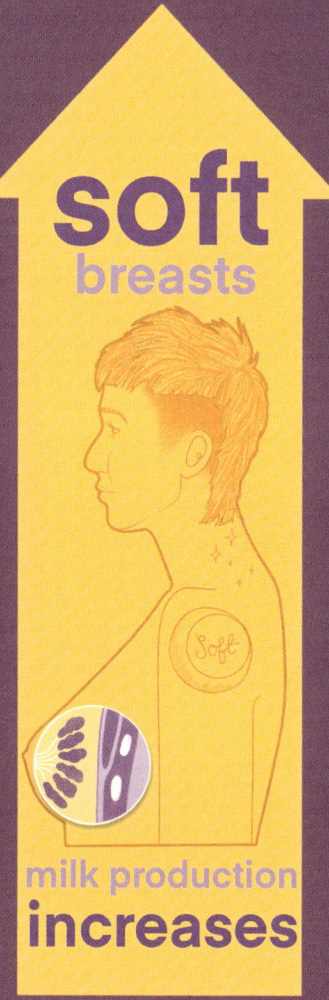

What is Colostrum?

Colostrum is the name given to the first milk that your breasts start to make during pregnancy. It contains lots of live cells such as secretory IgA and lactoferrin which help to support your baby's immune system. Colostrum also contains antioxidants, growth factors, and high levels of protein, vitamins and minerals. It is sometimes referred to as 'baby's first vaccine', a 'superfood' or 'liquid gold.' Even if you decide you do not want to breastfeed, you could consider hand-expressing some colostrum for your baby's first feed. You can do this antenatally or postnatally.

You continue to produce colostrum in small volumes for the first few days after you give birth to your baby, until your milk increases in volume (lactogenesis II). Mothers are often surprised at how small the volumes of colostrum they produce are. This may be something to do with growing up in a culture in which bottle-feeding is normalised and as a result many of us, without even realising it, have a visual in our heads of what a feed *should* look like. But in the first day or two of life, a baby needs a little and often. One feed could be the equivalent of around a teaspoon of colostrum. Try to visualise the size of your baby's tummy – at birth it is approximately the size of a marble and has a capacity of around 5ml.

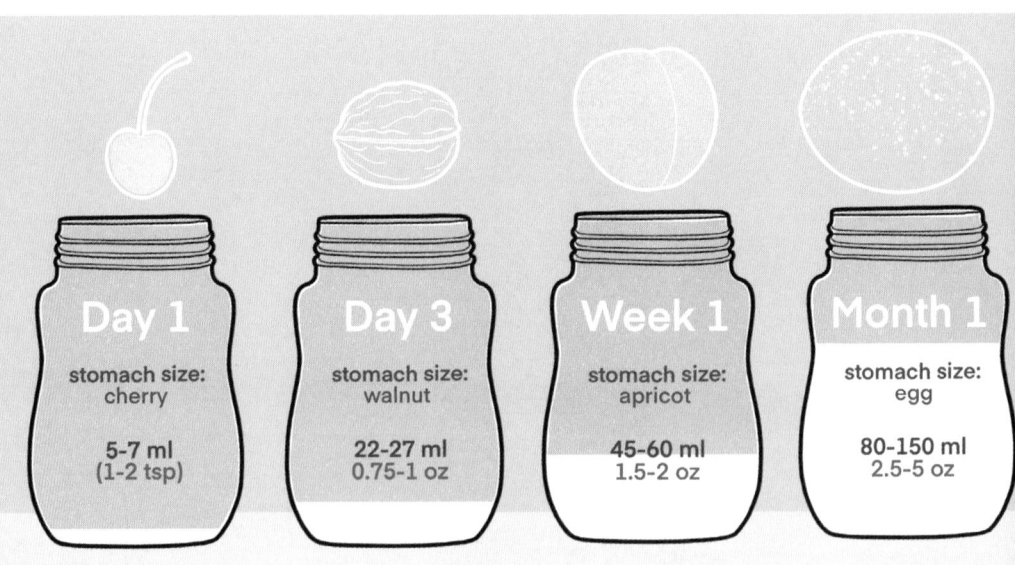

While colostrum does provide some nutrition for babies, it also has many other important functions such as

- acting as a laxative
- protecting the baby's intestinal lining
- establishing bifidus gut flora, the good bacteria in your baby's intestinal tract
- helping to prevent jaundice
- activating the baby's immune system
- protecting the baby against infection

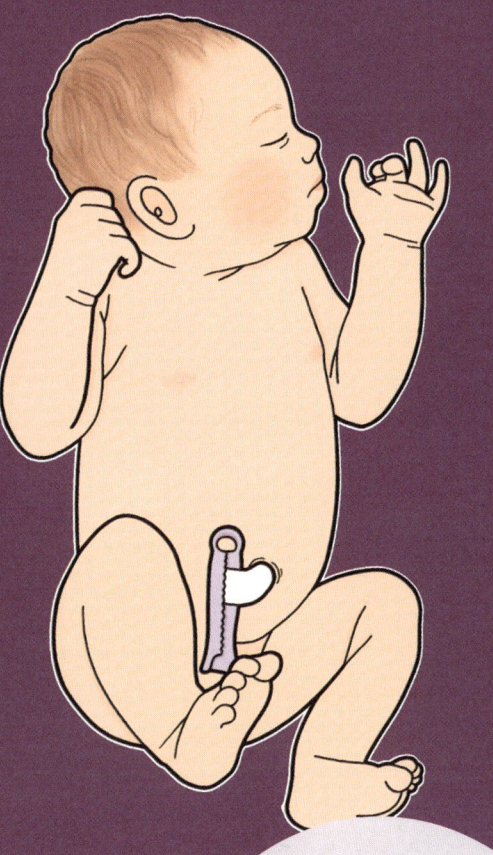

If you give birth to your baby prematurely, your colostrum will contain larger amounts of nutrients and immune factors. This provides them with extra protection against infections, particularly necrotising enterocolitis (NEC). NEC is a serious condition that can cause a baby's bowels to become inflamed. It is most likely to affect premature babies.

Just one teaspoon of colostrum contains millions of germ-killing white blood cells which help protect babies against infection.

Antenatal Expression of Colostrum

Some women choose to express colostrum towards the end of their pregnancy, but you don't have to. Many hospitals now recommend the practice antenatally to mothers who have type 1 or gestational diabetes, as the colostrum can be used to help stabilise baby's blood glucose levels after birth and reduce the need for supplementation with infant formula. Hand expressing and collecting colostrum in the antenatal period (sometimes referred to as *colostrum harvesting*) may also be recommended in other situations where breastfeeding difficulties are anticipated. For example, if a mother has risk factors for low milk supply or if a baby has a congenital abnormality such as cleft lip or palate. Antenatal expression is also quite commonly recommended for mothers who are having an elective caesarean section. The practice became quite popular following an Australian study called the DAME Trial which found that colostrum may be expressed safely antenatally from week 36 of pregnancy in diabetic women who have a low risk of complications. If you are interested in expressing colostrum antenatally, it is important to discuss it first with your midwife or obstetrician to determine whether or not it is safe and/or appropriate for you.

Some women find the practice of expressing colostrum antenatally empowering. It can help them feel confident about being able to breastfeed successfully and make milk. Expressing colostrum before birth also helps women learn how to hand express. However, antenatal expression may not be for everyone. For some women, the idea of trying to express colostrum antenatally causes anxiety and can be perceived as just another thing to do. Try to be guided by what feels like the right thing for you.

Not all women who choose to hand express antenatally manage to collect colostrum.

Not being able to hand express colostrum antenatally DOES NOT have any bearing on your ability to make milk once your baby is born.

Getting Started with Expressing Colostrum Antenatally

You can start expressing antenatally from week 36 or 37 of your pregnancy (depending on your maternity hospital's policy or on medical advice).

What do you need? You will need some very tiny containers to store colostrum. You may be able to get an antenatal expressing pack containing small syringes with stoppers and/or small plastic containers from your maternity hospital. If not, you may be able to buy a pack privately or order sterile syringes online. I recommend getting 1 ml and 2.5 ml syringes.

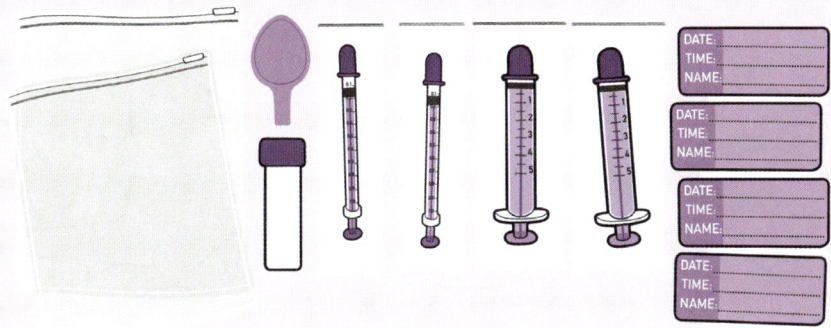

How often should you express? Two to three times a day if you can. The first couple of times you try, you may see only a tiny glistening of colostrum on the face of your nipple, or none at all. This is normal. It can take a little bit of practice to get the hang of hand expression.

How long do you express for? For a maximum of ten minutes - five minutes on each breast.

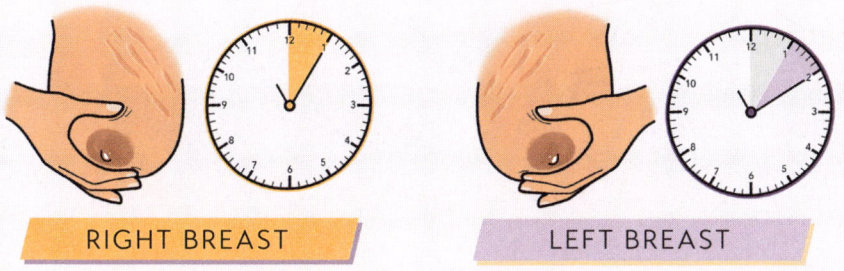

RIGHT BREAST   LEFT BREAST

How much colostrum can you expect to collect? It varies from woman to woman. Most women will collect small amounts, between 0.5 and 10 ml in total, while others will be able to collect more. Approximately one in four women will not get any colostrum from antenatal hand expression – so it is important to remember this if you struggle to get any colostrum when you hand express antenatally.

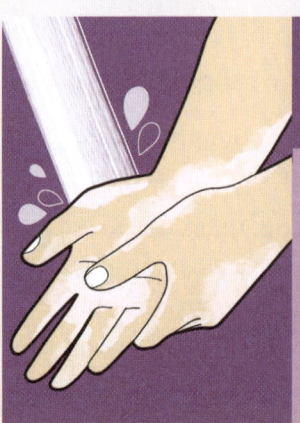

1 Wash your hands before you start.

2 Take some time to relax.

Many women find it helpful to have a shower first and/or to do some slow, mindful breathing. Warm compresses on your breasts, in addition to some massage (with warm hands!) can help to get that lovely feel-good hormone oxytocin flowing.

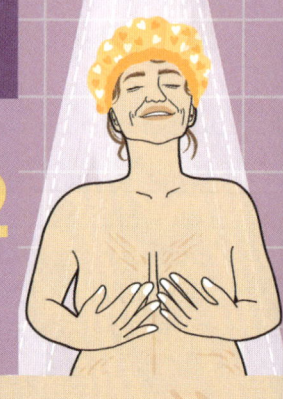

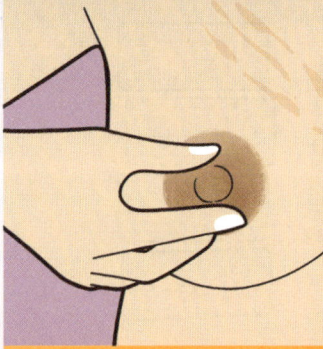 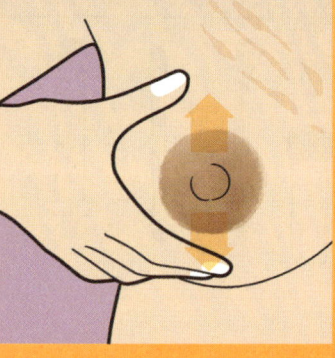 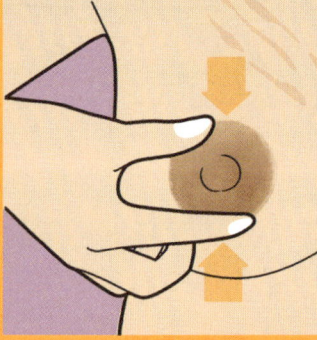

3 Place your thumb and forefinger on either side of the base of your nipple. Slide them back, away from the nipple, towards the outer edge of your areola. Apply a little bit of pressure and then slide the finger and thumb back towards the nipple. This should not hurt! It can take a little bit of practice to get the hang of this practice.

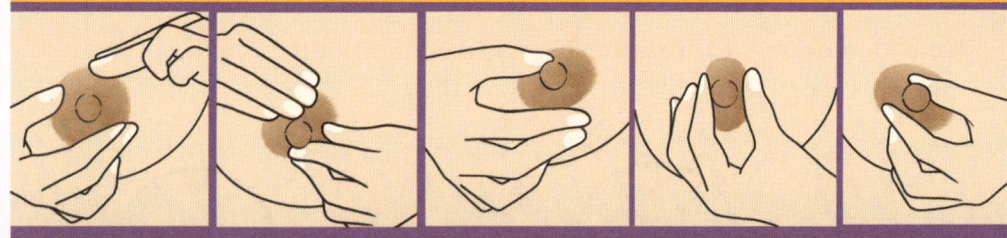

4 You can move your fingers around your areola or use different fingers – try to figure out what works best for you.

5 Many mothers find it easier to express drops of colostrum onto a clean teaspoon rather than directly into a syringe or container, and then draw the colostrum from the spoon into a syringe. Another option is to get some help – a second pair of hands could draw colostrum from your nipple with a syringe while you hand express.

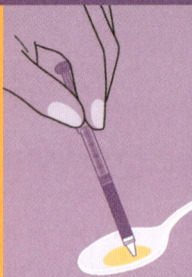

If you have been advised not to hand express colostrum antenatally.

Sometimes women are advised, for medical reasons, not to hand express colostrum antenatally. One example of a scenario where antenatal expression may be advised against is if a baby is in a breech position and the mother is having a scheduled C-section. If you have been advised not to hand express antenatally, you could request that you try some hand expression while you are being induced or being prepped for a caesarean selection.

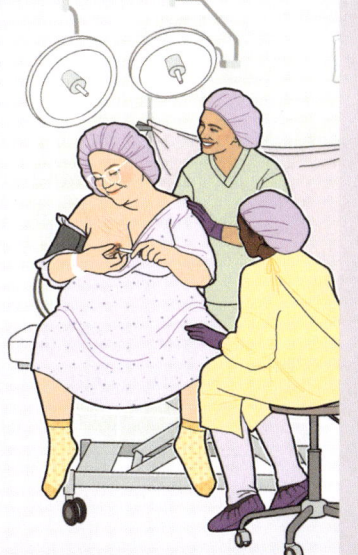

Storing Colostrum:

- Most containers and syringes come individually packed and are sterile. If you are using some other kind of container, make sure it is thoroughly washed in hot soapy water, rinsed with hot water, and left to air dry.

- Containers should be clearly labelled with the date, time, and your name.

- You can use the same container to collect colostrum for any hand expressing you do in a 24-hour period. Just keep the container in the fridge between one hand expression session and the next.

- When you are ready to freeze syringes or containers, place the stopper or lid on them, place them in a zip lock bag, and then put the bag in your freezer.

Going to Hospital

When you are going into the hospital to have your baby, bring your frozen colostrum in a freezer pack. As soon as you are admitted, give it to one of the

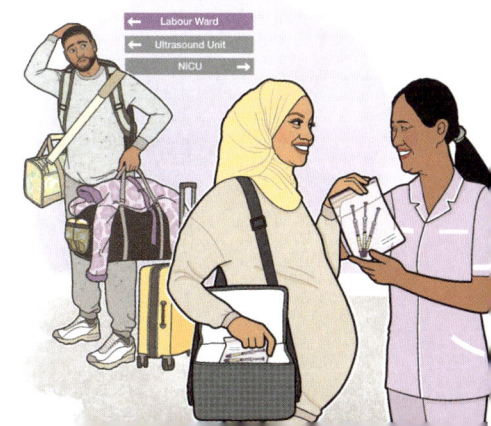

staff so that they can store it for you. If you have managed to express quite a lot of colostrum, you may not need to bring all of it with you into the hospital, particularly if you live a short distance away. Someone can always bring more colostrum into the hospital after you have had your baby, as and when you need it.

To defrost colostrum: Your maternity hospital will probably have its own policy on storing and defrosting colostrum, so ask staff what they advise. They may suggest defrosting colostrum by storing it in a fridge or by leaving it at room temperature. If necessary, you can defrost colostrum quickly by running the container under warm water.

When your Baby is Born

Your midwives will support you to give your baby your expressed colostrum. Usually, small volumes of colostrum are given to babies via a syringe as a *buccal* feed, whereby the colostrum is slowly squeezed one drop at a time inside the baby's cheek. If for some reason you are separated from your baby, ensure that staff know you have expressed colostrum for them.

The Benefits of Antenatal Hand Expression:

- You 'get to know the girls,' ie, become familiar with your lactating breasts and feel confident about touching them.
- You learn how to hand express.
- You may be able to collect and store some colostrum, so your baby will be less likely to need formula supplementation.'

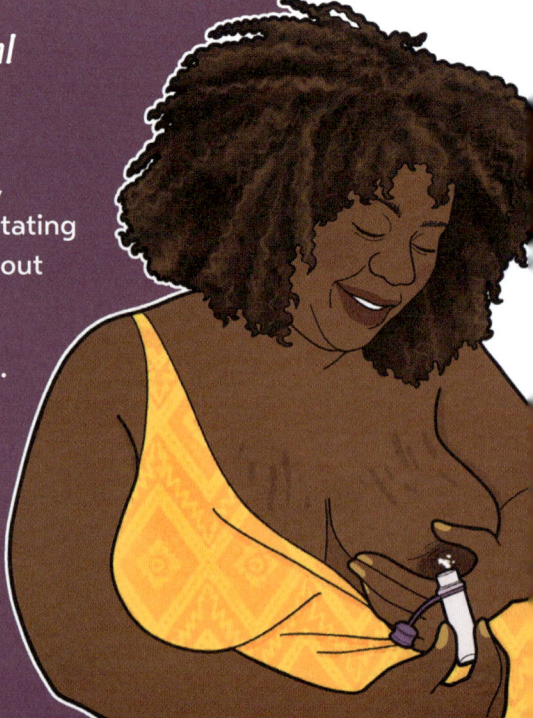

CHAPTER 3

Birth and the Golden Hours

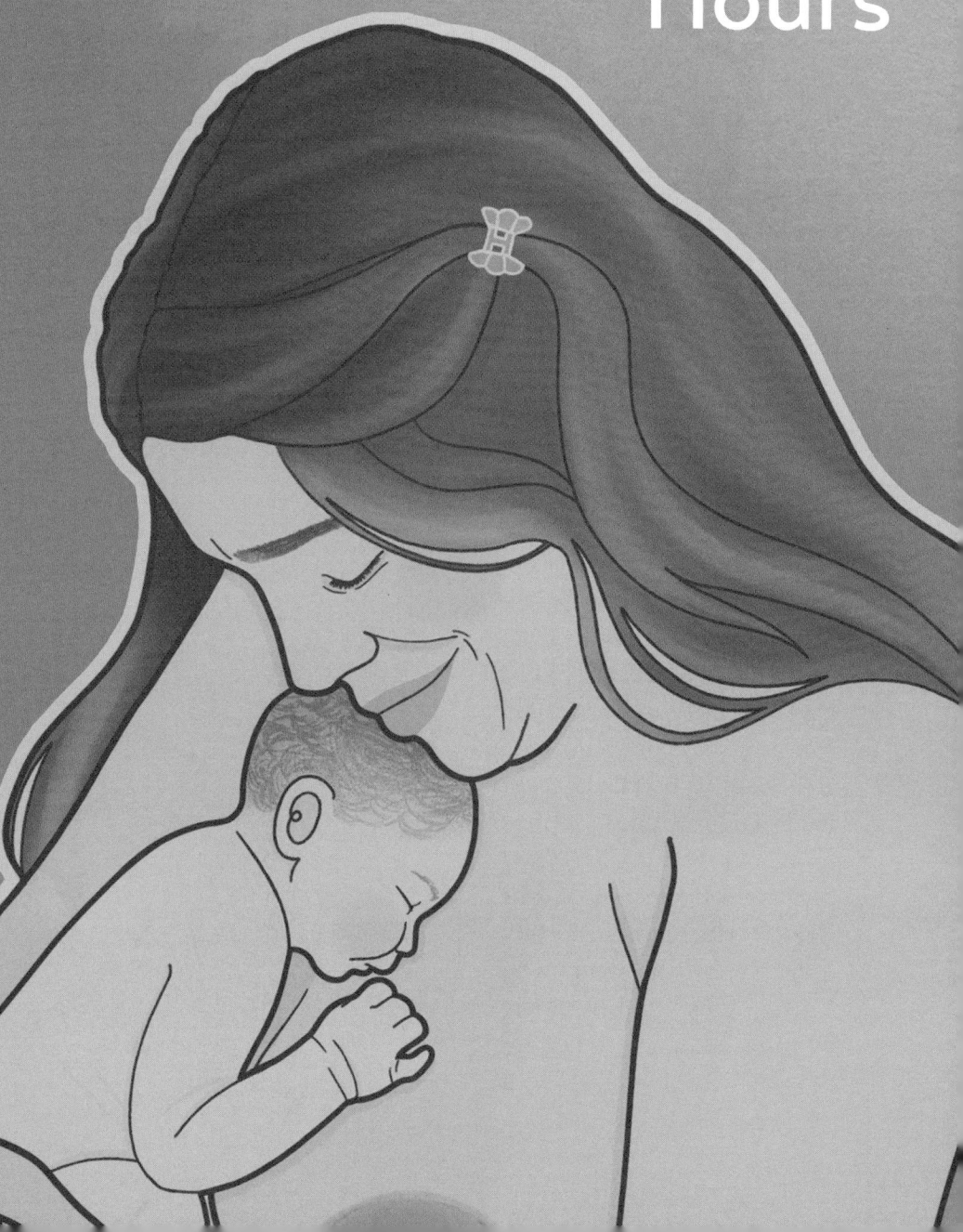

This chapter will give you the information and guidance you need to help you get breastfeeding off to the best possible start in the hours after you give birth to your baby, and what to do if things don't go according to plan.

Being in a Hospital

Most women and birthing people living in developed countries will have their babies in a maternity hospital. While there has been a small increase in the number of people having home births, the figures remain low, at approximately 1% in Ireland and 2.5% in the UK. Giving birth in hospital also means establishing breastfeeding in hospital. While there are some advantages to this, such as access to help from midwives and possibly lactation consultants, some aspects of establishing breastfeeding in hospital can be challenging.

A hospital is not a familiar setting for most of us. Hospitals are generally bright, noisy, and busy places, full of people and machines. If you are on a public ward, you may be sharing it with up to seven or eight other mothers and their babies, so you may not have a great deal of privacy — some women find this difficult. Conversely, if you are in a private room, while you might appreciate having your own space, you might also find it isolating. And the beds are probably not quite as snug and comfy as your bed at home. Hospitals will all have policies and procedures in place, rules and regulations, and boxes to be ticked at each stage of your admission, labour, birth, postpartum stay and discharge. Please note — this is not a criticism of maternity hospitals or the staff who work in them. This is simply how it is, and something that is worth giving some

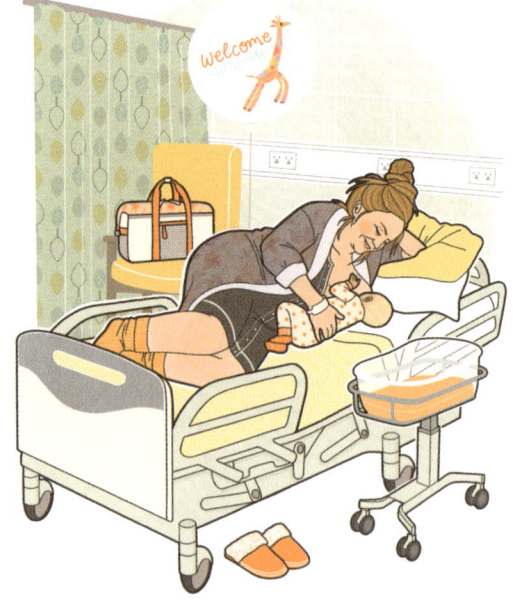

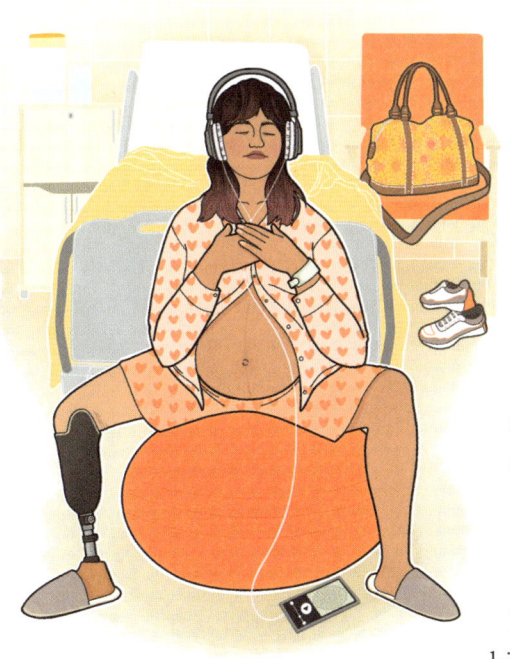

consideration to before you have your baby. This is one of the reasons why antenatal classes are recommended. They enable parents to think about the kind of birthing experience they would like to have and what they can do to help them adapt to being in hospital, for example, things like movement, listening to music or guided relaxation, hypnobirthing, massage, and warm showers. All of these things can help mothers and birthing parents physically and psychologically, and boost the flow of oxytocin, the 'love hormone' that we need lots of when birthing and when breastfeeding.

Most of the parents I see prepare thoroughly for giving birth in hospital. They often do both hospital and independent antenatal classes, learn hypnobirthing techniques and put time and effort into creating a birth preferences plan. But people tend to give less consideration to how they may feel about being in a hospital setting *after* giving birth, what things may be challenging for them, how they would like to be supported to breastfeed, and how they can advocate for themselves.

Hospitals, by and large, with their systems, rules and processes are patriarchal in nature. Many people feel cowed and afraid to speak up as patients, at a time in their lives when they are quite vulnerable. This is particularly true of people who have previously had negative experiences with healthcare professionals, or people who have concerns that they will be misunderstood or treated differently because of their ethnic background, sexual orientation or gender identity. In the United Kingdom Black mothers are, shockingly, four times more likely to die in pregnancy or in the first six weeks than white mothers. This is something to be aware of if you are a pregnant Black woman. Consider how you will advocate for yourself in hospital, and how you will ensure that your needs are communicated and understood.

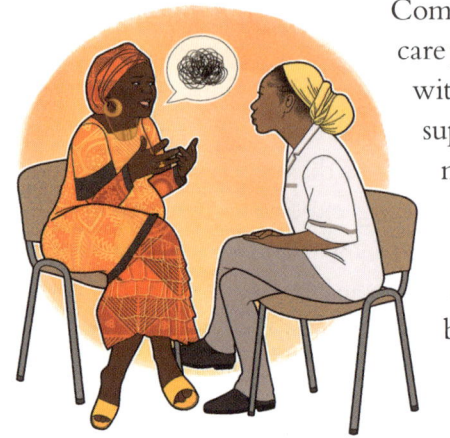

Communicating your concerns with your care providers will help them to provide you with sensitive and culturally appropriate support, and to better understand your needs. Hospital staff are there to help, support and care for you. Remember, your experience matters, how you feel matters and your voice should never be lost amid the noise and the busyness around you. You deserve to be treated with respect. It is YOUR body and YOUR baby.

The Golden Hours

The Golden Hours is a term commonly used to describe the first couple of hours of a baby's life, when they are kept in close skin-to-skin contact (SSC) with their mother. This time is also sometimes referred to as the *sacred* or *magical* hours. Uninterrupted SSC for the first couple of hours postpartum optimises the chances of getting breastfeeding off to a good start. When placed in SSC with their mothers, babies will usually initiate breastfeeding after an hour or two. Being in SSC contact triggers the baby's innate breast-seeking and feeding reflexes. The mother's body is a familiar place for the baby. The baby recognises the mother's smell, her familiar heartbeat and her rhythm of her breath and all of this helps them to feel a sense of security. The familiarity of the mother's body calms and soothes baby, and helps to ease their transition from womb to the world and get used to their new environment. The mother's body is this little mammal's natural habitat and the place where they feel safe.

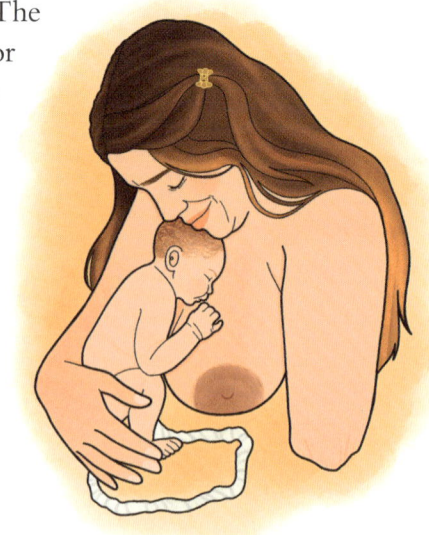

The golden hours are your baby's welcome to the world. Even if you do not intend to breastfeed, try to enjoy a couple of unhurried hours of skin-to-skin contact with your baby. Most hospitals will facilitate some quiet time for couples and their new baby after the birth.

Skin-to-skin Contact

Standard practice in most British and Irish maternity hospitals is to place a baby in skin-to-skin contact (SSC) on their mother's chest immediately after birth and support that SSC for at least one hour. Why has there been such a strong push internationally to implement and protect this first hour of skin-to-skin contact? In a nutshell, research conducted over the last 40 years has found that undisturbed SSC after birth:

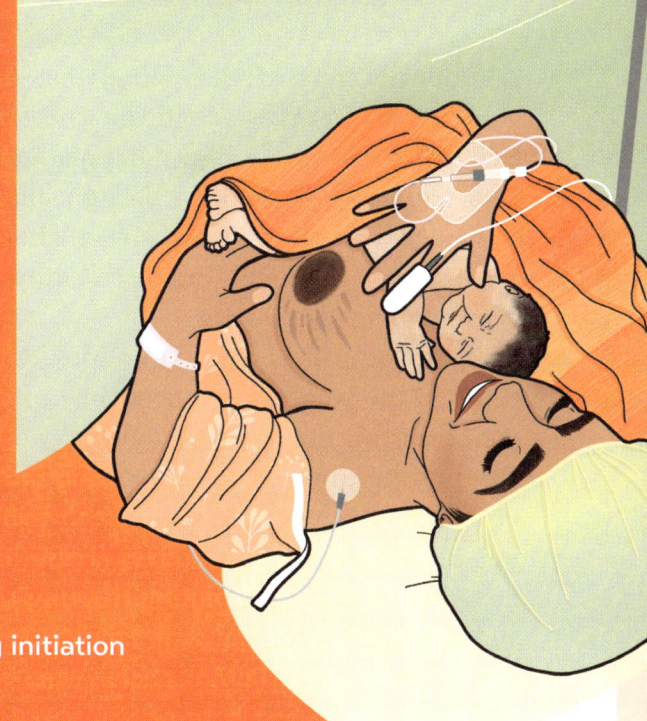

- keeps baby calm
- means less crying
- promotes physiological stability in the baby (heart rate, breathing, body temperature, blood glucose level and blood pressure stabilise)
- promotes mother-infant bonding
- improves breastfeeding initiation and duration rates
- supports optimal brain development

Studies have even found that newborns in SSC showed reduced pain. For a baby who has been born via a difficult instrumental delivery, immediate SSC with their mother may be even more important.

SSC also benefits the mother as it enhances the flow of oxytocin, often referred to as the 'love' hormone. This means:

- a deceased risk of post-partum haemorrhage
- a shorter third stage of labour
- the 'letdown' reflex which releases colostrum/milk is triggered
- an increase in mothering behaviours, bonding, facial recognition, relaxation and attraction to the newborn
- reduced maternal stress

Additionally, research has found that mothers who do SSC after giving birth feel more confident and empowered to care for their babies, breastfeed for longer durations and report less depression. SSC after giving birth improves breastfeeding initiation rates. It doesn't guarantee that you and your baby will be able to initiate breastfeeding without any problems. But it certainly optimises your chances of getting off to a good start.

Try to be patient with your baby. Give them time to adjust to being in the world. Give them time to explore your body and find your breast. It may take an hour or two before they start to suck so avoid trying to rush them – pushing them to the breast could upset or confuse them. Let them adjust to their new surroundings and to initiate breastfeeding themselves. Trust that your baby knows what to do. Also, if possible, avoid interrupting this special time – weighing and cleaning by hospital staff can wait until after your baby has had his first feed. And APGAR checks can be done while your baby is in SSC. Ideally, the first hour of SSC should be UNINTERRUPTED (assuming baby is physiologically stable and that there are no concerns for their health, and that the mother is well enough).

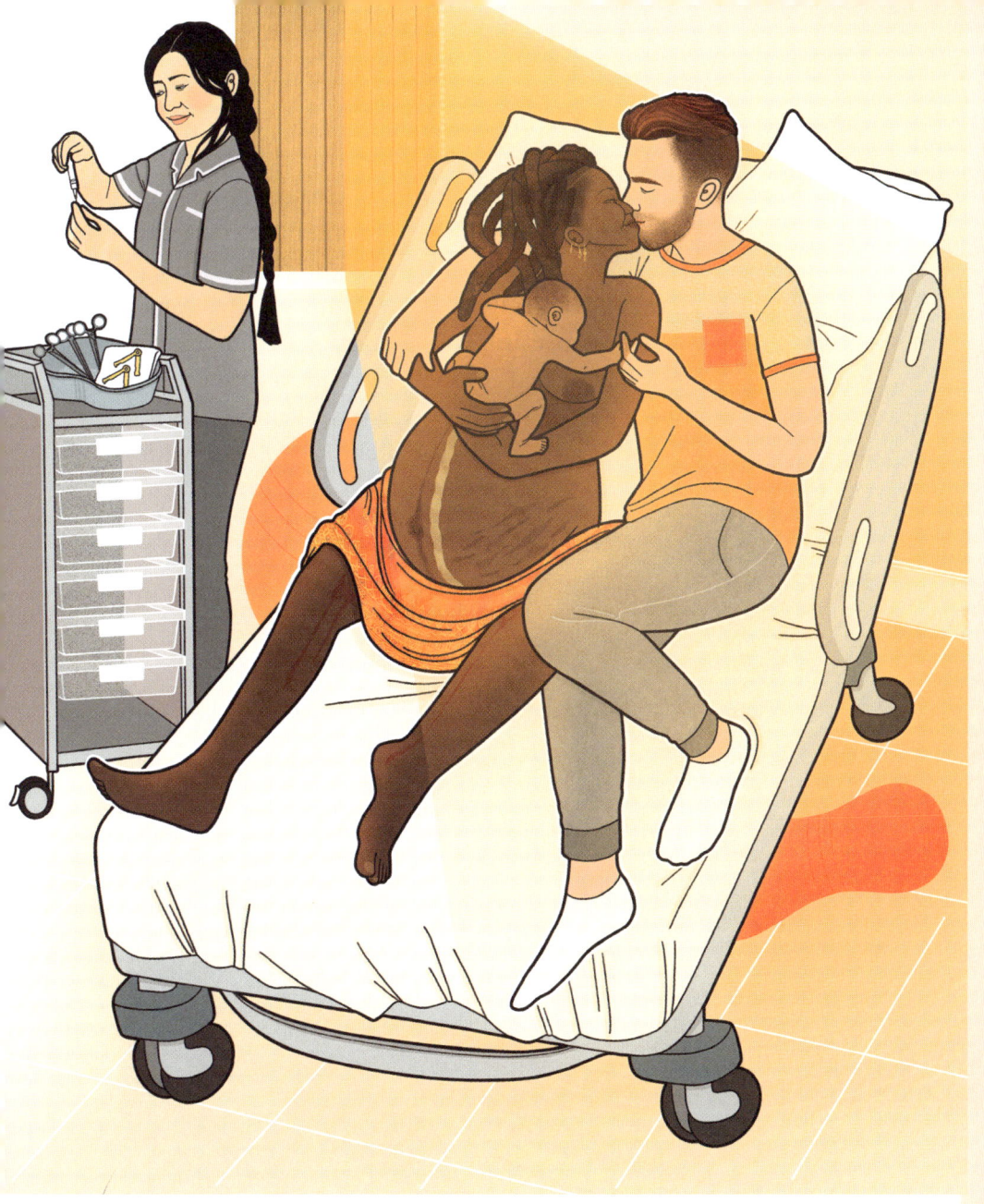

Enjoy the first hour – make it a gentle welcome to the world for your baby.

If your baby doesn't feed within the first hour or two (sometimes babies can be a little sleepy), don't hesitate to ask for help. You may need to wait until they are ready to feed at the breast. Your baby will need just a tiny amount of colostrum as their tummy has a capacity of only 5ml at birth. So every drop counts.

Missing out on immediate SSC with your baby in the hours after you give birth does not mean you cannot breastfeed or that you have missed out on an opportunity to bond with your baby. There are times when it may not be possible for a mother and baby to have SSC after the birth, for example, if a baby has to go to the neonatal intensive care unit (NICU) or if a mother is unwell. If separation is unavoidable, don't worry because you can make up this time later – your baby retains the newborn instincts and reflexes for a couple of months after birth, so even if they have spent time in NICU, it is not too late to do SSC and initiate baby-led latching. You and your baby can benefit from skin-to-skin at any time.

There may be times when a partner will do skin-to-skin contact with a baby instead of the mother, for example, if she

- Feels unwell
- Is in theatre and is not permitted to have her baby with her
- Does not want to do an extended period of SSC. Previous sexual trauma can make SSC difficult for some people.

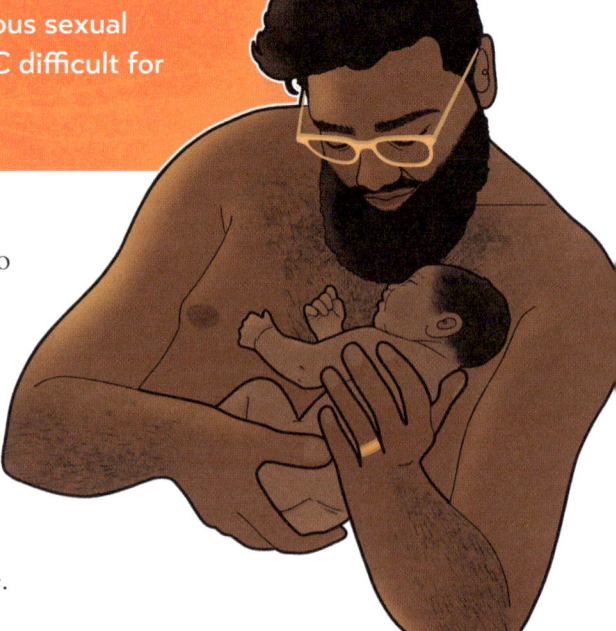

SSC with the partner is also very beneficial for babies as they are kept warm, experience physiological stability and are colonised with their family's bacteria. If you have a caesarean section, SSC should still be possible.

> *Bonding is not a single event that happens in the hours after your baby is born. It is a process that unfolds in the first six months.*

Within a minute of being born (and again five minutes after birth), babies are assessed using a scoring system called the Apgar Score. The Apgar score rates the following features:

A: Appearance (skin colour)

P: Pulse (pulse or heart rate)

G: Grimace response (reflexes and responsiveness)

A: Activity (muscle tone)

R: Respiration rate and breathing effort

Your baby will be given a score of either 0, 1 or 2 for each of the above components and these scores will be added together to give an Apgar score out of 10. A score of 7 or over is usually considered a positive sign of good health, while a baby who scores less than 7 may need some medical care. It should be possible to do Apgar checks while your baby is in skin to skin contact with you. Ask about it in your maternity setting or request in your feeding preferences plan that Apgar checks are done while your baby is on your chest.

The Nine Instinctive Stages

In recent years researchers have learned more about babies' innate behaviours in the hours postpartum. One well-known study conducted in the USA classified the behaviours that newborn babies' exhibit when they are placed in immediate SSC with their mothers after birth as 'The Nine Instinctive Stages' (more about the Nine

Instinctive Stages here www.magicalhour.org/aboutus.html). Most babies who reach full term will go through these stages when they are placed prone on their mothers' bodies after a straightforward birth. It can be tempting to intervene, especially in hospital where there may be pressure to get your baby latched within a certain timeframe. So, try not to rush this time, or put your baby under pressure to perform. Enjoy the golden hours, see what happens, and if your baby does not latch (after one and a half to two hours), ask staff for help. They will either provide assistance to help your baby latch or encourage you to hand-express colostrum.

Here's a job for your birth partner! Request that they observe and make note of the behaviours that your baby exhibits when they are in SSC with you. It can be really interesting to watch what they do. They may go through all nine steps or just some of them, and not necessarily in the exact order listed below:

Stage	Description
Birth Cry	Baby's lungs open for the first time during the initial birth cry. This crying helps to clear the airways of amniotic fluid (this is the liquid that surrounds and cushions your baby when they are in your womb).
Relaxation	Baby is placed in skin-to-skin contact with the mother. They have a little rest and take some time to settle in, feeling the warmth of the mother's body and hearing her heartbeat.
Awakening	Baby starts to become more active. They may make small movements of the head, arms, hands and mouth. They will gradually open their eyes.
Activity	Baby becomes even more active, moving arms and legs. They start to 'root' for the breast and stick their tongue out. They recognise the scent of their mother's breast from secretions of the Montgomery glands – the little bumps on your areolas). Babies also find the nipple by sight.
Resting	It is normal for babies to rest between stages - expect these little pauses. Try not to hurry your baby.

Crawling	With the help of their stepping reflex, baby will crawl or make their way from the centre of the mother's chest towards her breast. The stepping movement of the baby's feet may help with contraction of the uterus and expulsion of the placenta. Gently support and encourage your baby during this stage. It is a team effort.
Familiarisation	Baby familiarises themself with the breast by licking the nipple and areola area. This stage could last up to 20 minutes - again, try not to rush your baby. They are practicing oral-motor functions needed to breastfeed.
Suckling	During this stage, the baby opens wide, latches to the nipple/areola and breastfeeds.
Sleeping	Towards the end of the breastfeed, baby becomes sleepy due to high levels of a hormone called cholecystokinin (CCK). The mother's CCK levels will also be high at this stage, and she will probably also be ready for a nap.

Your Baby's First Feed

When a mother and her baby have unhurried, uninterrupted skin-to-skin contact (SSC) after the birth, the baby will usually exhibit breast-seeking behaviours which culminate in them latching and having their first feed. Think of the process as teamwork: you hold your baby in SSC so they get a chance to show off their innate breastfeeding behaviours, and you support and encourage them. Gradually your baby should make their way towards the nipple — this could take up to an hour and a half. Sometimes

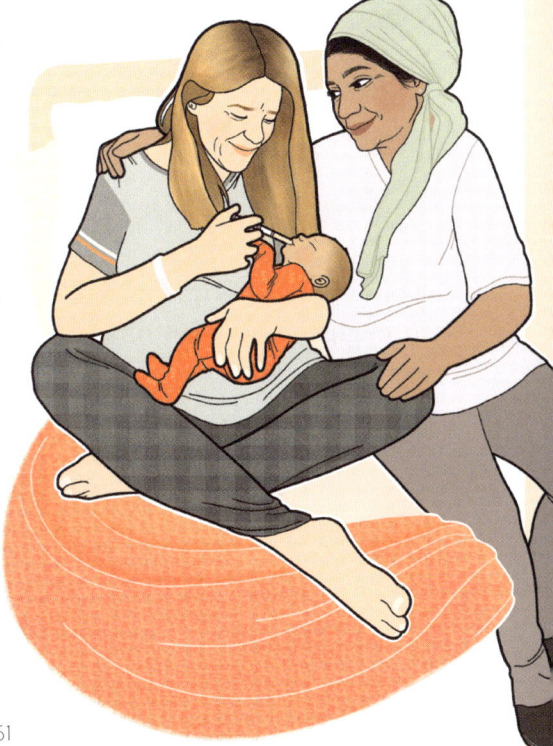

If your baby is sleepy, do skin-to-skin contact and hand express some colostrum.

a baby will latch without any assistance, but there are times when they will need a little bit of guidance from you, for example, a change to your position or baby's position. To latch, your baby will open their mouth wide and create a seal around the nipple and areola — sometimes it takes a few attempts. Remember, this is a new skill that your baby is trying to master. Try to be patient with them!

Your baby's first feed is often quite short — between five and twenty minutes — after which time your baby is likely to fall asleep. The volume of this feed may be as little as a teaspoon. Think of it not so much as food, because it is more about lining the baby's gut, immune protection and acting as a laxative.

If you and your baby are struggling to initiate this first feed together, ask for help! Midwives will either assist with latching or if your baby is not yet ready to latch and feed, they can help you to express colostrum and feed it to your baby. Sometimes babies will perk up and show more interest in direct breastfeeding after they have had some colostrum.

The small volumes of colostrum a baby drinks in the first few days enable them to practice breastfeeding without being overwhelmed by big volumes of milk.

If Your Baby Has to Go to the NICU

Doing skin-to-skin contact (SSC) and giving your baby time to go through the nine instinctive stages may not always be possible, for example, if you are unwell or if your baby has to go to the Neonatal Intensive Care Unit (NICU). Whether your baby goes to the NICU for a number of hours or for a longer time, it can be a very upsetting and anxiety-inducing experience. If you find yourself in this situation, try to remember that it is temporary and that you will be able to start over with SSC once you have your baby in your arms again. Babies retain the instincts and reflexes that they use in the hours after birth for months. It is never too late to do SSC!

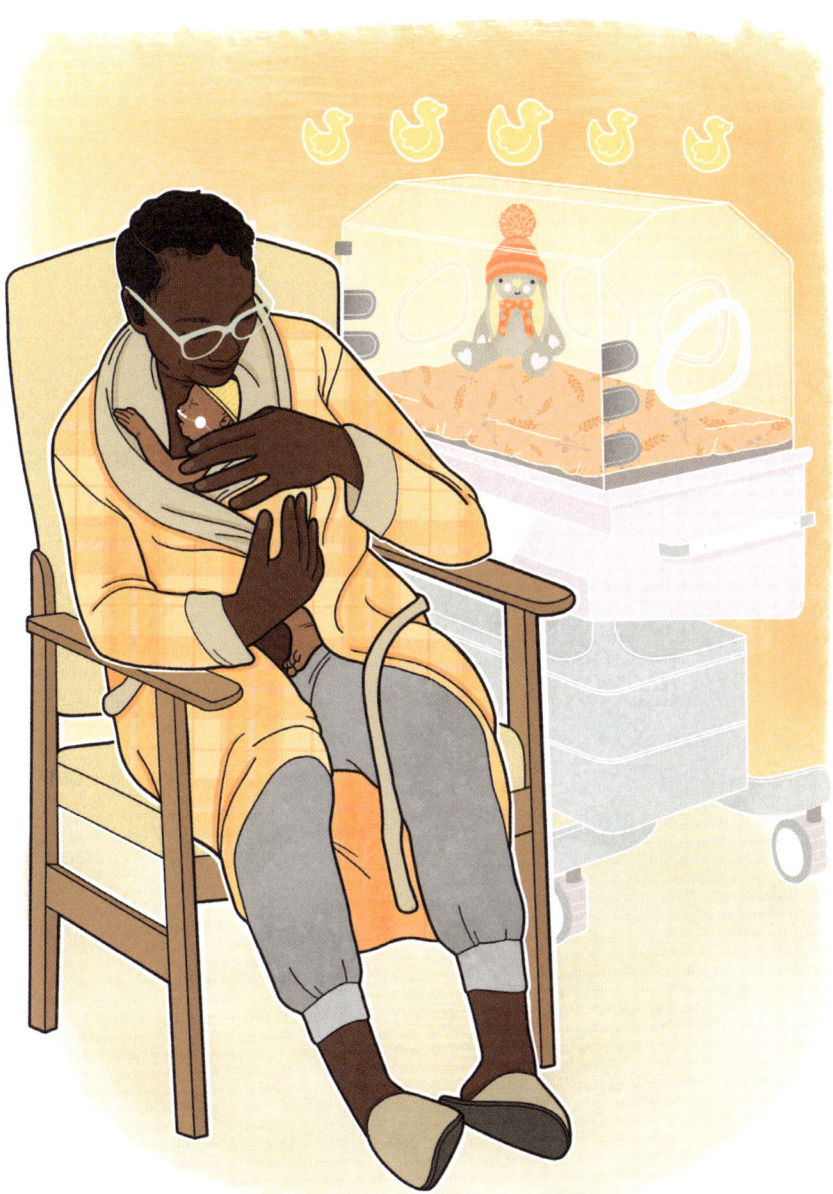

The one very important thing that you can do (that nobody else can do) while your baby is in the NICU, is to start hand-expressing colostrum. Your baby will need very tiny volumes to start with (remember that tiny newborn tummy). Ask midwives for help and try to hand express every two to three hours. Midwives will advise you when you need to start removing milk with a pump

Sometimes parents who have been unable to have SSC with their baby in the hours after the birth worry that this will affect bonding. This is not the case. Yes, SSC in the hours after birth helps to support bonding, but bonding is not a single event that happens during this time. Bonding is a process that unfolds in the first six months, and beyond.

Communicating with Hospital Staff

The care and support you receive in hospital should take into account your needs and preferences. Having a feeding preferences plan can really help staff understand how they can best support you. It can also be a good idea to think in advance about how you will communicate with staff when you are in the hospital. And if you will have a partner with you for the birth of your baby, it is important that they know what your feeding preferences are and understand what things are important to you. This enables them to advocate on your behalf. Also, consider if being in a hospital (not a natural environment for most people) will affect your ability to advocate for yourself. There is some research to suggest that women find it more difficult than men to assert themselves, consider themselves as authorities, or express themselves in public so that others will listen. I have found from working with women antenatally and postnatally, that preparing what to say in advance of giving birth and being admitted to the maternity hospital, and practicing those sentences, can help women feel more confident and empowered about speaking up for themselves. The key is having a voice and being confident about using it, without being combative. It is also important to trust your own inner knowledge, rather than just relying on the knowledge of those around you.

Are there any other reasons why communicating with staff in a hospital setting may be challenging for you? If you are a black woman, on the autism spectrum, or from a marginalised social group or a member of the LGBTQI+ community, you probably should give some thought to barriers to sensitive and inclusive care you may face and what you can do to protect yourself. For example, would you feel confident enough to ask that a different midwife cares for you if you did not feel comfortable or safe with someone? Could you face prejudice or racism? May hospital staff be more likely to make assumptions about you or about how you will feed your baby based on the colour of your skin, where you come from or your age? Do you anticipate that doing SSC or breastfeeding your baby, or even being in a hospital could present sensory challenges for you? Finding a way to communicate your needs and concerns can help staff provide individualised and sensitive care.

One of my clients, who I saw for an antenatal session prior to the birth of her second baby, created a feeding preferences plan and drafted some sentences that she planned to use in hospital to help her communicate how she wanted to be supported to breastfeed. This is what my client said about her experience of establishing breastfeeding in hospital:

> *When I arrived in the delivery suite and met my midwife one of the first things I asked her was, barring any medical interventions or mitigating factors, I would like at least one hour of uninterrupted skin-to-skin, and could we wait to weigh her until after that. I explained that I wanted to give myself and the baby a shot at starting breastfeeding in as natural a way as possible and see if we could figure it out together. She agreed that providing neither me or the baby needed any medical support after delivery, that was OK.*
>
> *I had a plan and a practised line in the event anyone wanted to intervene and try and "put my baby on" my breast. I used it quite a bit. "We're OK thanks, we're in no rush, just getting used to each other. We will get there."*
>
> *I felt it was important to have that as I knew when I was tired and in the ward on my own I needed a game plan.*

It can take time to learn how to get the baby to latch, for me several failed attempts at the start of each feed for the first week were the norm. I found when on the ward most midwives were quick to want to physically help, but from my perspective, they weren't coming home with me so if I didn't figure it out then I was just kicking the can down the road. I asked them to explain to me how to do it so I would figure it out myself before I was on my own with her in the middle of the night at home! "Could you come back in a few minutes, I'm just going to try myself for a while"

In advocating for those seemingly small experiences, I allowed myself and my baby space and time to figure it out and I didn't feel the pressure of having someone stand over me while I tried. Four months on I have a happy, healthy, chubby breastfed baby!

Birth and Breastfeeding

How you give birth to your baby and certain interventions that sometimes happen in hospital during labour and delivery can affect breastfeeding and lactation, especially in the first week postpartum. A little bit of understanding of how these practices can affect you, your baby and milk production can help you make informed decisions and be prepared for some challenges they may present. The first thing to keep foremost in your mind is that although some interventions and birth practices can make initiating breastfeeding a little more challenging, they do not (for the most part) prevent you from meeting your breastfeeding and lactation goals.

Instrumental Birth

During an instrumental birth instruments, such as a ventouse suction cup or a forceps, are used to apply some force to your baby's head during the

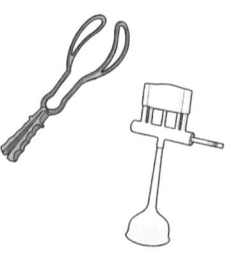

second stage of labour to 'pull' them out. They may be used if labour is not progressing, or a baby becomes stuck in an unfavourable position in the birth canal. Sometimes just a little force is required, sometimes more. If the birth of your baby is assisted using either ventouse suction or forceps, you may notice some red marks on your baby's head – a round haematoma in the case of ventouse suction and possibly some bruising or abrasion when forceps are used. If this is the case, be mindful that your baby's head could be a bit sensitive or sore to touch, and they could have a headache. So, when you are breastfeeding try not to touch their head or apply pressure (also request that midwives are mindful that your baby's head may be sensitive to touch). A semi-reclined position may work best in this scenario, or a side-lying position, especially if you had an episiotomy (a surgical cut made to your perineum during birth to make the opening to your vagina bigger) and stitches and are sore. Babies generally heal very quickly after an instrumental birth, often within days.

Occasionally, if quite a bit of force has been used during an instrumental birth, a baby could have a little bit of asymmetry through their body or *torticollis* – this is when your baby's head tilts to one side. Asymmetry or torticollis can affect breastfeeding by making latching a little more difficult for the baby or by making it difficult on just one side. Asymmetry or torticollis can also lead to latch-related nipple pain for you. If you think your baby has torticollis or you feel breastfeeding is more difficult on one side, seek some skilled breastfeeding support from someone who will be able to help you with positioning. You might also like to consider some bodywork for your baby with a trained professional such as a paediatric physiotherapist or a paediatric osteopath. They can do some gentle hands-on work to ease out birth-related tension and tightness your baby may have.

Postpartum Haemorrhage

There is always some blood loss after you give birth – anything up to 500ml is normal. However, sometimes the volume of blood lost is above 500ml. This is called a postpartum haemorrhage (PPH). This most commonly happens after a difficult vaginal birth involving the use of forceps. Studies have found that women who have had a PPH are less likely to initiate breastfeeding and that their babies are more likely to be supplemented with infant formula. This may be because after a PPH, SSC may need to be delayed, for example, if the mother is feeling unwell and cannot hold her baby. Another factor is that the mother may be somewhat incapacitated by an intravenous infusion in one arm, and they may be drowsy.

If you have a postpartum haemorrhage after the birth of your baby, your partner can do skin-to-skin contact with your baby while your PPH is being managed. You can do SSC as soon as the bleeding is under control and you are well enough. Ask for some extra support to get breastfeeding established or to do hand expression, and try to do as much SSC during your hospital stay as you feel able. Don't be afraid to ask for help at any stage. Sometimes some skilled support from someone in those first few days can make all the difference in establishing breastfeeding.

There is some evidence that a significant PPH (>1000ml), a sudden drop in iron levels and low blood pressure can result in lower milk production. So, if you have experienced a significant PPH, ask for lactation support in the hospital. If you are concerned about your milk supply after you have been discharged, seek out support from a lactation consultant as early as possible.

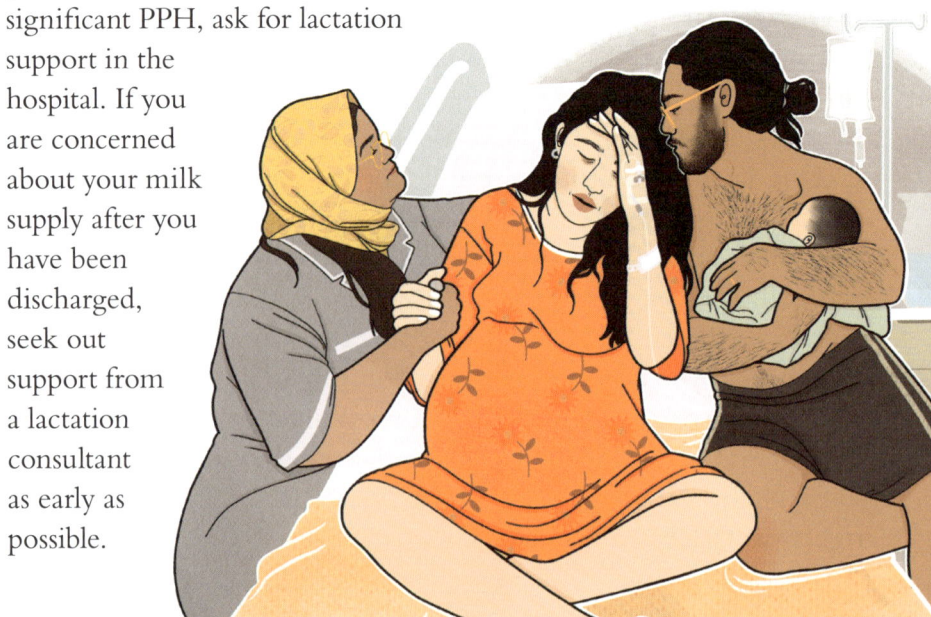

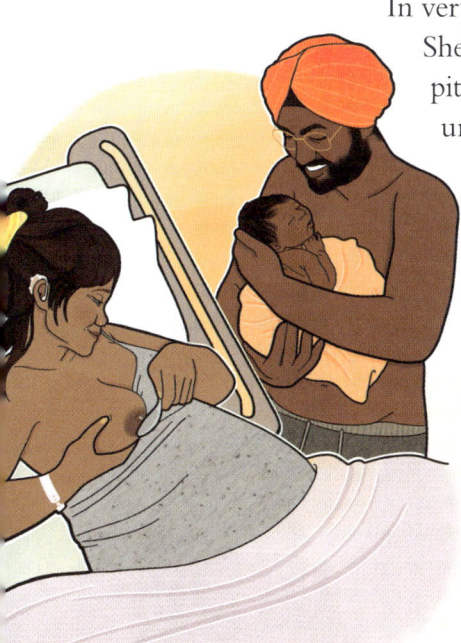

In very rare cases, a severe PPH can result in Sheehan's Syndrome, whereby the anterior pituitary gland is damaged such that it is unable to make the hormones required for milk production. Most women who develop Sheehan's Syndrome will not experience Lactogenesis II (milk coming in) and will be unable to breastfeed.

Please note: In my private practice work mothers who have had significant PPHs of up to 2000ml have successfully breastfed and made enough milk for their babies. Everyone is different and there are so many variables that can affect breastfeeding and lactation. The important thing is that you receive individualised support.

Pain Medications

While medications such as epidural anaesthesia and air and gas are commonly given for pain relief during birth and labour and are safe for mothers and babies, they can sometimes interfere with establishing breastfeeding by making a baby drowsy or causing a mother to feel sick (and possibly unable to hold her baby and breastfeed for a while). This could mean having to hand express colostrum (ask for help, especially if you are a first-time mother) until either you or your baby are ready to directly breastfeed. There is no strong evidence that receiving an epidural during labour has any impact on breastfeeding outcomes.

The use of another painkiller, pethidine, however, can be more of a problem. Pethidine can temporarily affect a new baby's ability to suck and effectively transfer milk at the breast, reduce the baby's alertness and inhibit their rooting reflexes. If you have pethidine and you experience difficulties with breastfeeding or you have concerns about your baby, insist on skilled and individualised support to help you overcome these challenges — because they can be overcome.

IV Fluids and Weight Loss

Intravenous (IV) fluids administered by tube to a mother during her labour can artificially inflate her baby's birth weight. The baby will pee the excess fluid out during the first 24 hours after the birth, and this can result in a higher-than-expected weight loss. Sometimes this weight loss will be flagged as a sign that there is an issue with breastfeeding (even if breastfeeding is going well) and supplementation may be suggested. If you have IV fluids and your baby appears to experience a big weight loss (losing more than 7% of their birth weight) on day two or three, it may be worth having a conversation with your care providers about the possibility that this weight loss is related to the IV fluids you were given.

IV fluids received during labour can also result in a delay in milk coming in, and this means an increased likelihood of supplementation with infant formula. Doing plenty of skin-to-skin and lots of breastfeeding in the first couple of days will help to encourage your milk to come in sooner.

IV fluids can also contribute to breast engorgement. This makes it more difficult for babies to get a deep latch, and sometimes they may not be able to latch at all. A shallow latch can cause nipple pain and damage. Doing reverse pressure softening before feeds can help to make the areola softer, thereby making latch easier.

Birth Trauma

Birth trauma is the term used to describe physical or psychological trauma experienced by a woman (and/or her birthing partner) during labour and delivery. Physical traumas include perineal tears or pelvic organ prolapse and psychological traumas could be caused by a feeling of being out of control, lack of informed consent, and disrespectful care. Whether the trauma experienced is physical, psychological or both, it can have lasting effects on a mother or birthing parent and/or their partner. Birth trauma can sometimes make establishing breastfeeding and bonding with your baby more challenging in the early weeks postpartum. If you experience birth trauma, don't be afraid to call it that, and ask for the help you need – partner support, family support, doula support, lactation consultant support or all of the above. Many women who have experienced birth trauma benefit from engaging in some kind of birth reflection session, either independently or through their maternity hospital. Another option for women who have experienced birth trauma may be birth trauma resolution therapy.

One of the things that I have found in my private practice is that women who have experienced birth trauma often feel very strongly about making breastfeeding work. Breastfeeding can actually become part of their healing journey, by helping them value themselves through their ability to provide for their baby.

Breastfeeding After a Caesarean Birth

Can you breastfeed after having a C-section birth? Yes, you can. However, there are a few factors that can make establishing breastfeeding in the first week a little bit more challenging:

Getting an extended period of uninterrupted skin-to-skin contact can be more difficult after a Caesarean Birth. A lot depends on the policies of the hospital you give birth in. Some hospitals allow for earlier and more prolonged contact after the procedure. Other hospitals can be reluctant to allow prolonged SSC for a mother and her baby after a Caesarean. This can result in a delay in breastfeeding initiation. So, what can you do to protect SSC with your baby after a Caesarean birth? Discuss with your care providers your intention to breastfeed and your desire to have as much uninterrupted SSC as possible following the birth of your baby. This discussion can take place before giving birth if you have a scheduled Caesarean birth or during or immediately after the procedure if you have an unscheduled section. Explain that you would like for your baby to get an opportunity to latch and have their first feed while you are in theatre. If for whatever reason this is not possible, seek help with hand-expressing colostrum while your birth partner does SSC with your baby. This ensures that your baby receives colostrum for their first feed and it can help you to feel more confident about establishing breastfeeding.

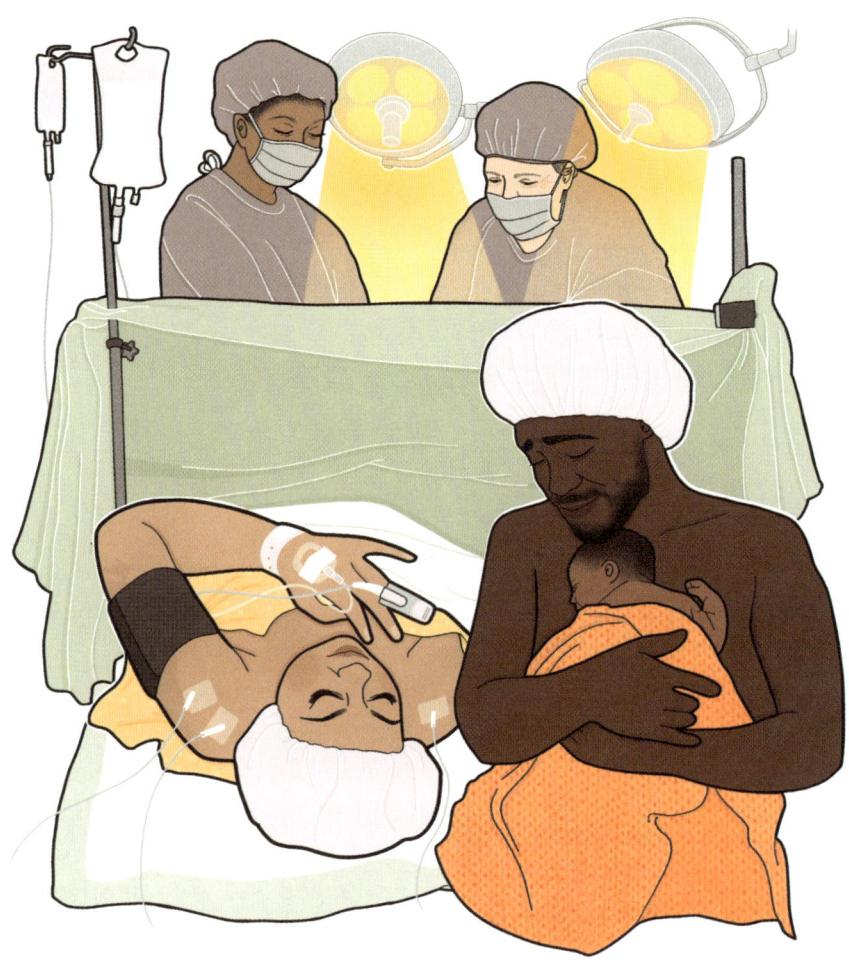

Having a Caesarean Birth limits your mobility in the first 24 hours after the procedure and can leave you feeling tender during the first week postpartum. This can make picking up your baby difficult and comfortable positioning more challenging. Let your care providers know that breastfeeding is important to you. And ask for help with positioning that avoids causing you discomfort, for example, sitting semi-reclined and placing your baby across your body so that their feet do not kick against your caesarean section wound. Also, don't be shy about asking for help to lift your baby out of their bassinet (cot) every time they need to feed, even if this means ringing the bell every two hours! Getting the help and support you need during these few days after your Caesarean birth is crucial. Remember – a Caesarean birth is major surgery. If you are having a scheduled Caesarean, discuss with your care providers the level of support that will be available to you in the hospital. Ask them how long your partner will be able to remain with you after the procedure, and what kind of flexibility they give to women who have had Caesarean births (who by definition, require more help). In an ideal world, your partner would be allowed to stay in the hospital with you for the first few days, but this rarely happens in Irish and British maternity hospitals.

Having a Caesarean Birth is a risk factor for a delay in your milk coming in, and therefore increases the likelihood that your baby will require supplementation with infant formula. Sometimes after a Caesarean birth, a mother's milk will only start to come in on or around day five or six. Two things you can do to help avoid this delay in your milk coming in are to do as much skin-to-skin contact with your baby as you can and breastfeed your baby frequently (every two-three hours).

Experiencing pain after a caesarean birth can get in the way of comfortably breastfeeding, so do not hesitate to let your care providers know if you are in pain.

Gentle or mother-centred Caesarean birth: A gentle or mother-centred Caesarean section puts the mother at the heart of the procedure and aims to make one as much like vaginal birth as possible. Healthcare providers who facilitate a gentle Caesarean birth aim to give the mother greater autonomy by giving her options, for example, choosing to have the drape lowered so she can see her baby being born. Once the baby is born, the HCPs will endeavour to place them in immediate skin-to-skin contact on their mother's chest, and to keep them there while the surgery is finished off. This enables the baby to latch and have their first breastfeed within the first hour.'

There may be times when a mother is unable to hold her baby – if she is feeling unwell or has had a general anaesthetic. In these situations, the next best thing for the baby is for the Dad or partner to hold the baby skin-to-skin until the mother is well enough to do skin-to-skin herself.'

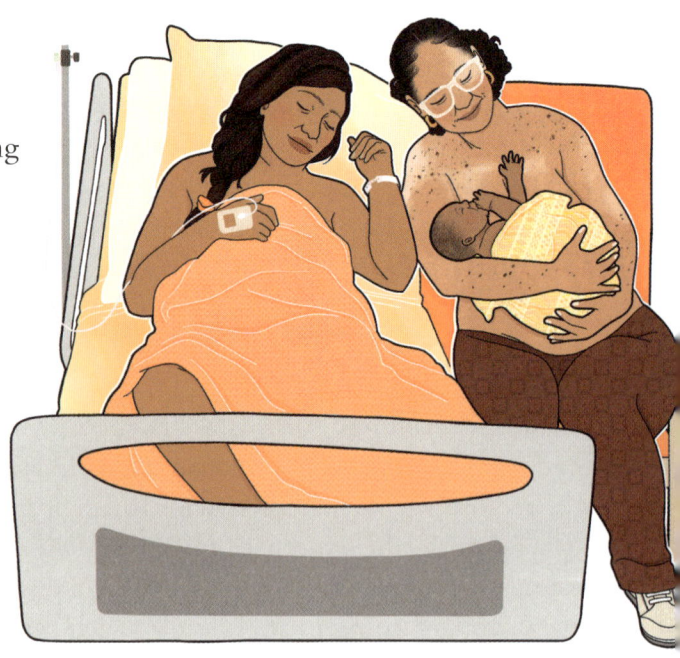

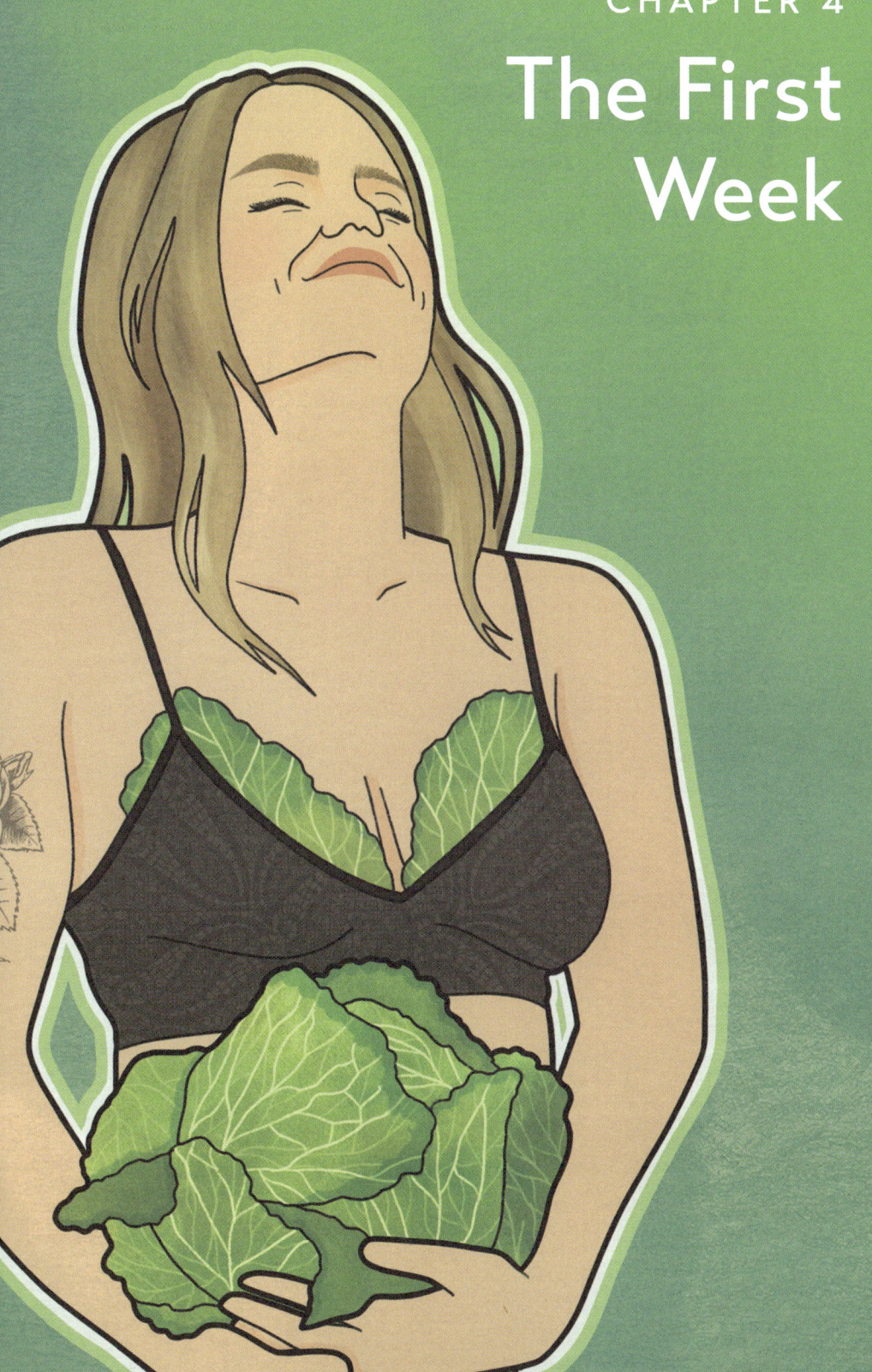

CHAPTER 4

The First Week

During the first week, you and your baby learn how to breastfeed. In the first few days you produce small volumes of colostrum and then your milk increases in volume (comes in), usually around day three but sometimes a little later. Your baby loses weight initially and then if they are feeding well, they start to gain weight towards the end of the week.

The First 24-48 hours

It's normal for babies to sleep quite a lot in the first 24 hours. During this time you should try to rest as much as possible. Keep your baby close and offer your breast to them every two to three hours. Ask for help if you are struggling to get your baby latched or having difficulty waking them up. If your baby is not yet ready or able to latch and directly breastfeed, you can hand express small volumes of colostrum and give it to them using a syringe or spoon. Half a teaspoon or just a few millilitres could be enough for a full feed for your baby!

During the first 24-48 hours, babies will have two or three wet nappies and will pass meconium. This is your baby's first poo. It is a greenish-black colour and quite sticky. Small, frequent colostrum feeds act as a laxative and help your baby pass meconium from their digestive tract.

It is normal for mothers to experience a drop in the volume of colostrum between the hours 12-27 postpartum. So, if you are hand-expressing and notice a decrease in volume, don't panic! The milk volume will probably start to increase from around 30 hours postpartum.

Your Baby's Second Night

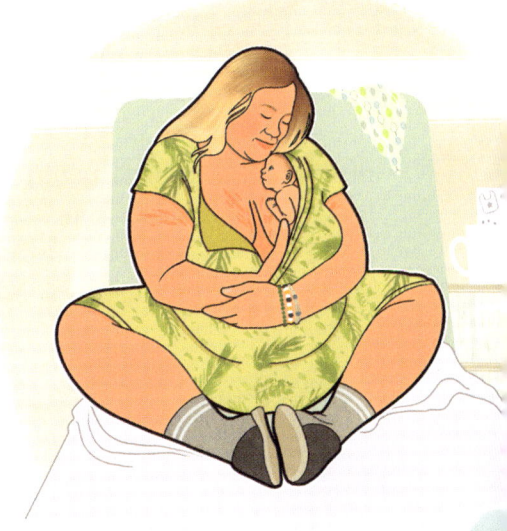

If you Google 'Baby's Second Night' you will find a plethora of articles on this phenomenon. So, what does it mean? After a relatively calm and sleepy first twenty-four hours, during which babies usually sleep off the exertion of being born and propelled into an entirely new environment, they start to perk up a little. They start to realise that they are in an unfamiliar setting and this may feel scary and overwhelming. Think about it from their perspective – they have spent nine months in your womb, surrounded by fluid, snug and warm, constantly being jostled around and hearing the sounds of your body, feeding continually, and buffered from the world. And then all of a sudden they are born and everything is unfamiliar. The sounds are louder and it's bright. Everything is different. Even the sensation of feeling air on their skin is a new experience. Now, imagine how lying alone in a bassinet may feel for your baby. Naturally it's going to feel a little bit scary and lonely. Instinctively babies crave reassurance and a feeling of security, and the place where they find it is your body. Being on your chest, snuggled in close, gives them a feeling of calm and a sense of safety, reassurance that everything is OK. They feel the warmth of your body, they hear all the familiar sounds of your breathing, and your voice and they are comforted by your smell. The other thing that gives them comfort is the close proximity to your breasts. They can latch and suckle whenever they want. This is bliss for your baby.

Your baby's first bath can wait! Studies show that delaying a baby's bath by up to a week helps to support breastfeeding. Another reason to delay the first bath is that the protective coating on babies' skin (vernix caseosa), has antimicrobial, anti-inflammatory and antioxidant properties which protect them from infection.

To let you know that they need to be close to you, babies cry. This is their only way to communicate. But very often increased crying on the second night is misinterpreted as hunger, or a sign that something is wrong. You feed your baby, put them in their bassinet, and they cry. This cry may not necessarily mean that they are still hungry. It is more likely to be their way of way of saying to you

 Mum, please don't leave me on my own. I'm scared. I need you. Please hold me close.

It is normal for babies to feel like this on the second night. The intensity of their need to be close to you and to feed can feel exhausting but it will pass. Not every night is going to be like this! Here are some suggestions to help you and your baby get through the second night:

- Your baby is exhibiting normal newborn behaviour. They are not being demanding or unreasonable They are simply responding to an instinct to be close to you.
- Keep your baby close to you. Many mothers find the easiest thing to do is to snuggle their baby in beside them, in a side-lying position.
- Give your baby unlimited access to your breasts. It is normal for them to feed a lot during the second night.
- Ask for help when you need it, for example, with latching your baby or with positioning.
- Be mindful of how you are feeling – if you are in pain, consider asking for pain medications.
- Sometimes an infant formula supplement will be suggested during the second night. If it is, consider if this is something you really want. Does your baby need a supplement, or are they just behaving in the way most babies do on the second night?

Keeping your baby close during the second night and giving them unlimited access to your breasts not only helps to make them feel calm and secure, it also hastens your milk coming in. In contrast, mother-baby separation at this stage can delay milk coming in.

> Your body is your baby's natural habitat.

Latch and Positioning

Sometimes in hospital, when staff are busy, the focus is on getting your baby latched to your breast. This is of course necessary for them to be able to breastfeed. But what can be missed, is both your physical comfort and your baby's physical comfort. Both of these things are important to get right first, *before* you focus on your baby's latch. So, think of each breastfeed as a three-step process:

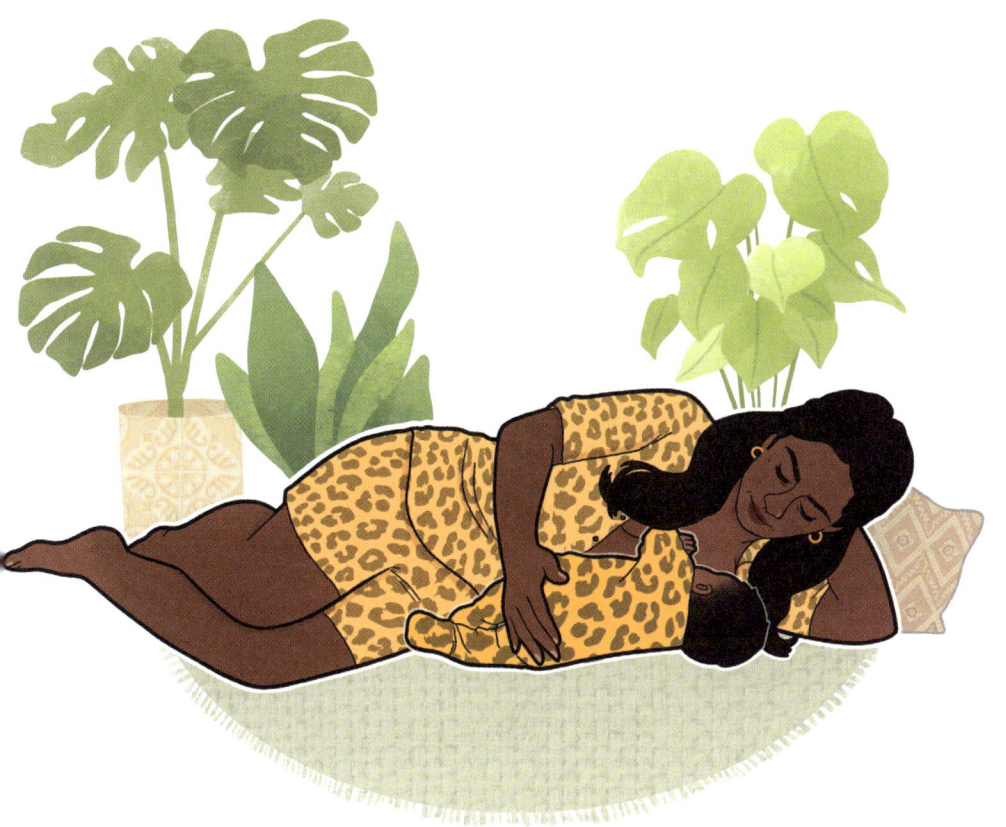

1. *Your Body:* Get yourself comfortable! Whatever that takes. You may need pillows behind you, something to rest your elbow on. Just take a few moments to check in with your body to ensure you're feeling supported and at ease. Many mothers find that a semi-reclined position works well, but it's not a one-size-fits-all.

2. *Your Baby's Body:* Place your baby on your body and give them time to get comfortable and find their bearings. For babies to feel secure and relaxed, they need a lot of contact with your body. Try to use gravity, so that you are supporting your baby with your body rather than taking their weight on your arms and shoulders.

3. *The Latch:* Observe what your baby does. They may mooch towards one of your nipples or start moving their head from side to side and making mouthing movements. They may need a little help from you to wriggle a little closer to your nipple – ideally, you want them coming up to your nipple rather than face on, so that when they latch they take in more of the lower part of your areola into their mouth. Avoid pushing your baby's head in towards your breast. Babies tend not to like this as their little heads are quite sensitive, especially if you had an instrumental birth. Also, pushing your baby's head towards your breast can be counterproductive as it limits your baby's neck extension and therefore their ability to open wide and get a good latch.

More often than not babies will latch themselves or with a little bit of help from you if you follow the above steps. Sometimes mothers will need to shape their breast into a *breast sandwich* for their baby, or provide more guidance for their baby. There is no one correct breastfeeding position that will work for everyone. Be patient with yourself and with your baby. Sometimes babies need a few attempts at latching before they get it right. And some women will need to try different positions until they find one that works best for them and their baby. Remember, your baby is learning a new skill, and so are you. If you are struggling with latch and positioning, ask for help from a midwife or lactation consultant.

When your baby latches it is important that they create a seal and that they can remain attached. If the initial latch feels sore or uncomfortable, give it a few moments – babies often shimmy their way on, so the initial soreness or sensitivity can ease once the milk starts flowing.

If the initial soreness does not ease, you could probably do with a little bit of skilled breastfeeding help from a midwife, breastfeeding counsellor or lactation consultant. Often, a change to positioning can help your baby get a deeper latch – try bringing your baby in closer, ensure they are able to open wide, and see if shaping your breast helps. If a change to positioning doesn't help, ask for help to figure out what is going on. It could be that there is some degree of *oralur-boobular* disproportion (big nipples, small mouth!), or that your baby is struggling to open wide due to birth-related tension, or that your baby has a tongue tie. Getting skilled help will help you figure out a way to keep feeding your baby, protect your milk supply and figure out how to overcome whatever problem you're facing.

There are lots of different positions you can try. There is no one right way to breastfeed your baby, because there are so many variables – breast size and shape, body shape, anatomical variations, your and your baby's preferences, your baby's needs etc. Ultimately all you need is to find one position you can use confidently. You certainly don't need to master a range of breastfeeding positions! See Chapter 5 for more on different breastfeeding positions.

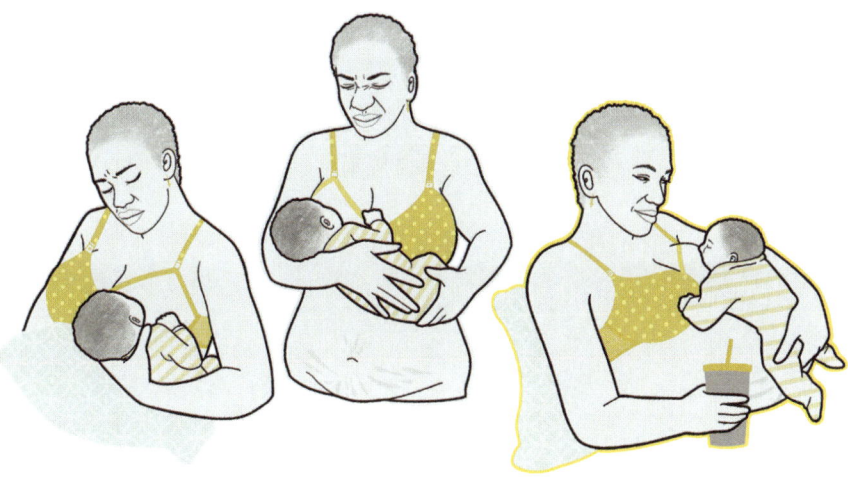

> ***Rusty Pipe Syndrome,*** whereby a little bit of blood-tinged milk discharges from your nipples, can occasionally present in the first few days postpartum. It is a benign condition and generally clears within a couple of days.

Is the latch good?

Firstly, does it feel comfortable? If yes, that is probably a sign that your baby is latched well to your breast. Secondly, can your baby create a seal and remain attached? If yes, these are also signs of a good latch. Thirdly, what does your nipple look like after your baby has fed? A normal, rounded shape suggests that the latch was good, while a flattened nipple is a sign that your baby's latch was shallow, ie, that they were attached to your nipple rather than your breast.

Usually, when babies are latched well, their chin, cheeks and nose will be touching (or be very close to) your breast. Even if your baby's nose is touching your breast, their curved nostrils allow for airflow. Babies prioritise breathing over feeding so if they need to come up for air they will!

Common misconceptions about latching

- Your baby's lips (particularly the upper lip) do not need to be flanged out like a blowfish, for them to have a good latch! The important thing is that they create a seal.

- Your baby does not need to have ALL of your areola in their mouth – just a good mouthful of breast tissue rather than your nipple.

Focus on how the latch *feels* and how well your baby is feeding, rather than on what the latch *looks like*.

Latching Tip and Tricks

Sometimes little tweaks and adjustments can help you and your baby find a more comfortable or a deeper latch.

The Flipple Technique

Hold your breast so that your fingers are on the underside and your thumb presses down just above your areola, so that your nipple points upwards.

Bring your baby in close to your breast, with their chin touching the lower part of your areola.

Just as your baby latches release your nipple so that it 'flips' into your baby's mouth, giving them a deeper latch (hopefully!)

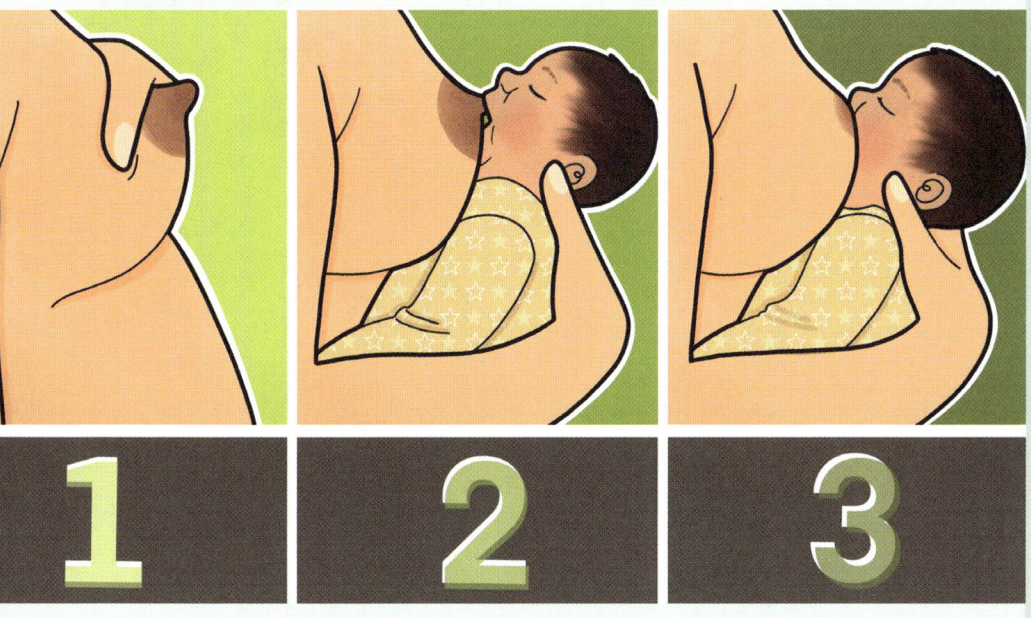

Create a 'Shelf'

Place your index finger underneath your breast to create a *shelf* of breast tissue and nipple that baby can latch on to. The nipple may be slightly pointing downwards.

Bring your baby in close to your breast. Ensure your fingers are not too close to your nipple.

When baby opens wide and is about to latch, direct your nipple into their mouth, as if pouring it in.

Make a Breast Sandwich

With this technique you use your hand to slightly flatten the breast tissue around your nipple. This creates a 'sandwich' that your baby can more easily latch on to.

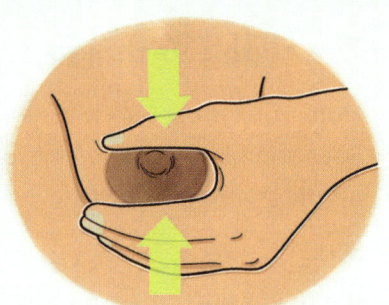

Scissor Hold

This is very similar to making a breast sandwich. This difference is that you use your forefinger and middle finger to shape your breast.

Baby's Head Tilt

Whatever position you are feeding your baby in, they should be able to tilt their head back easily. This enables them to open wide when latching. When you pull your baby in close to you, do so by applying gentle pressure to their back. Doing this causes their head to naturally tilt back.

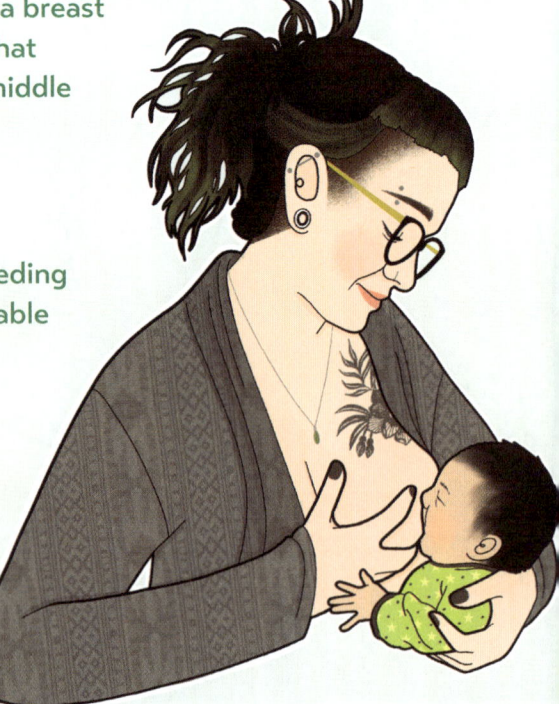

Drop Baby's Hips

If your baby's latch does not feel comfortable, try leaning back slightly and dropping baby's hips down a little bit, so that you are taking their weight on your body and they can stretch out.

Ensure Your Baby is Close You

Recline and use gravity so that there are as few gaps as possible between your body and your baby's body.

> *Many babies will have lip blisters in the early weeks. This is normal. However, if you are concerned about how your baby is feeding, seek support.*

Breastfeeding with Larger Breasts

Latching and positioning can be more challenging for mothers with larger breasts. Some tips that may help include

- Using a rolled-up towel or muslin wedged under your breast to bring your nipple higher, or make it visible to you.
- Shaping your breast can make latching easier.
- Some mothers opt to use a scarf to make a sling to lift and support their breast.
- Laidback or side-lying positions that use gravity can often work well.

- Rugby hold, with your baby well supported on a feeding cushion or even a table, can also be a good option for some mothers.

- Sometimes you need to be creative. One mother I worked with found that the position that worked best for her was sitting cross-legged on her sofa, with her baby wedged in between her breast and her leg.

- Get help from a breastfeeding supporter or an IBCLC and remember that latching and positioning will get easier as your baby grows and develops more head control.

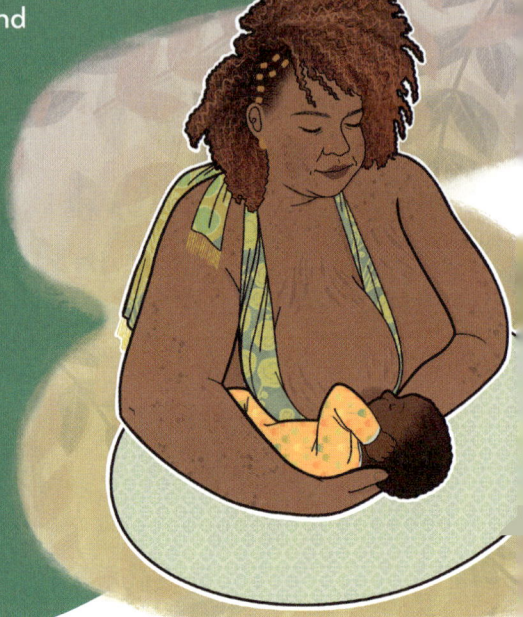

Mothers with larger breasts often feel more self-conscious about feeding their babies in public. It can feel like more of a palaver to get your boobs out and get your baby latched. If the idea of feeding in public seems daunting, investigate places that have comfortable seating, bring a friend with you and throw a scarf over your shoulder while you get your baby latched (if you're self-conscious). A good place to practice and build your confidence is at a face-to-face breastfeeding group.

Lactogenesis II – Your Milk *Coming In*

Lactogenesis II, or *milk coming in* as it is more commonly known, is when your breasts start to produce bigger volumes of milk. It is triggered by the expulsion of your placenta from your body. When this happens, levels of the hormone progesterone drop, and this allows your body to start making more milk. Lactogenesis II usually happens on around day three postpartum but can happen any time during the first week.

Usually, mothers notice their milk coming in as their breasts go from feeling soft, to feeling significantly bigger and heavier. And the breasts will also have noticeable veining due to an increase in blood flow to the area (milk is made in the breasts using constituents from the bloodstream).

The important thing when your milk comes in is to keep your baby feeding regularly on both breasts. If your baby is not feeding enough, your breasts can become very full or engorged and this can make latching more difficult for your baby. Because the breast is harder and the areola is more full of fluid (milk, blood and lymph fluid), your baby may struggle to get a good mouthful of breast tissue into their mouth. They may seem like they are bouncing their head against your breast in an effort to latch or they may latch onto your nipple. This is something you want to avoid as it is likely to hurt. If your baby is struggling to latch after your milk comes in, or their latch becomes painful, you could try *reverse pressure softening*.

Reverse Pressure Softening

This technique helps soften your areola and make it easier for your baby to latch on to. Before you feed your baby, recline, place your fingers either side of the base of your nipple and push down. Hold for a few minutes. Doing this helps to move fluid from your areola into the breast, thereby softening it and making it easier for your baby to latch. A softer areola is easier to latch on to than a firm areola that is full of fluid.

Delayed Lactogenesis II

Milk usually *comes in* or increases in volume on around day three postpartum. However, sometimes it can be delayed. If your milk has not come in on day three, do not panic! Factors that could lead to a delay in your milk coming in include having had a caesarean section, mother-baby separation, birth trauma, a delay in starting breastfeeding, oedema (fluid retention), high blood pressure, diabetes, and obesity. Milk could also be slower to come in if your baby is not feeding effectively or is preterm.

If it seems like your milk is slow coming in, doing plenty of skin-to-skin (where possible) and lots of frequent breastfeeding (or pumping if your baby is not feeding directly at the breast) will help. Ensure you get some skilled breastfeeding support. Your baby may require supplementation until you are producing adequate volumes of milk for them.

Occasionally, milk coming in can be inhibited if some fragments of your placenta have been retained in your body. These fragments, even if they are very small, keep progesterone levels high and prevent the onset of full milk production. If there is absolutely no sign of an

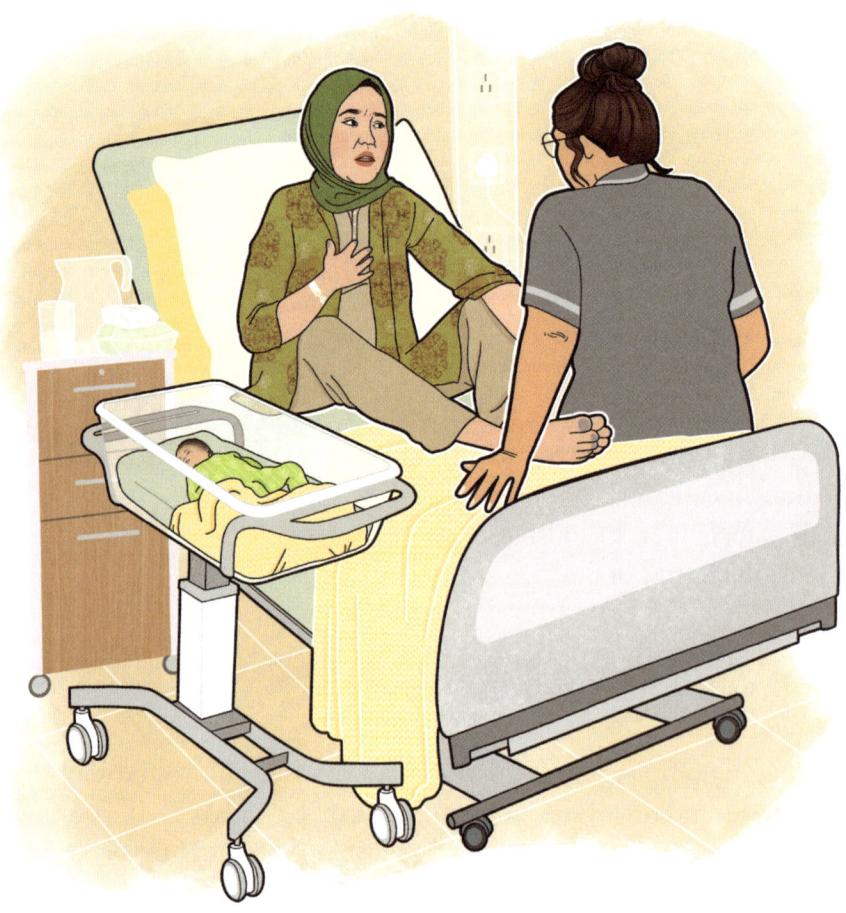

increase in milk volume after the first week, you need to discuss this with a healthcare professional who will try and figure out what is going on. If retained placental products are identified in an ultrasound, removing them generally results in an increase in milk volume. Retained placenta is sometimes accompanied by abdominal cramping, abnormal lochia or signs of infection such as a high temperature.

Engorgement

Sometimes breasts can become engorged in the days after your milk has come in. The engorgement is caused not only by a big volume of milk, but also by an increased flow of both blood and lymph to the area. Engorgement can make it difficult to get milk out – think of it as a traffic jam. The area is so congested that nothing can move. Engorgement can also flatten your nipple and make it more difficult for your baby to latch. If you experience engorgement you can help to relieve it using the following measures:

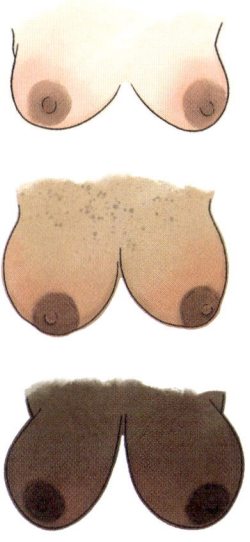

Therapeutic Breast Massage: Doing this before breastfeeding helps to move blood and lymph away from your breast. This reduces pressure in the breast and makes it easier for the milk to flow.

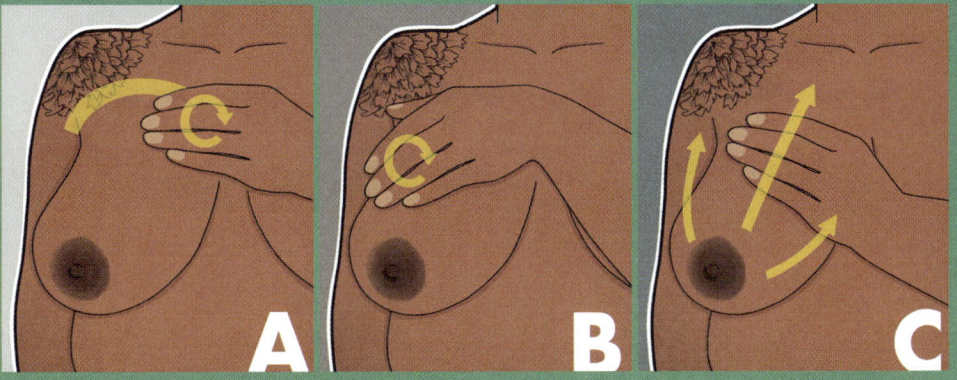

- Recline and try to relax. A few long slow breaths may help.
- Warm your hands up by rubbing them together, and start very gently massaging and rolling your breasts (no firm pressure).
- You can make small circular movements with your first two fingers all around your breasts and make light tapping movements on the breasts.
- Also, massage gently from the nipple radially outwards towards your armpit. This movement helps with lymphatic drainage.

Hand Expression: Sometimes it may be necessary to remove a little bit of milk using hand expression before breastfeeding, just to help you feel comfortable and make it easier for your baby to latch.

Cold Compresses or Cabbage Leaves after feeding: Applying cold to your breasts after feeding can help to reduce the signs of engorgement. Cabbage leaves have actually been found to be more effective in relieving engorgement than cold gel packs. Keep them in your freezer and pop them into your bra after you've fed your baby.

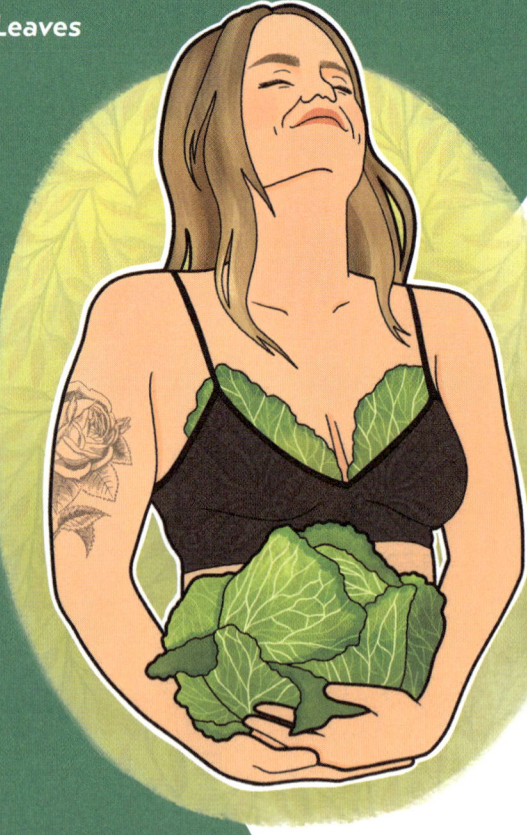

Common anti-inflammatory medications: such as Ibuprofen can help relieve the pain of engorgement (and are safe to take when breastfeeding).

Keep breastfeeding your baby as often as they want to be fed.

Milk Ejection Reflex (MER) – The letdown

The Milk Ejection Reflex (MER), more commonly known as the *letdown*, happens when your milk starts to flow in response to your baby's sucking or stimulation of your nipple. It happens like this:

your baby latches and starts to suck

the sensory nerves of the nipple send a signal to your brain's pituitary gland

the pituitary gland triggers the release of the hormone oxytocin

oxytocin causes milk in your breasts to start flowing towards your nipples, via the ducts

Your baby continues to suckle and this keeps the milk flowing. Several letdowns can happen in one feed.

It is easier for oxytocin to flow when you are relaxed. Stress hormones can inhibit the flow of oxytocin and delay or stop your milk from letting down.

Some women feel the letdown as a tingling sensation or pain in their breasts, while others do not feel it at all.

If you look at your baby feeding you will probably be able to notice the point at which your letdown happens, because their sucking pattern will change. It will switch from being fast and fluttery (baby stimulating the nipple to initiate a letdown), to being slower and deeper (baby drinking) – look for longer jaw movements and swallowing sounds.

How Often Should your Baby Breastfeed?

Small babies breastfeed a lot – just how often they feed often comes as a surprise to new parents. It can be helpful to bear in mind that their tummies are tiny, and that breastmilk has a gut transit time of approximately 50 minutes. Healthcare staff may sometimes suggest that your baby should feed every three hours (I hear this regularly from parents) but think in terms of feeding them *at least every three hours* instead. It is important that you don't try to stretch out the times between feeds, and that you put your baby to the breast whenever they show feeding cues. This is called *responsive feeding*. If you're not sure, put them to the breast anyway! Most babies will need to feed between eight and twelve times per 24 hours. All the frequent feeding is ensuring that your baby is getting sufficient milk and that you will be able to produce enough milk for you baby in the future. Suckling turns on prolactin receptors, which allows for optimal milk production.

You can hold your baby as much as you want

Another helpful way of thinking about breastfeeding in the early days is to think of feeds as being like three-course meals: baby feeds for a short while on one breast, then has a snooze, wakes up and feeds on the other breast, snoozes again, and then wants another little bit of dessert! And there may be times when your baby decides they want the *all you can eat buffet!* You may be advised that your baby needs to feed for '15/20 minutes on each side.' This is not good advice. In the first week babies often feed for shorter durations. Sometimes they will feed from both breasts and sometimes one will suffice. The number of minutes they spend at the breast tells us nothing about the

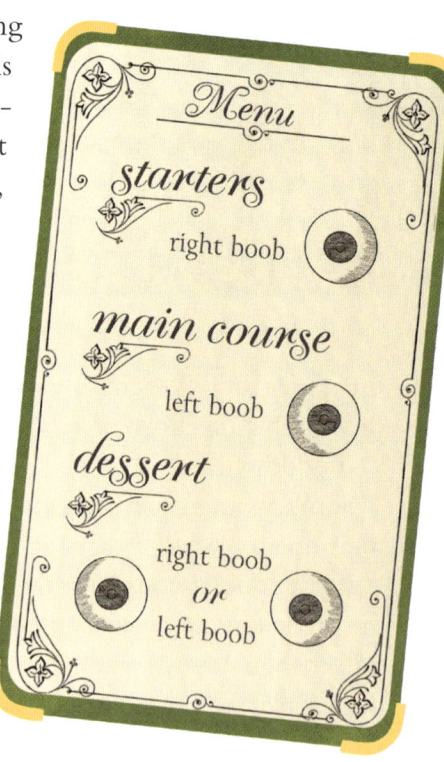

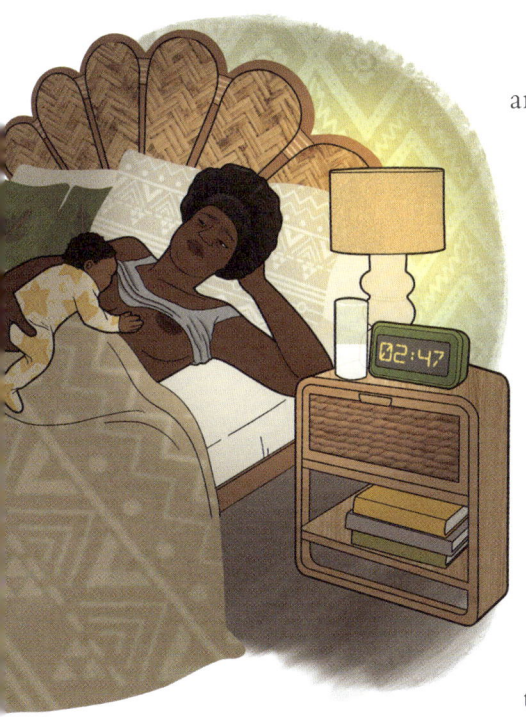

amount of milk they are getting. Instead, it is more helpful to look at your baby feeding, determine if they are actually drinking, and consider other signs that they are getting enough. It's an old adage, but *watch the baby, not the clock*. There may be times during the day when your baby feeds more frequently – most parents find evening time or night-time is when their baby does more breastfeeding – and other times when they want to sleep more. The important thing is that they are getting enough milk per 24 hours.

Breastfed babies do not generally feed according to a schedule, and this means that every day will be a little bit different. Your baby is growing and developing so fast that their feeding needs can change from day to day. Most parents find that they will eventually settle in a sort of feeding rhythm with their baby. Just give it time and trust that you and your baby will figure things out.

> *While broken sleep during the night can be difficult, nighttime breastfeeds while establishing your milk supply are important as prolactin concentrations are highest during the night. Prolactin is the main hormone involved in milk production.*

Is your Baby getting enough Milk?

There are a number of different indicators that can tell us if a baby is getting sufficient milk from breastfeeding:

DAY	WET	DIRTY	POO COLOUR
1	1	meconium	(black)
2	2	2+	(black)
3	3	3+	(green, green)
4-5	6-7	3+	(brown, brown, brown)
6-7	6-7	3+	(yellow, yellow, yellow)

1. Nappy Output

What goes in must come out, and at no time is this saying more apt than during the first few weeks of your baby's life. There is no gauge on your breasts to tell you how much milk your baby is getting, but keeping an eye on nappy output is usually a good indication of their intake. Once your milk comes in, you should expect to see six to seven wet nappies and at least two or three dirty nappies per day.

2. Your Breast is Softer after Feeding

Feel your breast before and after breastfeeds. Is it softer after your baby has fed? What does this tell you?! If it is noticeably softer, your baby has more than likely transferred milk while breastfeeding.

3. Is your baby drinking?

Look at your baby when they are breastfeeding. Are they actively feeding? Can you hear them swallow? Can you see some big jaw movements? Often you will see a few short jaw movements followed by a longer downward movement of the jaw – this is a swallow.

4. Does your baby seem content after feeding?

How does your baby seem after they have breastfed? Relaxed? Content? Sleepy? These are all signs that they have taken sufficient milk at the breast. But do bear in mind that feeds are often like three-course meals, and that it is quite normal for babies to have a short snooze between breasts.

5. Your Baby's Weight

Your baby's weight can be a good indicator of their milk intake. Following an initial drop in weight, a baby's weight will often plateau for a few days (days 4 – 5), and then start increasing from day 6 or 7.

Please note: It is important to consider all of the above indicators when trying to determine if your baby is feeding efficiently and getting enough milk. If you are not sure about anything or if you have any concerns, do not hesitate to ask care providers for help.

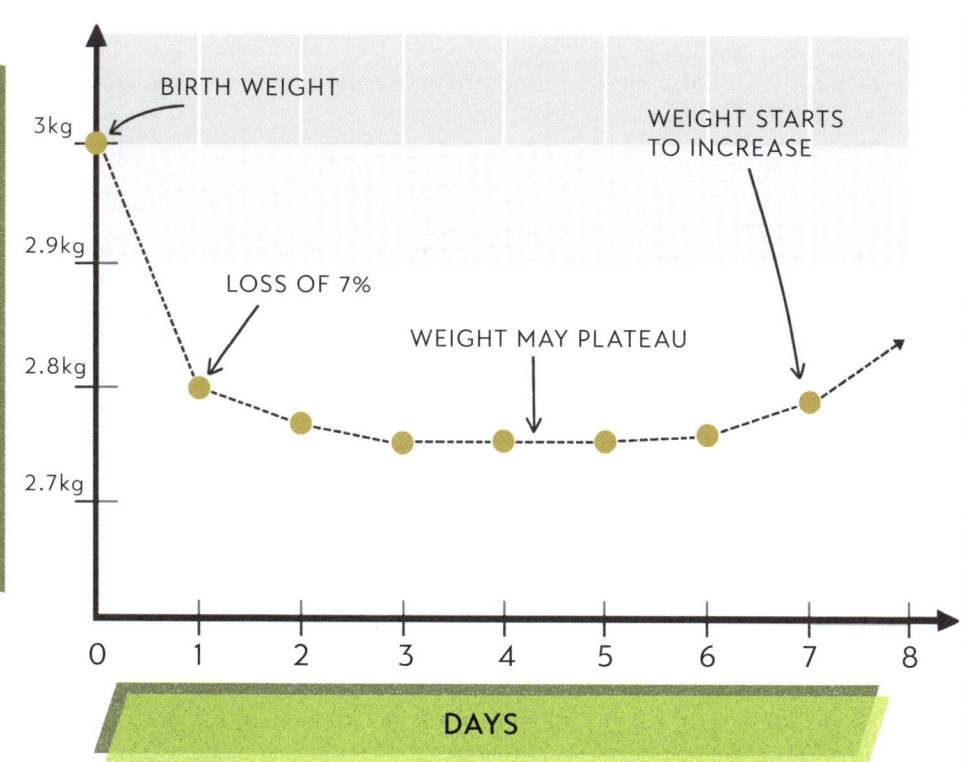

Your Baby's Weight in the First Week

There is usually quite an intense focus on your baby's weight, especially in the first couple of weeks. One of the first questions people will always ask you after you have had your baby is 'What weight were they?' Everybody wants to know, we're obsessed. Whatever your baby's birth weight is, it will probably drop within the first few days postpartum – this is normal. Most babies will lose between seven and ten percent of their birth weight. They poop out the meconium that was in their tummy at birth and this naturally means weight loss. After this drop babies' weight is expected to stay the same for a few days. By day six or seven after your milk has started to increase in volume, we expect that babies who are breastfeeding well will *start* to gain weight.

Day 1 – 3	7 – 10% drop in weight
Day 4 – 5	No weight gain
Day 6 – 7	Weight starts to increase

What if your baby loses more than ten percent of their birth weight?

This suggests that your baby may not be getting enough milk. But other factors could influence a weight loss of more than 10%. For example, if you had IV fluids during your labour, your baby could be born with a slightly elevated weight. After they are born, they pee out all of the excess fluid they had taken on, and this results in a bigger drop in weight. If your baby's weight loss is more than 10%, talk to your care providers about your wish to continue breastfeeding. They may suggest continued breastfeeding, with or without supplementation. If supplementation is suggested, you could ask to supplement with expressed milk. And if this is not possible, you may need to supplement with a small volume of infant formula (or donor milk if that option exists wherever you had your baby – most maternity units only give donor milk to preterm babies).

If you do supplement with formula, this does not mean the end of breastfeeding. The important thing is that your baby is fed, you keep breastfeeding and protecting your milk supply, and you get whatever breastfeeding support you need.

Potential Challenges

Low Blood Sugar Level (*Hypoglycaemia*)

Low blood sugar in a baby is often given as a rationale for suggesting infant formula supplementation. However, it is important to remember that it is normal for babies' blood sugar levels to drop immediately after birth, and to rise gradually over the following few days. Most term babies who are breastfeeding well and doing plenty of skin-to-skin contact with their mothers will not require intervention for low blood sugars. Staff in maternity units will generally monitor a baby's blood sugar level where a mother has type 1 diabetes or had gestational diabetes, or if the baby has some clinical risk factor for low blood sugars, such as being small for gestational age (in the bottom ten percent for weight), large for gestational age (in the top ten percent for weight), or preterm. Staff will usually also check a baby's blood sugar level if they show some clinical sign of having low blood sugars, the most common of which is jitteriness. Babies' blood sugar levels are checked by pricking their heel and putting a drop of their blood on a glucose meter test strip.

Different maternity hospitals may have different policies around neonatal hypoglycaemia, and different thresholds for intervention, but most will suggest some kind of action where a baby has a blood sugar level lower than around 2.5 mmol/L. The action suggested will depend on other factors, but the goal in all cases will be to increase the baby's blood sugar. The kinds of actions that may be suggested include

- Continued frequent breastfeeding
- Supplementation with expressed breastmilk
- Continued monitoring of blood sugar level every 2 – 3 hours

- Treatment with Dextrose gel (a gel that is rubbed into the inside of baby's cheeks)
- IV glucose solution
- Supplementation with infant formula or donor milk

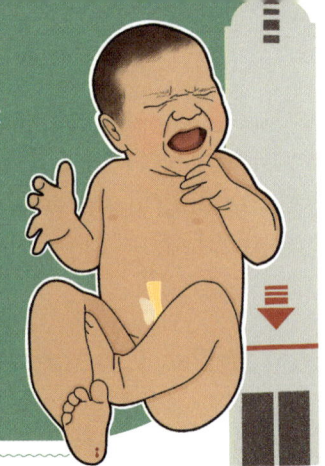

Whatever course of action your care team suggest for you and your baby, ensure that they know that breastfeeding is important to you. If infant formula supplementation is advised, ask if you can express some of your own milk to supplement your baby with instead. And keep breastfeeding and doing skin-to-skin where possible. Doing skin-to-skin for 70 to 90 minutes has been shown to raise blood sugar levels by 0.6 mmol/L, and this could be the difference between a baby needing intervention and not requiring intervention.

Jaundice (Hyperbilirubinemia)

Jaundice is the yellow colour that babies have when they are born, and it is very common. In fact, most babies will experience some degree of jaundice in the first week. Jaundice is caused by bilirubin, an orange-yellow pigment which results mainly from the breakdown of red blood cells. During your pregnancy, your liver does the job of removing bilirubin, but once your baby is born, their liver must do that job. However, your baby's liver is not fully developed at birth, so it may struggle to process all the bilirubin This excess bilirubin is absorbed back

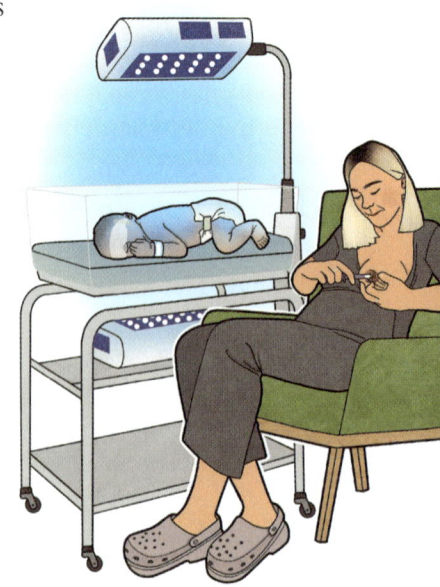

into the body and presents as yellow skin. Bilirubin that your baby's liver has been able to process is excreted in your baby's poos as bile. Jaundice can be harder to see if your baby has darker skin, but you should be able to notice a yellowing of the whites of their eyes.

If your baby is getting enough milk through breastfeeding, their jaundice levels will probably be within normal range. Hospital staff will sometimes want to check a baby's bilirubin levels if they appear particularly jaundiced and/or if they are not breastfeeding well. They will measure your baby's Total Serum Bilirubin (TSB)*. If this test reveals a value above the range of normal they may suggest any of the following interventions:

- Increased breastfeeding
- Increased skin-to-skin contact
- Hand expression or pumping to provide extra milk for supplementation
- Phototherapy treatment

Sometimes hospital staff will recommend supplementation with infant formula when a baby has high TSB levels. This is only recommended if you are unable to provide expressed breastmilk or if donor milk is not available. So, if you are advised to give your baby infant formula, first ask if it would be possible to give your own expressed milk instead.

Whatever interventions are advised, continuing to breastfeed directly is usually still possible, even if your baby must spend some time under phototherapy lights.

***Please note:** Some rare conditions can contribute to abnormal levels of bilirubin in babies. These include biliary atresia (whereby the duct that connects the liver and the intestine is blocked) or Gilbert's syndrome, a genetic condition that is characterised by the liver's inability to process bilirubin. In these instances, your baby will need medical treatment, while you continue to provide breastmilk for them.

Jaundice beyond the first weeks:

Many breastfed babies will continue to have a tinge of jaundice for up to 12-15 weeks after they are born. Assuming they are feeding well and do not have any underlying conditions, this is normal and is referred to as *breastmilk jaundice*. This type of jaundice is seen in around two-thirds of newborns.

> Newborn Jaundice is normal! It acts as an antioxidant helps to protect babies against sepsis. It also helps babies adapt to breathing for themselves.

Urates in Your Baby's Nappy

Urates, or *brick dust crystals*, are little pink specks that can appear in a baby's nappy. They are a waste product found in the bloodstream and are excreted in urine. Urates in your baby's nappy in the first couple of days postpartum are normal and not a cause for concern. However, urates after the first couple of days should be investigated as they may suggest that your baby is not getting enough milk. Your healthcare provider may suggest increased breastfeeding, breast compressions, skin-to-skin and/or pumping and supplementation with your milk, and then continued monitoring of your baby's nappies.

Sore or Cracked Nipples

Sore or cracked nipples are usually caused by a suboptimal latch and/or position, and very often coincide with your milk coming in. Often small adjustments can enable a baby to get a little more of your breast into their mouth and enable both of you to feed comfortably. If adjustments to latch and positioning do not help, there could be some other cause of the pain and/or damage, for example, a tongue tie, a high palate or a recessed chin. A lactation consultant will help you determine what is going on and they will also help you figure out how to manage the pain, how to treat damaged nipples and how to feed your baby and protect breastfeeding. See Chapter 8 for more information on managing nipple pain and damage.

Non-latching Baby

There are many reasons why your baby may not be ready or able to latch and feed directly at the breast in the first week. It could be that they are preterm or late preterm and not developmentally ready. It could be something to do with your nipples – for example, your baby may struggle to latch on to your nipple if it is flat/short or inverted. Or your baby's difficulty with latching could be something to do with their oral anatomy (tongue tie and/or high palate). Whatever the cause, it is important that you get skilled support to determine what the issue is and to ensure that you protect your milk supply and continue providing breastmilk for your baby. This may mean a combination of hand expression and/or pumping until such time that your baby is able to latch and feed well. If you are exclusively pumping, it is important that you double pump at least eight times per 24 hours, using a multi-user pump. Your care team will advise where you can rent one of these pumps.

The B.R.A.I.N Technique

B.R.A.I.N (an acronym that stands for Benefits – Risks – Alternatives – Intuition – Nothing) is a technique that can help in evidence-based decision-making. It can be helpful for accessing breastfeeding help and support in the early weeks after birth. Using BRAIN can help you determine what questions to ask staff, give you some time to understand what is happening, and it may help you avoid potentially unnecessary interventions such as supplementation with infant formula, stopping breastfeeding and pumping.

1. Benefits – Ask how the suggested intervention will be helpful. Also ask about duration. For example, if you are being advised to pump or triple feed (breastfeeding, pumping and bottle feeding), ask for how long.

2. Risks – Also ask if there are any risks to the suggested intervention. Do the risks outweigh the benefits or vice versa?

3. Alternative – Is there an alternative? For example, if you have been advised to supplement with infant formula, could you supplement with your own milk instead?

4. Intuition – Does the suggested intervention feel right? Is it supporting your wish to breastfeed? What is your gut telling you? Would you benefit from a second opinion?

5. Nothing – Is doing nothing an option? What happens if you do nothing, or if you wait and see – even for an hour or two?

Something else you could do when presented with a proposed intervention which may be helpful, especially if you are neurodivergent, is to write things down.

You and your baby are entitled to the best possible evidence-based care when you are establishing breastfeeding. Unfortunately, it's quite common to receive conflicting advice, so remember to trust your instinct and don't let yourself be put under pressure to make a decision on the spot.

Don't be shy about asking questions. Even if going through the B.R.A.I.N. steps results in you agreeing to the proposed intervention, you will probably have a better understanding of why you are doing it and what the goal is. And you may just have greater confidence that you are doing the right thing for you and your baby.

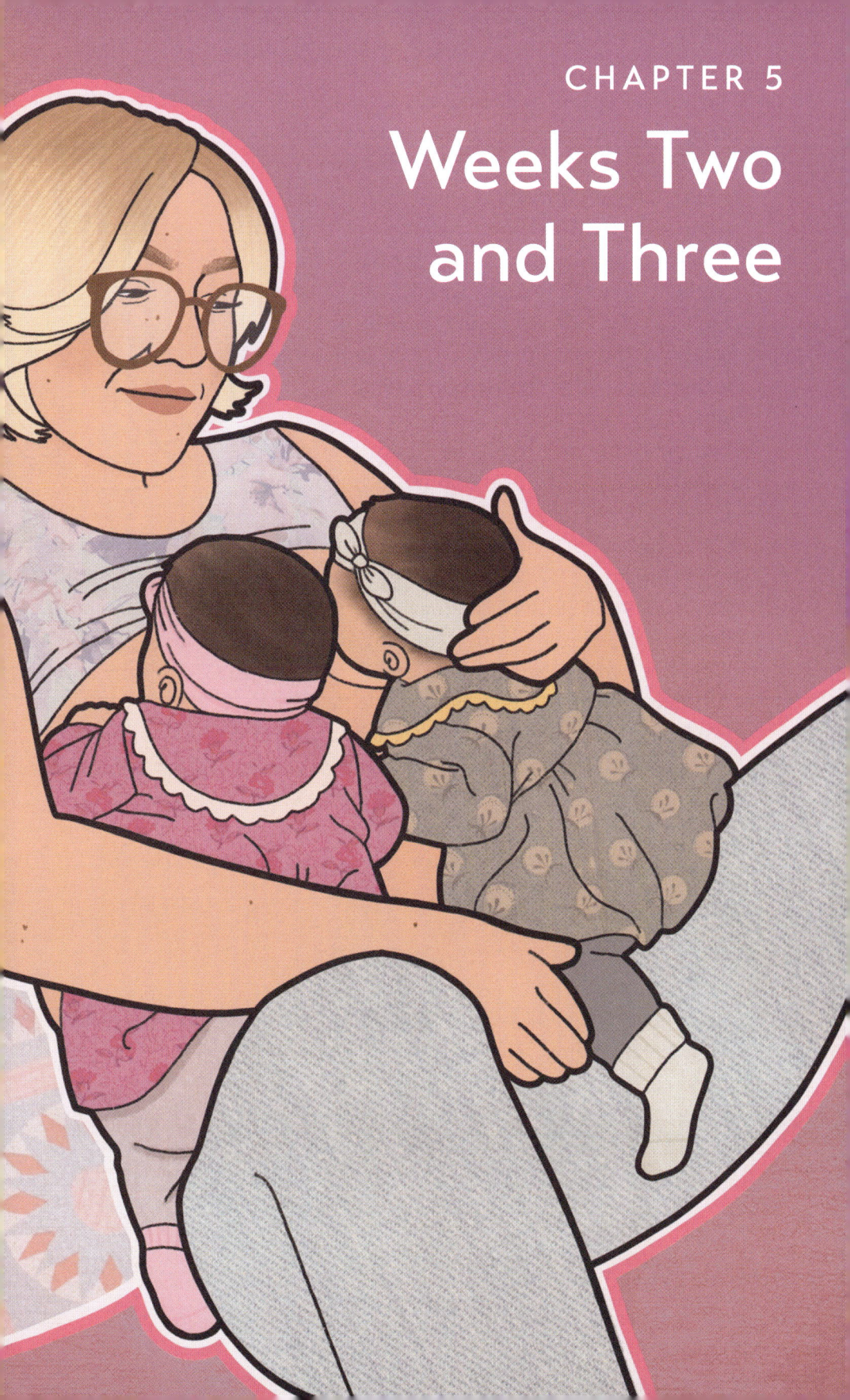

During the second and third week, your milk production will continue to increase, as will the volumes of milk your baby drinks when breastfeeding. These bigger volumes of milk mean that your baby should start to gain weight at a rate of approximately 30g per day. This relatively rapid increase in weight will usually result in your baby regaining their birth weight by the end of week two, or sometime during week three. Please note: Some babies may be a little bit slower to regain their birth. In cases like these, linking in with skilled breastfeeding professionals is important.

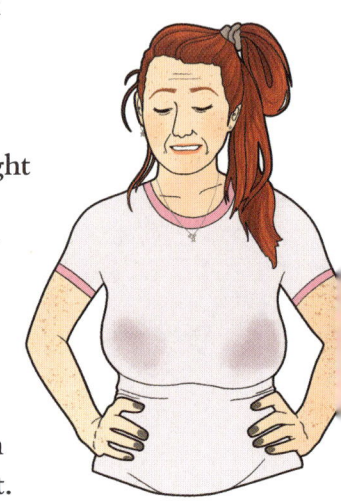

While your milk is increasing in volume, it can take your body a little while to figure out just how much milk to make for your baby. This means that at times you may experience intense fullness in your breasts and perhaps leaking. And the big volumes of milk may be difficult for your baby to cope with. This is normal. Give it time and trust that your milk production will settle down.

You and your baby are still probably trying to figure out how to breastfeed and what it is going to look like for you. It's OK at this stage if you are not sure how you feel about breastfeeding, or if you feel like you have no idea what you are doing. Try to keep yourself in the moment and take one feed at a time. You are very much learning on the hoof.

Breastfeeding Positions

There is no one right way to position yourself and your baby when you're breastfeeding. The main things are that

- you are comfortable
- your baby is comfortable
- your baby is able to latch and feed well

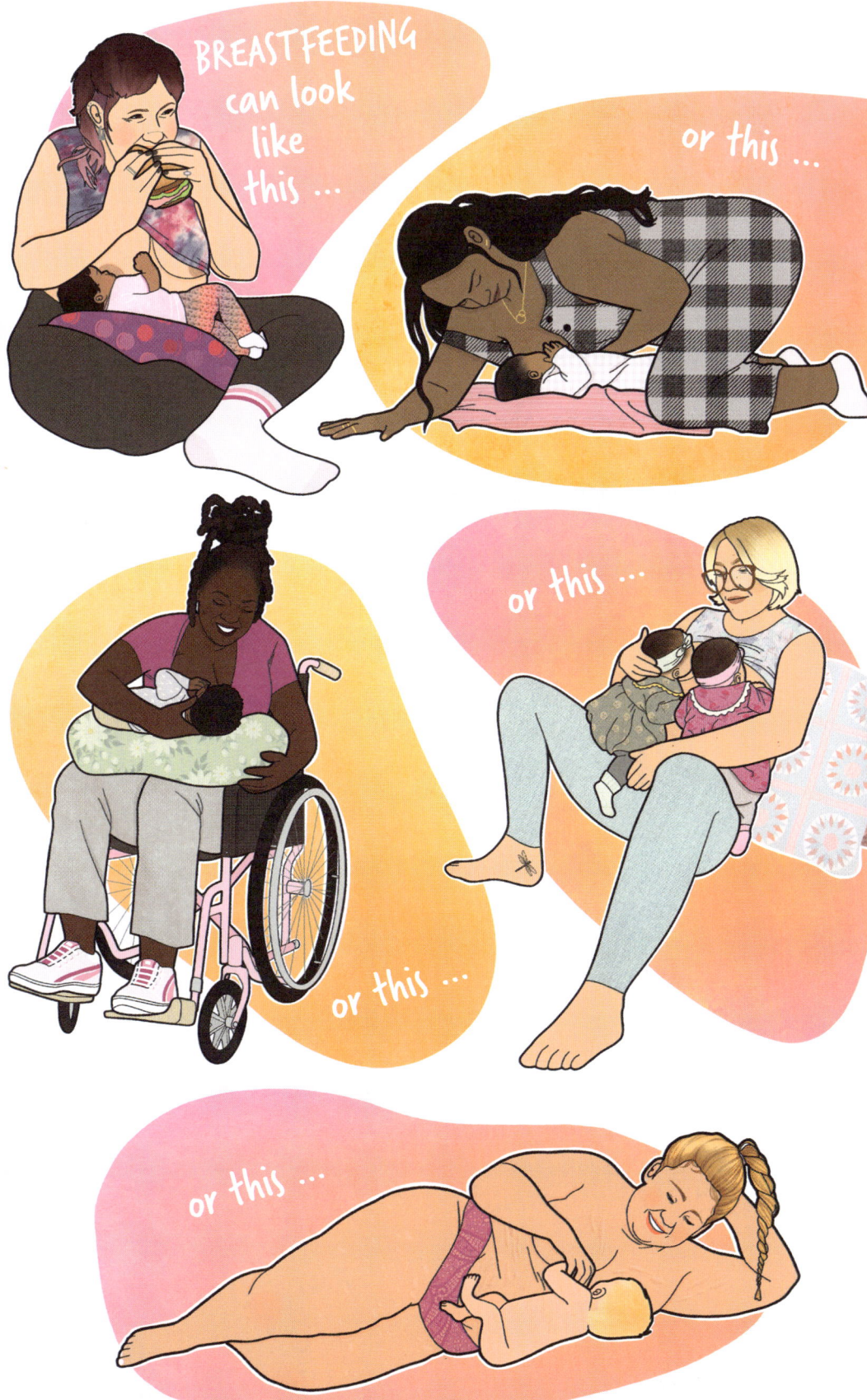

Being Responsive to your Baby's Needs

I mentioned the term *responsive feeding* in Chapter 4 – it means feeding your baby whenever they show feeding cues. But being responsive is not limited to breastfeeding. Being responsive to your baby in a more general sense is also important – responding when you smell a dirty nappy, when your baby seems to have wind, when your baby cries or gurgles, and to your baby's facial expressions. More often than not, the response they seek is to be put to the breast, but there are also times when they are seeking touch, rocking, movement, your physical presence, the sound of your voice, or a nappy change.

> Compared to other primates, human babies are born premature. This means that they are unable to cling to their mother's body, unable to keep themselves warm, unable to move around on their own, unable to control their bowels, and unable to communicate their needs except by crying.

Being responsive to your baby's signals plays a role in the development of many important biological processes:

- Helps your baby's nervous system develop and mature

- Builds a strong immune system

- Helps your baby to develop a robust stress response

- Grows your baby's brain and develops their ability to retain information, process emotions and learn impulse control

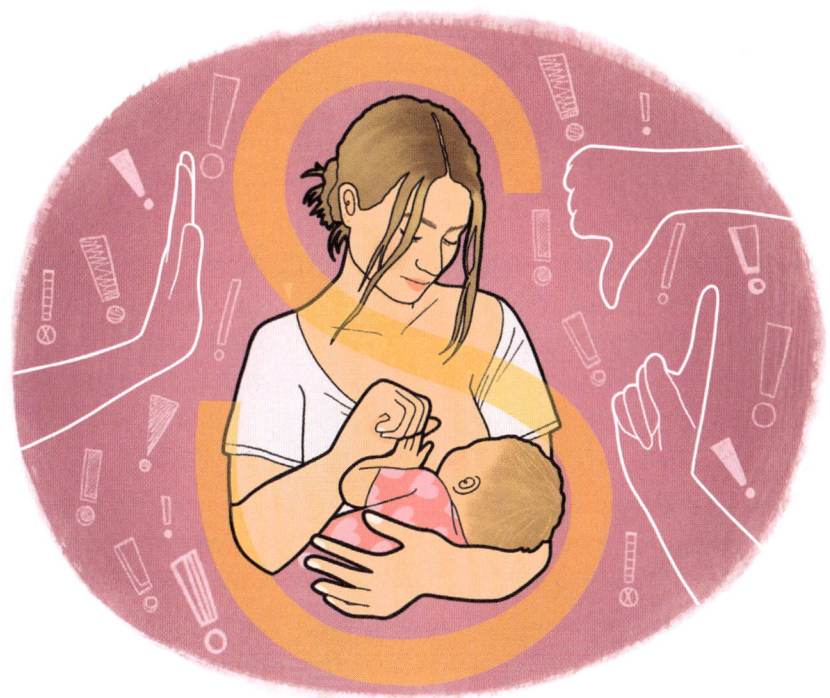

It is stressful and confusing for your baby when you don't respond in some way.

When you respond to your baby, they receive the message 'I am here for you, you are safe' and that expressing themselves is worthwhile. They learn to trust in their ability to communicate their needs and they learn to trust you and other people caring for them. This kind of responsive care in infancy forms the bedrock for secure attachment (confidence in others' availability to provide emotional support) and emotional wellbeing in adulthood and shapes how babies respond to stress in later life.

You may have people tell you that your baby needs to learn how to *self-soothe* or that they'll become too attached to you. In fact, the opposite is true. Being responsive and giving unlimited cuddles) is the foundation for independent, confident individuals with a capacity to form healthy relationships with others.

You may not always know what need your baby is trying to communicate to you. There may be times when they don't even know themselves. But respond in some way and reassure them that they are seen and heard.

The Four S's of Secure Attachment:

Feeling SAFE, SEEN, SOOTHED and SECURE

Your Baby's Weight Gain

If breastfeeding is going well, your baby will probably regain their birth weight by the end of the second week. However, there are a number of factors which can result in babies being slower to regain their birth weight. If your baby is not back to their birth weight by two weeks, the most important thing is that you are supported by a skilled breastfeeding professional to figure out what's going on. It could be that your baby is not feeding as frequently as they should be or that they are not feeding efficiently, but with some help and guidance it should be possible to increase your baby's intake of milk. Things like breast compressions, switch nursing and more frequent breastfeeds can help.

Equally, there may not actually be a problem with breastfeeding if your baby has not regained their birth weight by two weeks. It could be a case that your milk was slow to come in, and that this has had a knock-on effect on the timing of your baby's weight gain. Or it could be that you had IV fluids during labour and your baby's weight dropped by 10 or 11%, which could result in your baby needing a few extra days to regain this weight. Either way, it is important to look at the big picture and take into account your baby's lowest weight (usually a day or two after their birth) and use it as a baseline for assessing their weight gain.

Switch Nursing involves switching sides more frequently during a breastfeed. When your baby's sucking has slowed down or stopped or your breast has softened, move them to your other breast – this enables them to get the letdown on that side (the initial, big volume of easily available milk). Switching your baby a couple of times during a feed increases the volume of milk they get and helps to increase your milk supply.

Compressions help your baby get more milk during a breastfeed. Watch your baby as they feed. Whenever they stop sucking and/or become sleepy, give your breast a little squeeze and hold for a few moments. This pushes some milk out and encourages your baby to start sucking and actively feeding again. You can repeat each time your baby stops sucking. This is an early days hack and you should not have to continue doing it beyond the first few weeks.

Three-Course Meals

You may have been told by someone that your baby should breastfeed for 15 or 20 minutes on each breast. This is not the case. How many minutes your baby spends at the breast is not indicative of how much milk they drink. All babies are different and while some will feed quite quickly, others will need more time. But what most babies have in common at this stage, is that their breastfeeds are often like three or four-course meals. For example, your baby may feed on one breast (starter), then snooze for a few minutes and wake up deciding they want more. So you offer them the other breast (main course). They feed and again eventually come off and fall asleep. Just as you go to move them, they signal that they want more, so you offer the first breast again (dessert). And sometimes they even want a second helping of dessert! Each feed can be different to the last feed. It can be confusing, but this is all very normal. It's just how breastfeeding works.

Your Baby's Digestive System

Your baby's digestive system is relatively immature and inefficient compared to that of an adult, with a gut transit time of approximately 50 minutes. This means that after a breastfeed, they will probably have either a wet or a dirty nappy within the hour. Your baby may even poop or pee while they are feeding. There is a spectrum of digestive-system related behaviours that babies exhibit, and for the most part these behaviours are normal. They include:

- Spitting up/Posseting (Reflux)
- Silent reflux
- Farting
- Hiccupping
- Burping
- Explosive nappies
- Squirming due to digestive discomfort/wind
- Fussiness
- Grunting or straining when trying to pass a poo
- Poos that are varying shades of yellow and green

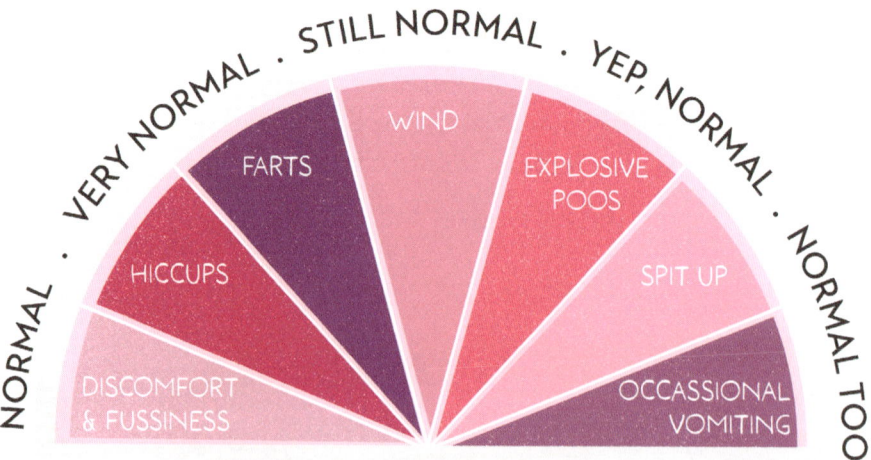

SPECTRUM OF INFANT FEEDING BEHAVIOURS

Spitting up milk after a breastfeed is a common concern for parents. It is usually your baby's way of making themselves comfortable. The little ring of sphincter muscle at the opening of your baby's stomach is quite weak, so when their stomach is very full, the muscle will release and allow some milk to be regurgitated. Sometimes milk moves from the stomach up into the oesophagus, without being regurgitated. This is referred to as silent reflux. 40 to 60% of babies will shows some symptoms of reflux.

Usually, **comfort measures** will help your baby if they are experiencing digestive discomfort or if are inclined to get reflux. Try to figure out what helps your baby:

- Holding your baby upright and rubbing their back
- Putting your baby in a sling and walking around with them
- Bicycle legs – with your baby on their back alternately bend their knees towards their tummy
- Keeping your baby upright after feeding
- Calming touch can help to soothe and relax your baby
- Sitting your baby on your lap and moving their torso in circles
- Putting baby back to the breast
- Giving your baby short frequent feeds

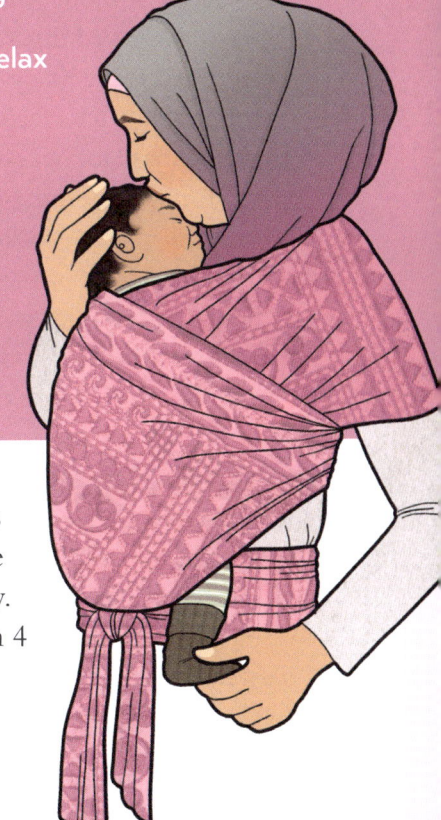

Remember, your baby's digestive system is growing and developing all the time, so these symptoms and behaviours are temporary. Babies very often grow out of them between 4 and 6 months.

When is reflux not normal? Sometimes the volume of milk that babies regurgitate is so large (and sometimes projectile) that it can affect their ability to gain weight. It can also cause significant pain and discomfort. Your baby may cry, arch their back, gag while feeding and have difficulty sleeping. This is called Gastroesophageal reflux disease (GORD) and is a medical problem. You should see your doctor. It may also be helpful to work with an IBCLC to help you find a way to keep breastfeeding.

If you are worried about your baby or suspect that any of their digestive system-related behaviours are not normal, reach out for support. There may not always be a quick fix, but skilled and empathetic help will help.

Winding Your Baby: Yay or Nay?

Most of us are probably conditioned to think that babies need to be winded after feeds. This belief is probably reinforced by some healthcare professionals and baby care books. But babies do not always need to be winded after a feed. If they are allowed to snooze or relax in a comfortable position after feeding, their little digestive system is likely to sort itself out without you actively getting involved. A relaxed and calm baby means relaxed digestive muscles, which in turn means a digestive system that is more likely to work very well. If your baby cries or seems uncomfortable after a feed, they will need you to do something, but that something may not necessarily be winding. They may want to go back to the breast to do some comfort sucking or to have some dessert. Or they may need to be rocked or cuddled. The only way to find out is to try different things and see what works, but don't assume it's wind.

There may be times when your baby *does* need some help to get wind up and out. But before you start jigging them around and patting them on the back, try putting them to the breast and if that doesn't work try cuddling or walking around with them. Try to keep yourself in the moment and read your baby's cues, rather than automatically winding them straight after a feed. Give them a chance to rest and digest and see what happens if you do nothing. There are lots of countries in the world where it's not customary to wind babies after feeds. It's more of a Western notion that probably came about due to the widespread use of infant formula, which is not as easily digested as breastmilk.

Cluster Feeding and Growth Spurts

Cluster feeding is a term that describes the way breastfed babies feed frequently for a period of time, usually a few hours, when they are going through a growth spurt. For example, a baby may want to breastfeed every thirty minutes for three hours. This is normal, and usually happens in the late afternoon or early evening. Often after an intense few hours of cluster feeding, babies will have a long sleep.

Typically, babies go through two to three days of cluster feeding during the following times:

Between Day 7 and Day 10

Between week 2 and week 3

Between week 4 and week 6

Four months

Cluster feeding is not limited to these times – it can take place any time during the first few months. It is not always associated with growth spurts.

Cluster feeding can be exhausting and overwhelming. When you feel trapped under your baby and they are hopping from one breast to the other and back ad infinitum, it can be difficult to understand the intensity of their need to feed. But this behaviour is completely normal! It is a sign that your baby is doing what they need to do to get the extra milk required for optimal growth. In addition, the frequent feeds stimulate your milk supply. Try to go with it, let your baby feed as much as they want, and remind yourself that it will pass!

It is common for parents to interpret cluster feeding behaviour as a sign that they are doing something wrong or that their baby needs more milk than the mother can provide. This is not the case. With each feed, your baby is getting milk that is higher in fat than milk produced at other times of the day, and consequently higher in calories. So, hang in there! A lot of parents will find it easier to deal with cluster feeding by setting themselves up for the evening, perhaps watching a movie or a favourite box set, and just feeding baby whenever they ask to be fed. Think *path of least resistance.*

But wouldn't giving a bottle of formula or expressed milk in the evening make things easier?

Not necessarily. I'm often asked this question by parents and I understand the logic – that giving baby a bottle would mean a break for the mother. However, it can actually mean more work for her and has the potential to interfere with breastfeeding at a time when establishing milk supply is important. If you want to supplement with expressed milk, that means making time to pump and wash pumping parts and bottles. And then if you give your baby a bottle feed in the evening, you could end up with a situation where your baby sleeps for a longer period and isn't ready for a breastfeed when your breasts are! With very full breasts and a baby who is not interested in feeding, you may need to pump again to feel comfortable. You have to ask yourself then, how this is making life easier for you.

If you do decide to give a bottle in the evening, consider giving a supplement (eg, 20 – 40ml) rather than a full replacement feed. This smaller volume is less likely to interfere with milk supply and responsive feeding.

Note: While periods of cluster feeding are normal, feeding constantly all the time is not, especially when there is scant nappy output. If you are concerned that your baby is feeding all the time, seek skilled support to help find out what is going on.

Babies often start to cry a little bit more in week three. This does not mean that there is a problem or that your baby has reflux. It is probably just that your baby is becoming more vocal and expressive. Crying usually peaks at around six weeks. It isn't always possible to figure out why your baby is crying, but you can try different things to soothe them – breastfeeding, carrying, putting them in a sling or a stroller, movement, talking to them or exposing them to white noise.

Should You Follow a Feeding Schedule?

You and your baby are still getting to grips with breastfeeding, your baby is growing very fast (hence the need for frequent feeding), your milk supply is still increasing, and your baby is only beginning to adjust to life out of the womb. Their needs are quite simple – milk, cuddles, warmth, nappy changes, sleep – but one thing they are not remotely concerned with just yet is sticking to a schedule or a routine. This can be challenging for new parents and it can feel chaotic, especially for more left-brained people. In a way we all crave security and love the certainty of knowing what to expect and what each day brings - such is human nature. But with the birth of a baby comes *'thrownness.'* This is a philosophical term which means being thrown suddenly into an especially unfamiliar, confusing and challenging situation and it is apt to describe the process of becoming a parent. Probably without realising it, we are conditioned to think that routine/schedule is something to strive for in the postpartum period. But for now, see if you can just roll with the madness and the unpredictability of each new day with your baby. Have little cat naps when you can and try not to let the clock govern your day. You will both eventually settle into a unique rhythm together.

There isn't any book that can tell you exactly what that rhythm will look like – it is for you and your baby to figure out.

Sometimes a little bit of mindfulness can help you when the chaos of life with your new baby feels overwhelming. Take a moment for yourself, settle your body, and be aware of physical sensations. Let your breath settle, and gently observe three long, slow in breaths and out breaths. Feel yourself in the moment and remind yourself that everything is exactly as it should be. You may find it helpful to repeat a little mantra to yourself, something like 'I embrace this chaos. Everything this is as it should be' or 'I am gentle with myself.'

> *Scheduling or trying to space out breastfeeds has the potential to affect your milk supply, and this can have a knock-on effect on your baby's weight gain.*

Growing Your Baby's Brain

Your baby's brain will double in size in their first year of life. Much of this growth and development is dependent on the experiences they have – caring touch, skin-to-skin, making eye contact, being responsive and attuned, being breastfed in response to hunger cues, the reassuring presence of your body, talking and singing to your baby – all these things help to grow your baby's brain. Even when you are simply holding your baby, you are helping to create new connections in their brain. The other thing you are doing with this kind of nurturing care is building the foundations for good mental health in later life.

> *Social interactions in infancy build social brain circuits and stress regulation circuits in the prefrontal cortex.*
>
> The Nurture Revolution, Greer Kirschenbaum 2023

Approximately 75% of the breastmilk that your baby drinks fuels brain growth and development (in adults it's 20-30%), so another way to think about breastmilk is as *brain juice*. Every drop helps to form new neural connections.

Why Breastfeeding is Hard and Why Support is so Important

If breastfeeding is natural, why do so many mothers find it difficult and why do parents need so much support to make it work? Shouldn't mothers just instinctively know how to breastfeed? For most other mammals, feeding their babies is relatively easy. They don't require help to get their young to latch and don't need to be taught how to breastfeed. However, primates are the exception to this rule as they usually need a period of learning to be able to breastfeed successfully (remember the mother gorilla in the zoo from Chapter 1?). There is a theory that this learning may be a trade-off between the reliability of innate and instinctive behaviours and the power of a big, learning brain. So, the more we evolve, and the bigger our brains get, the further we move from our innate knowledge and behaviours. Our big brains get in the way of our innate breastfeeding behaviours. There are other reasons why breastfeeding is difficult for humans, one being that we are born very immature compared to other mammals – we are *altricial*. Human babies are helpless at birth, needing parental care for feeding, protection and warmth. They are sometimes referred to as an 'external foetus.' Newborn babies come with innate feeding behaviours, but they need assistance and support if they are to make it to their mother's breast. The mother needs to be actively involved in ensuring her baby makes it to her breast, holding or supporting them and gently guiding them. She may also need support and assistance from people around her at the time of the birth. But either way, human actions are required if the baby is going to breastfeed successfully. It doesn't just magically happen.

Many new parents today may not have grown up seeing breastfeeding in their families or communities. It is possible that the only type of infant feeding they have been exposed to (in real life and through the media) is bottle-feeding. This lack of exposure to breastfeeding and lack of opportunities to learn about normal breastfed baby behaviours can act as a big barrier to establishing breastfeeding. Our ancestors would have lived in large groups where children would see breastfeeding happen among family members. They would have indirectly soaked up knowledge about how breastfeeding works. And new mothers in these communities would have had a kind of wrap-around practical and socio-emotional support due to the practice of *alloparental care*, meaning that other people in the community would be involved in the care of the baby and the mother. In contrast many new parents today are relatively isolated and the modern societal expectation tends to be on the mother to take on the responsibility of caring for her baby. So, when we consider all the factors that make breastfeeding difficult for humans, we begin to understand why breastfeeding support is so important.

Social support to breastfeed helps new parents learn how breastfeeding works, understand normal newborn behaviour and develop greater self-confidence as a new parent. No one is meant to be able to do it on their own. You are not meant to parent alone and you are not expected to instinctively know how to breastfeed and care for your baby. We have evolved as humans to need other humans around us to support and encourage us as parents and to teach us about breastfeeding.

FAQS

What about fore milk and hind milk? At the beginning of a breastfeed, your milk is high in lactose – the main source of carbohydrate in your milk. It quenches your baby's thirst, helps with the absorption of zinc, calcium and magnesium, supports gut health, and plays an important role in brain development. This milk is sometimes referred to as *fore milk*. As your baby feeds, the amount of fat in your milk increases. The amount of fat in your milk is also determined by the time since the last breastfeed – it is changing all the time. Fat contains fatty acids which are essential for growth and development and plays a role in the regulation of inflammation. This fattier milk is called *hind milk*. The idea that a mother needs to feed for a set number of minutes on one breast so that her baby 'gets the hind milk' has been debunked. It is now accepted that speaking in terms of fore milk and hind milk as if they are two different types of milk is not helpful. If you feed your baby responsively, they will get as much of everything that they need from your milk.

Should I give my baby a pacifier/dummy/soother? Both the National Health Service (NHS) in the UK and the Health Service Executive (HSE) in Ireland advise against the use of soothers for breastfed babies, especially in the first few weeks postpartum. The rationale for this advice is that using a soother can result in less breastfeeding and this can have a knock-on effect on your milk supply. It can be easy to miss a baby's feeding cues if they are sucking on a soother. If you do decide to use a soother

- Try to wait until your baby is a few weeks old and breastfeeding is established.
- If your baby cries, offer your breast first to see if your baby is hungry before you give them the soother. The soother should not replace a breastfeed.
- Remove the soother from your baby's mouth after they have fallen asleep.
- Don't use the soother to stretch out the time between feeds.

Should I Swaddle my Baby? It depends. Do you want to swaddle your baby? Does your baby seem to enjoy being swaddled? If the answer to both of these questions is yes, then swaddle your baby. If you don't want to swaddle your baby, don't. It's really a matter of personal preference and trying to determine what is the right thing for your baby. Some babies love the sensory experience of being swaddled while others dislike it and are not shy about letting you know. Just a note of caution: swaddling can potentially reduce feed frequency and lower milk production, and this can have a knock-on effect on your baby's weight gain. So, if you do swaddle your baby, ensure that they are breastfeeding frequently and that you are not missing feeding cues (especially in the early weeks when your milk supply is establishing).

A few other important points to note about swaddling:

- Swaddled babies are at a greater risk of overheating, especially important to bear in mind if you live in a hot climate. Use thin swaddling materials and ensure that your baby is not overdressed.

- Tight swaddling where the baby's legs are extended and hips are in extension and adduction increases the risk of developmental dysplasia of the hips. Therefore, a 'hip-safe swaddle' where your baby's legs can remain in a froggy position is recommended to reduce the risk of hip dysplasia.

- Co-sleeping with a swaddled baby is advised against by The Lullaby Trust www.lullabytrust.org.uk

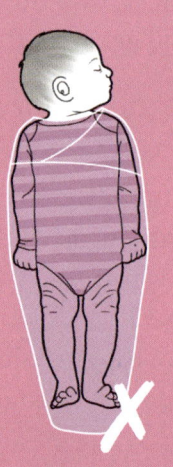

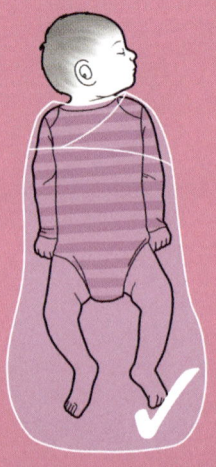

CHAPTER 6

Life in the Fourth Trimester

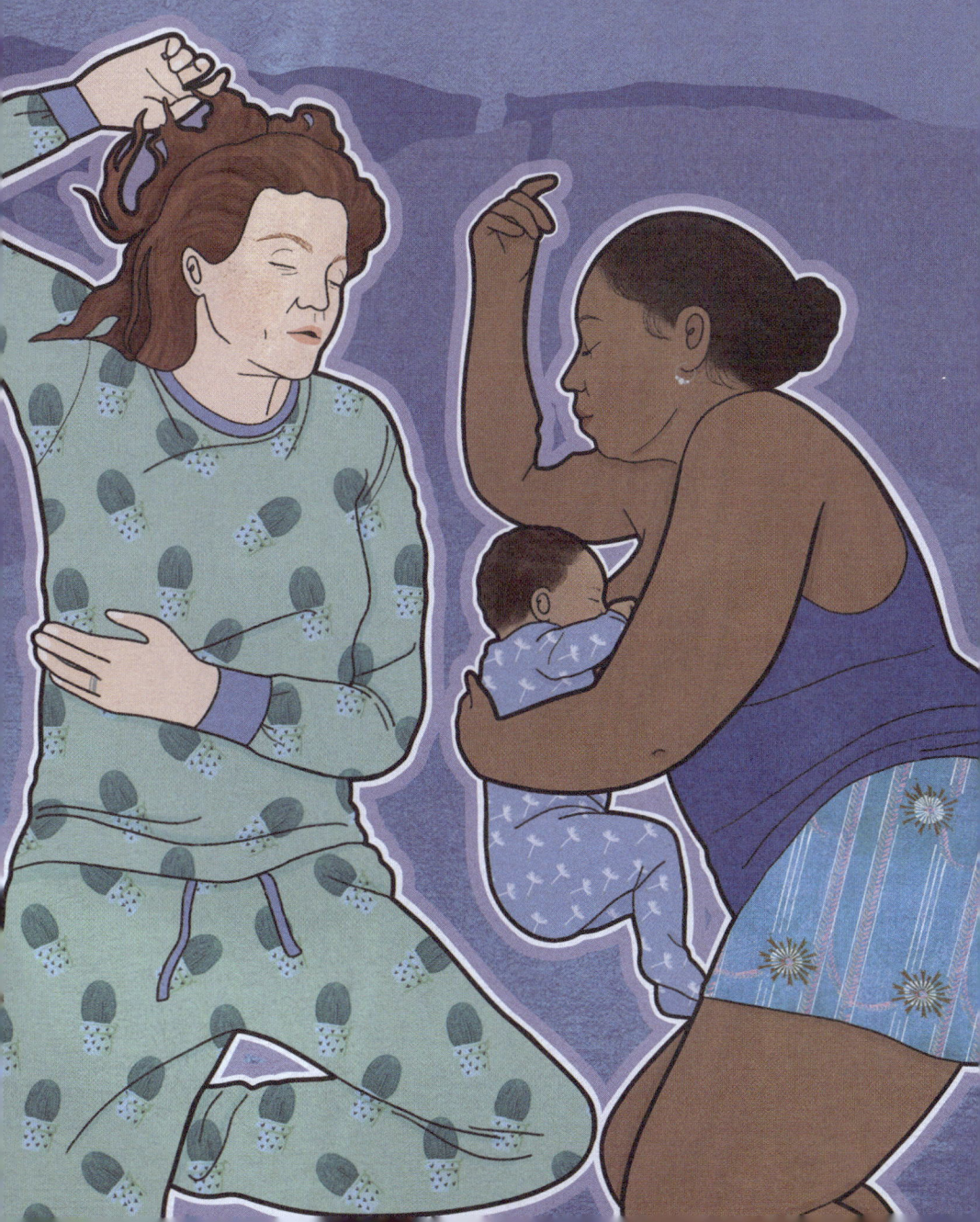

As you reach the end of week three you will hopefully be starting to feel a little bit more confident about breastfeeding, and perhaps you're even thinking about attending local support groups or feeding out and about. This chapter provides some information on life in the fourth trimester and addresses common concerns that parents may have during this time.

What is the Fourth Trimester?

'The Fourth Trimester' is a term that is commonly used to describe a baby's first three months of life, after they have been born. Trimesters one, two and three take place in the womb and then the fourth is the three months after birth. This is a time of huge transition for your baby when they are required to adapt to being in the world, having just spent nine months in the warmth and safety of your body. The first three months postpartum are also a time of massive transition for you as you come to terms with being and becoming a mother and having a tiny little person so entirely dependent on you. There will be times when it can all feel very intense and overwhelming, or when you feel like you're flailing, or struggling with breastfeeding

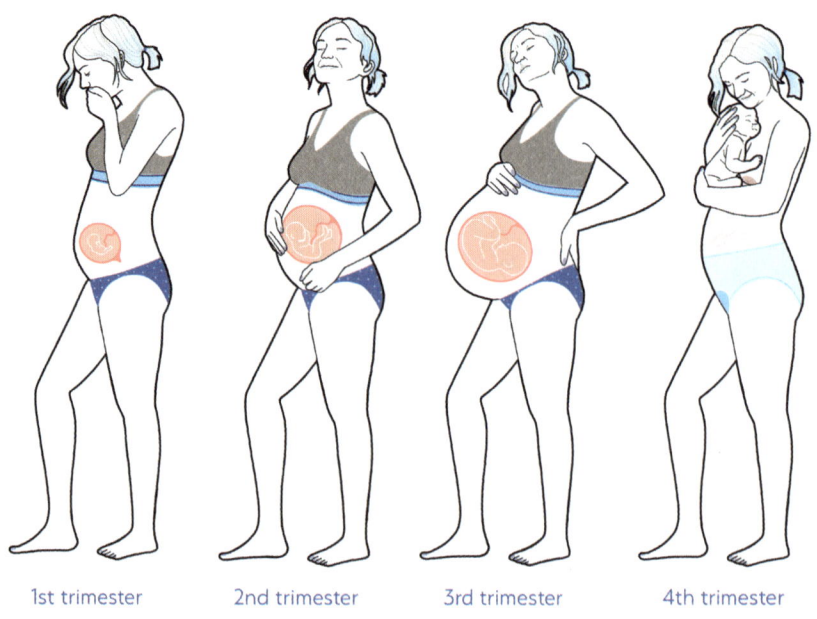

1st trimester   2nd trimester   3rd trimester   4th trimester

– that's normal! There will also be times when you feel immensely joyful, grateful that you are a mother and like you're a natural-born breastfeeder. As the cliché goes, it's a *rollercoaster of emotions* that are heightened and that can feel overwhelming.

Being aware of this concept of the fourth trimester can help you to see things from your baby's perspective and better understand their behaviour. It can also help you to be gentle with yourself as a new mother doing her best to navigate a challenging new chapter of her life.

Fussy Evenings

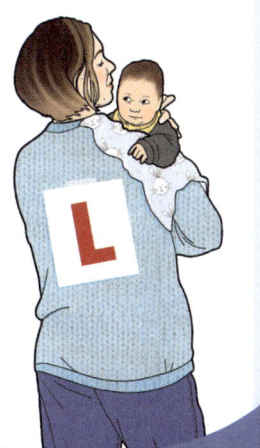

It is very normal for babies to be fussier in the evening and want to breastfeed more frequently, for example, every half hour to an hour, for a few hours. It doesn't mean that you are not providing enough milk for your baby, even if your breasts feel soft. Reasons why babies cluster feed and fuss in the evenings include the following:

- Your baby may need extra milk due to a growth spurt or developmental leap

- Your baby may feel a little bit *discombobulated,* or be feeling some degree of sensory overload after a busy day of just being a baby

- The frequent feeds help to increase milk production

- Milk flow may be a little bit slower in the evening, which could be frustrating for your baby but it does *not* always mean that you don't have enough milk

- Fussy evenings can be exhausting, and also frustrating when you can't pinpoint exactly why your baby is fussing. The following tips may help you cope:

- Remember that fussy evenings and frequent feeding are normal!

- Your baby will not have fussy evenings forever. This is a temporary stage and is normal.

- Try to surrender to your baby's needs and let go of any notion that your baby needs to be *put down* in their cot for the night.

- Get your feet up and watch a movie or your favourite box set.

- Carrying baby in a sling can sometimes help to soothe them.

- Let your baby sleep on your or your partner's chest between feeds. It is very common for new parents to play 'pass the baby' in the evenings.

- Talk to your baby. Even if they are crying, the soothing sound of your voice will help them to feel safe and reassure them that you are there for them, no matter what. Talking to your baby can also help to keep you calm.

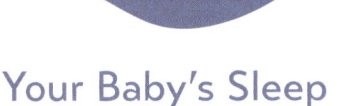

Your Baby's Sleep

Babies wake frequently at night and need to be fed. It can be exhausting. But it's normal and healthy. Think of your baby waking at night, mooching for a feed, as them being clever and simply doing what they are supposed to do to thrive – waking to get the milk they need to grow, and in particular, to grow their brain (remember, 75% of the milk that babies drink is used to fuel brain growth). Frequent night feeds, especially in the early weeks, also help to build your milk supply.

Babies spend most of the night in light sleep phases. This enables them to wake frequently to feed. But breastfeeding is not the only reason babies wake at night. They wake to be cuddled and touched, and to be reassured that you are close to them and that they are safe.

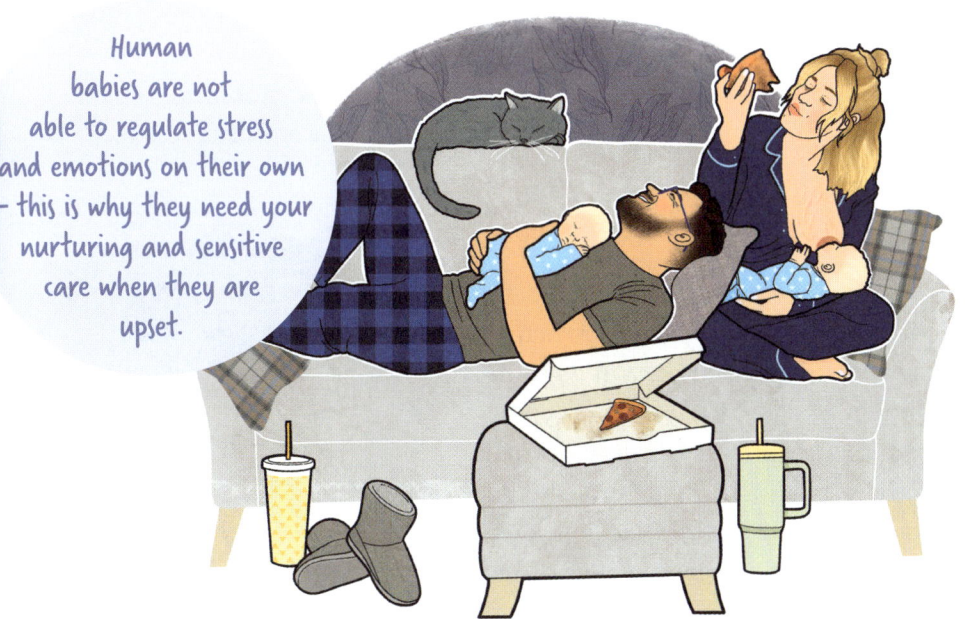

Human babies are not able to regulate stress and emotions on their own – this is why they need your nurturing and sensitive care when they are upset.

How many times exactly should your baby wake during the night? That depends on a number of different factors –your baby's nutritional needs, their personality/disposition, developmental leaps, and brain growth. No two babies are the same, so they will all exhibit slightly different patterns of waking during the night. And these patterns can vary from night to night. They like to keep things interesting for you! It is not uncommon for babies to wake every two hours during the night to feed. Some babies will go for longer stretches and some babies will wake even more frequently. Understanding that nighttime waking is normal can help you to cope with the exhaustion of it all.

Breastsleeping

American anthropologists, Dr James McKenna and Lee Gettler, coined the term *breastsleeping* to describe the behavioural continuum of sleep and breastfeeding that babies and their mothers exhibit at nighttime when they share the bed. The basic concept is that breastfeeding and sleep do not happen in isolation from each other. Breastfeeding can happen while both the mother and her baby are half asleep, and one does not have to stop for the other to begin. The big positive in looking at night times in terms of breastsleeping is the understanding that frequent breastfeeding does not necessarily mean a lot of periods of wakefulness. Breastmilk contains hormones (melatonin, prolactin and cholecystokinin), which play a role in helping your baby fall asleep towards the end of a breastfeed.

Safe Bedsharing

Most breastfeeding parents, whether they intended to or not, will do some amount of bedsharing or co-sleeping with their babies. It is a very normal practice but some guidelines should be adhered to ensure that you keep your baby safe – see Chapter 12 for Safe Sleep Guidelines.

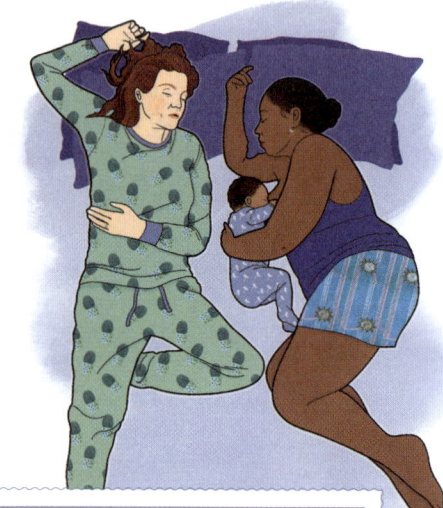

> ...a baby needs its mother even more during the night than during the day, and even more in the dark than in the daylight. In the dark, the baby's predominant sense – sight – is at rest. Instead, the baby needs to use its sense of touch through skin-to-skin contact, and its sense of smell.
>
> Michel Odent, Primal Health

Breastfeeding Support Groups

Breastfeeding support groups provide social support and help with common breastfeeding problems. They are an important aspect of building your confidence and they provide you with an opportunity to learn from other parents. People sometimes make assumptions about these groups – that you must have a problem to attend or that the groups are only for mothers who are exclusively breastfeeding. This is not the case. Breastfeeding support groups are for all parents who are providing milk for their babies, whether directly at the breast or via pumping.

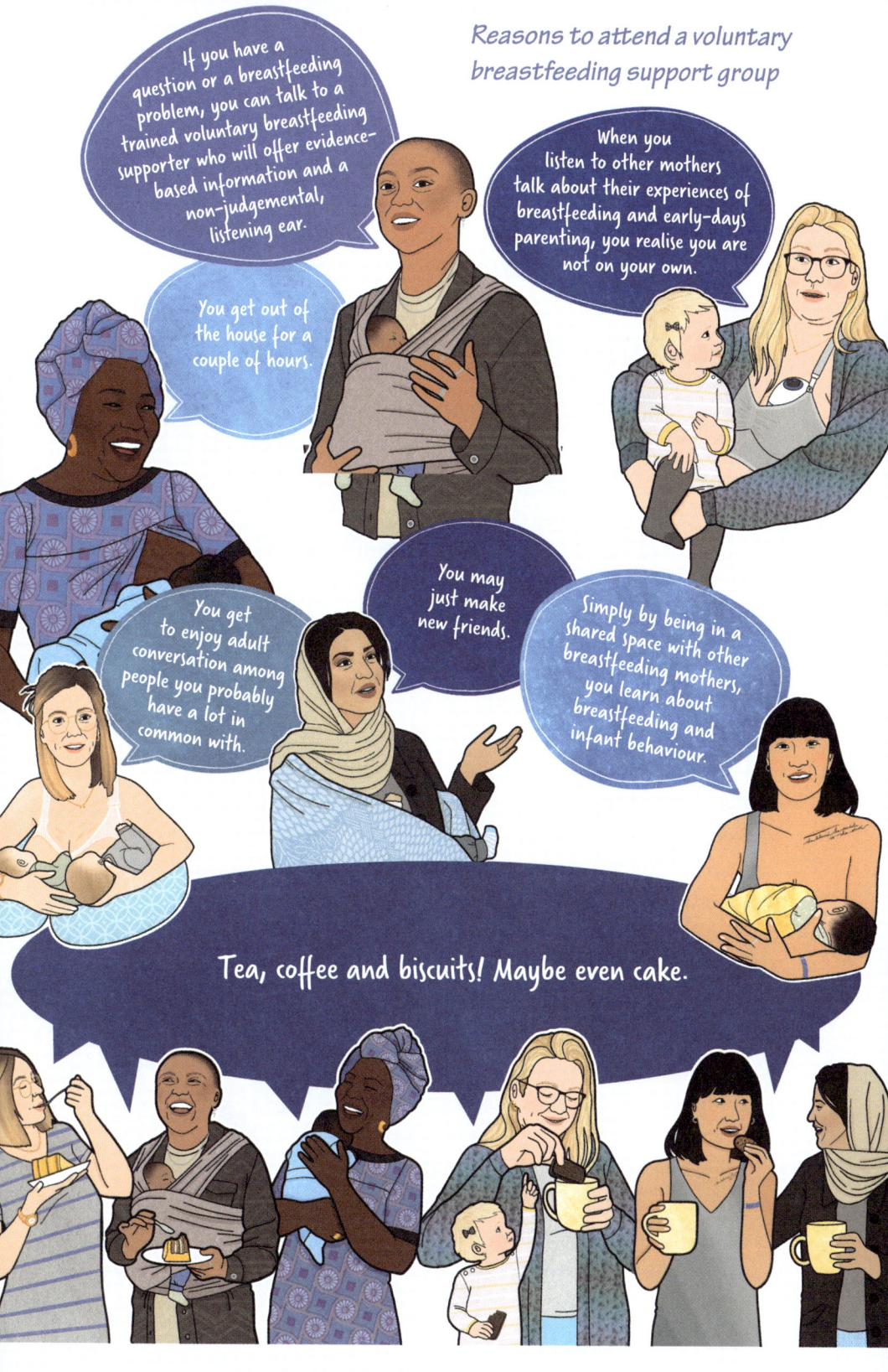

Organisations that facilitate face-to-face and/or online breastfeeding support groups in the UK include the Association of Breastfeeding Mothers, National Childbirth Trust, The Breastfeeding Network, and La Leche League. In Ireland, groups are run by Cuidiú, La Leche League and Friends of Breastfeeding. You may need to attend a few groups until you find one that feels like a good match.

> *You can have good days and bad days with breastfeeding. There will be times when it feels never-ending and all-consuming. It's okay if sometimes you don't love it. It's also OK to sometimes hate it!*

Unhelpful Advice and Unsupportive Comments

You will probably receive lots of unsolicited advice from people you know (and people you don't know) on all things baby feeding and sleep during the fourth trimester. People mostly mean well. They want to share something with you of their own parenting experience that worked for them, and perhaps even validate the parenting choices they made. Some of the advice you receive will be useful, but some of it will be rubbish, irrelevant and undermining. It can help during this time to have an approach to dealing with unwanted and unhelpful advice. When someone tells you that introducing formula enabled their baby to sleep through the night or that too much cuddling can spoil a baby, you could just nod, smile (or grimace) and say 'Yes, thank you, that's so interesting' – rather than wasting energy trying to defend your parenting choices.

Breastfeeding is an emotive topic. Everyone has something to say about it and people who have no experience of it probably do not understand that it

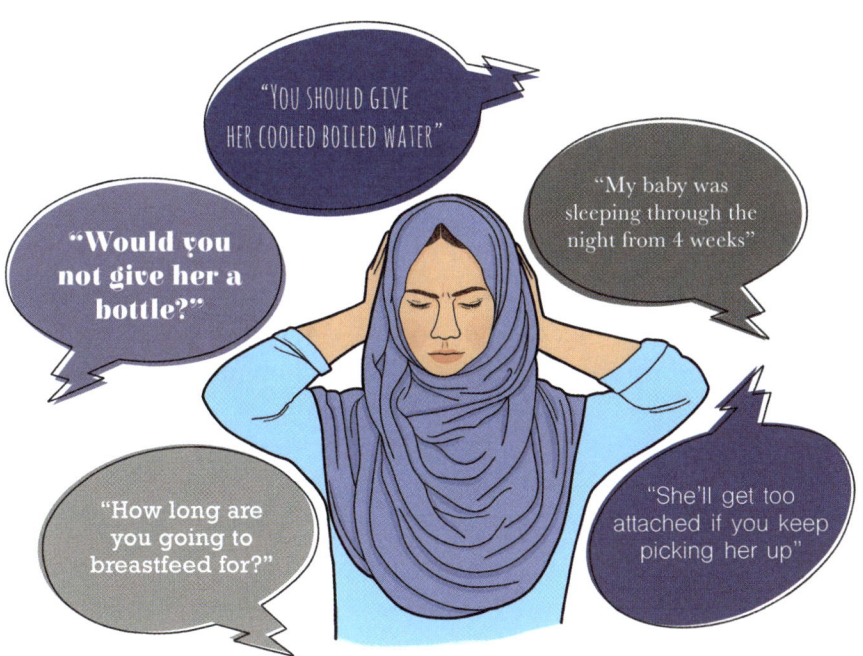

is about more than just feeding your baby. Women who never got to breastfeed themselves (my mother was one of those women – in 1970s Ireland most mothers formula-fed their babies) may find it a bit triggering to see you breastfeed. Perhaps it brings up feelings of guilt or regret that they missed out on something beautiful with their own babies. A reaction to these feelings may be a barbed or loaded comment about breastfeeding, like 'Is she feeding *again*?!!' – the implication being that you or your baby are doing something wrong. Comments like these are unacceptable and can be hurtful, but having a little bit of understanding of where a comment is really coming from, may help you deal with it calmly, without feeling undermined.

There will be times when you have to set a firm boundary. For example, if there is someone close to you, a friend or family member, who is persistently giving you unhelpful advice or making unsupportive comments about breastfeeding, you may need let them know that you don't want to hear any more. When you're feeling vulnerable or at a low ebb, these kinds of conversations can be especially difficult, so you could ask your partner to speak on your behalf. Either way, you do not have to tolerate unwanted comments about breastfeeding (or any other parenting choices you've made) and you have a right to stand up for yourself and say 'enough!'

'Listen to what [is] useful and ignore the rest.'
— Alice Walker

There may also be times when you receive unhelpful or incorrect advice from healthcare providers (HCPs). Not all HCPs will have the same level of breastfeeding and lactation education or the same amount of experience supporting breastfeeding families. So, if you are given information or advice from a HCP that you are unsure about or that is not supportive of your feeding goals, don't assume that they are right and you are wrong. Ask questions, ask to be directed to evidence and further information and/or seek a second opinion from a trusted source. Remember, your instinct is rarely wrong.

Your Baby's 2-Month Vaccinations

Your baby will be vaccinated when they are two months old. These vaccinations include

- the '6 in 1' vaccine for diphtheria, tetanus, whooping cough, polio, hepatitis B and hib (haemophilus influenzae b)
- Meningococcal B vaccine
- Rotavirus oral vaccine
- PCV (pneumococcal conjugate vaccine) – this vaccine is given in Ireland but not the UK

There is evidence that breastfeeding your baby while they get their injections can give them some pain relief. Inform the nurse who is giving the vaccines know that you are going to breastfeed your baby while they do so. Sometimes babies can be a little bit out of sorts and fussy in the 24 hours after they receive their vaccinations. They may want to breastfeed more frequently.

To Pump or Not to Pump

Most new mothers are advised not to start pumping until their babies are six weeks old, unless they need to pump (for example for a non-latching or preterm baby). The rationale is that it's better to just focus on establishing breastfeeding and to keep things simple. However, this doesn't mean that you can't or that you shouldn't start pumping! What do you want to do? You may need to pump and store milk for times that you will be away from your baby or you may want to pump for a period of time to help increase your milk supply. Another reason to pump is so that you can donate milk to a human milk bank. Milk banks provide lifesaving donor milk to neonatal and sick babies. You can find more information about donating milk and the closest milk bank to you here https://ukamb.org/.

Many parents I talk to feel that a breast pump is something they have to buy, and that pumping is something they need to start at some point in time., another box to tick on their list of parenting milestones. But actually, it's OK to never pump, or to wait until such time that you really need to. Pumping does not necessarily go hand in hand with breastfeeding. For more information on pumping, see Chapter 10.

Breastfeeding Out and About

The idea of breastfeeding in public for the first time can be daunting. What if you flash your boob at a stranger in a coffee shop, or worse still, spray someone in the eye with milk?! (not a likely scenario). Here are a few pointers that may help:

- Bear in mind that it is your legal right to breastfeed your baby whenever and wherever you want to. You don't have to ask for permission. It doesn't matter what anyone else thinks. The law is on your side.

- Most people don't even notice when mothers breastfeed in public. If they do, they are likely to look away, ignore you, or smile and make a positive comment.

- It can feel awkward at first. You may feel self-conscious. But over time your confidence will grow.

- A good place to breastfeed in public for the first time would be a face-to-face breastfeeding support group, surrounded by other breastfeeding parents and volunteer supporters.

- If you decide to breastfeed at a café, choose one with comfortable seating. And bring a friend or family member along for moral support!

- If you are self-conscious about feeding in public, you could throw a scarf or a wrap over your shoulder, or buy a nursing cover. Alternatively, you could investigate places that have dedicated nursing rooms.

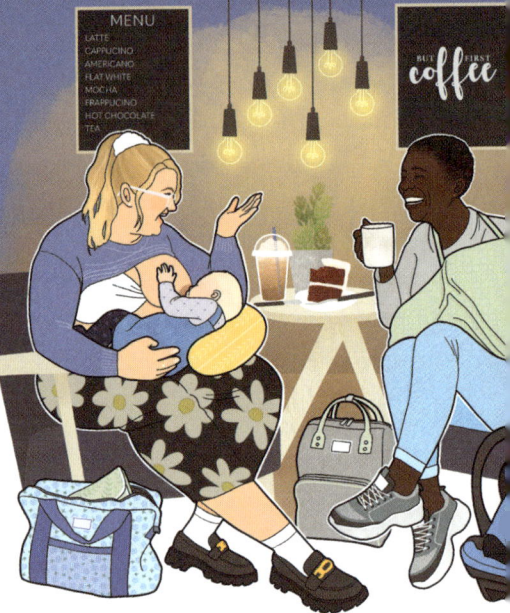

Remember, every time you breastfeed in public, you are helping to normalise breastfeeding and possibly inspire others to breastfeed. Be proud of yourself!

Lactational Amenorrhea Method (LAM)

LAM is an effective method of birth control that breastfeeding mothers can use, but only if they meet the following criteria:

- Baby is less than six months old.
- Their periods have not returned.
- They are exclusively breastfeeding day and night whenever the baby wants to be fed.

It is also recommended that you limit the use of soothers. According to the World Health Organisation, the risk of pregnancy when using LAM is less than one percent. LAM works because of the way your baby's sucking at the breast releases hormones that stop your ovaries releasing an egg.

If your periods return before your baby turns six months, LAM will no longer be as effective.

Is LAM effective if you are exclusively pumping? There isn't enough evidence to say how effective LAM is in mothers who are exclusively pumping. But it is probably less effective than direct breastfeeding as it means less frequent nipple stimulation (eight times a day versus on-demand feeding).

FAQS

How much milk should I leave for my baby if I am going to be apart from them? The general rule is that you leave 1oz or 30ml of expressed milk for every hour that you are going to be away. If you can time it so that you feed your baby just before you leave and as soon as you come home, your baby may not even need a feed while you're gone. If you are going to be away from your baby for more than three hours, you will probably have to express milk while you are away so that you protect your milk supply and avoid getting uncomfortably full.

Should I introduce a bottle to my baby? Many of the mothers I see are given to believe that there is a certain window of time (sixish weeks) during which they should give their breastfed baby a bottle, and that if they miss this window their baby won't ever take a bottle. This is not true, so it is important that you don't put yourself under any pressure to introduce a bottle or feel that doing so is a box that has to be ticked. Try to keep yourself in the moment and decide what is going to work for your family. Some breastfeeding parents never give their babies bottles, while others choose to introduce a bottle of expressed milk or infant formula at some point along the way. There is no 'should' about it.

Will giving my baby a 'dream feed' make them sleep for longer?
A dream feed is a feed that you give to your baby around the time that you are going to bed yourself, without fully waking them. The concept is usually associated with bottle feeding rather than breastfeeding. The goal of the dream feed is to give your baby a big feed that will fill them up and result in them sleeping for a longer stretch. Giving a dream feed does not give you any guarantee that either you or your baby will get more sleep. Dream feeding is kind of at odds with the baby-led nature of breastfeeding, whereby you feed your baby when they give you signs that they are hungry. That's not to say you can't dream feed if you are breastfeeding. Some parents swear by it while others will tell you that it makes no difference whatsoever to their baby's sleep.

Should I give my baby probiotics? Probiotics are live bacterial cells, 'good bacteria', in your breastmilk that help to establish a healthy gut microbiota in your baby and protect them from gastrointestinal infections. Probiotics also play an important role in the development of your baby's immune system. If your baby is exclusively breastfed, they will get all of the probiotics they need in your milk and you do not need to give them a probiotic supplement. In recent years many companies have started marketing infant probiotics to both parents of breastfed and formula-fed babies, making claims that they 'support health' and a 'balanced microbiome.' There is very little independent research to support these claims. If you are concerned about some aspect of your baby's health, chat to a healthcare provider before you decide to start giving your baby a probiotic supplement.

Is it possible to overfeed a breastfed baby? Not really. If you feed your baby whenever they show feeding cues (that is, responsively) they will regulate the amount of milk they drink. Lots of breastfed babies are chunky – this is normal! There is no evidence that chunky babies turn out to be chunky adults. Sometimes a very big milk supply can result in a bigger than usual weight gain in a baby. This is not something to be concerned about. However, if you are worried or if oversupply is making breastfeeding difficult, seek support from a lactation consultant or breastfeeding supporter.

CHAPTER 7

Using Social Media

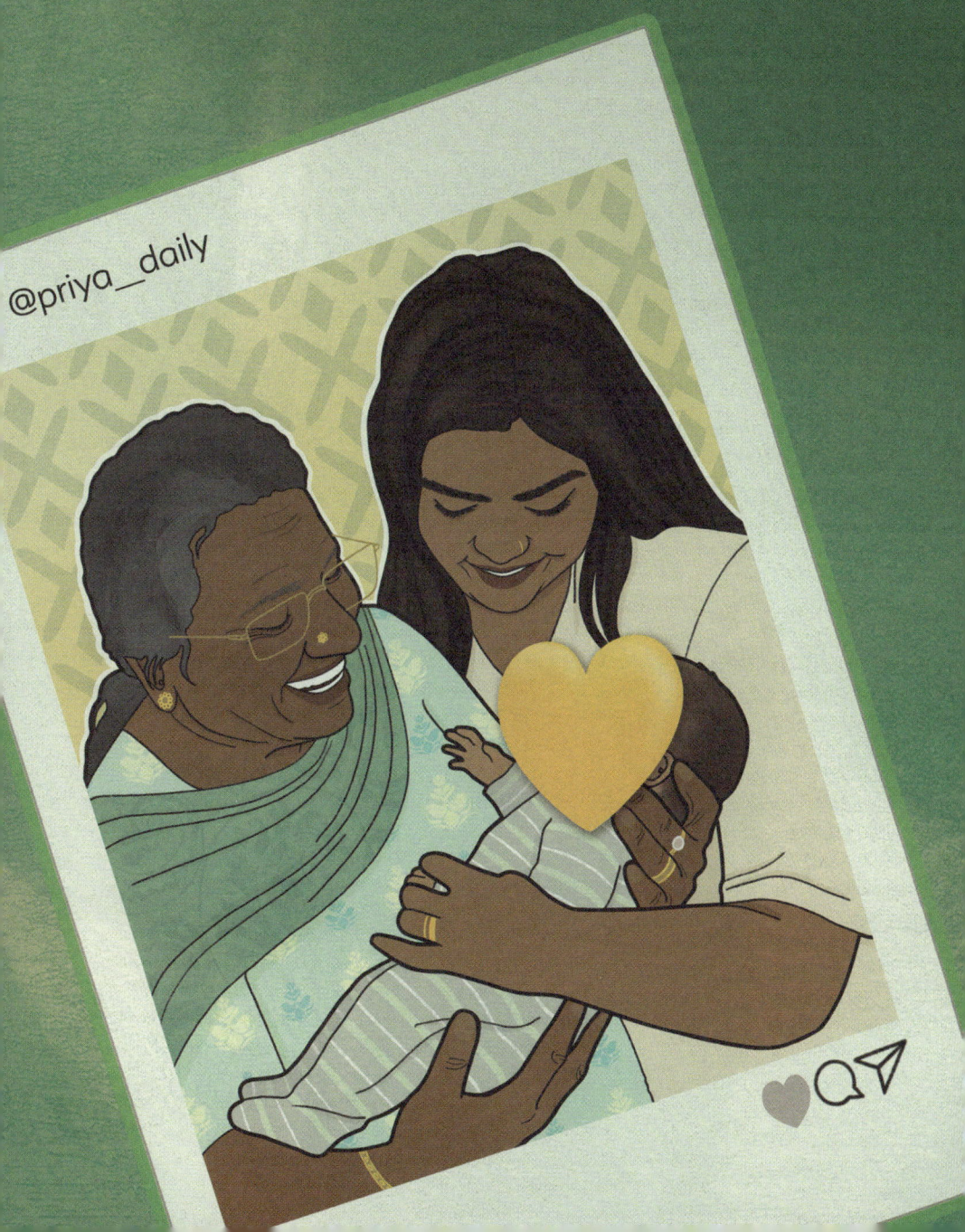

New parents are increasingly using social media platforms such as Instagram and TikTok to access information about infant feeding and parenthood. There are lots of positives in using these platforms and plenty of great accounts that share useful, evidence-based information. Benefits of using social media for new parents are:

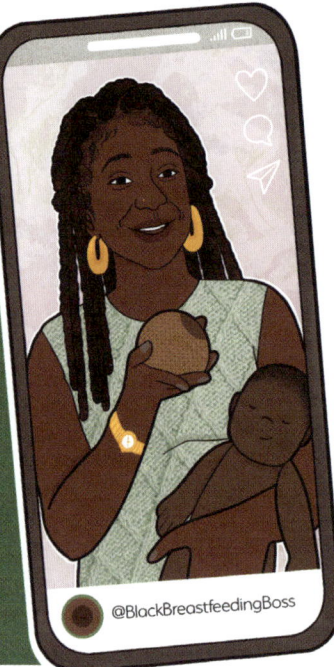

- Access to useful information on breastfeeding and lactation and support with breastfeeding challenges

- A sense of community and connection with other mothers, and the reassurance that you are not alone in navigating the challenges of new parenthood

- Connecting with others of shared cultural backgrounds (research has found that Black mothers experience social media platforms as a 'safe space' to connect with other Black mothers)

There is even some research which shows that women who access social media support groups breastfeed for longer and have a greater sense of breastfeeding self-efficacy. These positive aspects of using social media platforms are important, particularly if you don't have family support or friends around you who have breastfed or don't have access to skilled breastfeeding support. However, there are also a number of pitfalls in using social media to be aware of as a new parent.

Misinformation

It's no secret that social media platforms are awash with misinformation, disinformation and pseudoscience. This is due in large part to the fact that anyone can post anything on social media. So, the challenge for you as a parent is to try and figure out what is true and what is utter nonsense, and it is not always easy! There is so much conflicting information, especially around infant feeding and sleep. Here are some tips to help you navigate social media and know what posts to bin or what accounts to unfollow:

If you see posts on social media that seem a little bit dubious (for example, if you saw an *untrue* statement like 'Drinking carbonated drinks can make your breastmilk fizzy'), I suggest that you Check Your Sources:

- Who is behind the account?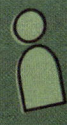

- Are they qualified to post about breastfeeding or whatever it is they are posting about? Do they have International Board Certified Lactation Consultant (IBCLC) accreditation and/or experience helping breastfeeding families? Are they accountable to a professional governing body?

- Have they provided evidence or citations to support their post?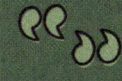

- Is the statement an opinion or a hypothesis?

- Does the person posting have any kind of vested interest? Are they trying to sell you something?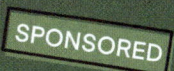

- Finally, where is the poster located? Context matters where breastfeeding is concerned. What may be appropriate in one country, may not be relevant somewhere else.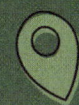

Not everything that professional-seeming accounts on social media post is true. A large number of followers does not guarantee that an account's posts will be reliable.

Exposure to Picture-perfect Motherhood

When you go on to social media, you are going to see a lot of images and portrayals of motherhood. Some of the portrayals you will see are real, honest (and sometimes very funny) depictions and accounts of messy motherhood, with unfiltered photos of real postpartum and lactating bodies. When you are struggling yourself or just having a bad day it can be reassuring to know that there are lots of other people out there just like you, just about managing to survive early parenthood. But in addition to these real-life accounts, you will also probably come across accounts presenting picture-perfect representations of motherhood. Many of these types of accounts are mother influencers*, *momfluencers* who partner with companies to market all manner of products and services, from infant formula to cosmetic surgery, and from household appliances to make-up. Momfluencer accounts tend to be carefully curated and present a beautiful version of motherhood. Many momfluencers have a particular type of aesthetic – slim, tanned, long hair, beautiful skin, fabulous clothes – a kind of perfection that is enhanced by filters. You may quite enjoy having a little glimpse into these influencers' lives, or perhaps you have no interest in them, but being exposed to picture-perfect representations of motherhood can negatively affect your mental health. Research has found that comparison with momfluencers on social media

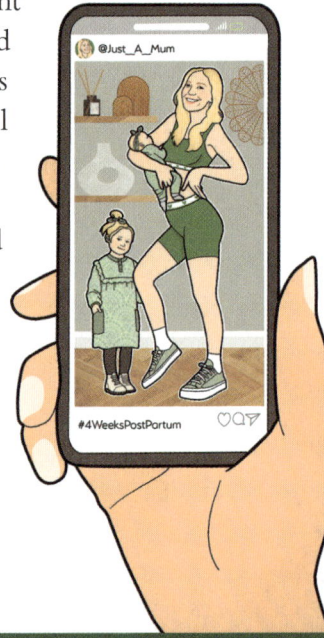

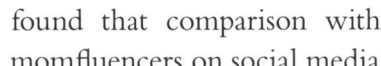

- can make you feel anxious, frustrated, stressed, guilty, and sad
- can reduce your sense of confidence in your parenting ability
- is linked to higher levels of depression in mothers

If seeing particular types of social media content makes you feel in any way anxious or sad, or like you just don't measure up as a mother, know that you are not the only one who feels like this and that you can always choose to unfollow.

* Influencers are people on social media who have a large following and who have the power to shape user attitudes and purchasing choices.

Predatory and Exploitative Marketing

Almost as soon as you become pregnant, or even before you conceive, the companies that market products on social media to new and expectant parents will also know. Remember, everything you do online (every Google search you make, every post you linger over for a few seconds longer, every Like, every link you click) is tracked and this information is used to target content and advertising to you. Big business knows that you want to do parenthood 'right' and that you will want the 'best' for your baby, and they capitalise on that. In recent years companies have become very clever in the way they use social media to market their products. They prey on parents' vulnerabilities and exploit parents' emotions with tactics that seek to make you feel that you are somehow deficient, and that purchasing their product will make parenting easier. Some of these big businesses even present normal infant behaviours as problems that need to be fixed – by using their product or service.

Infant formula companies have become adept at marketing their products across social media, using influencers to good effect, along with various other techniques to try to convince you that using their product will lead to less stress, more sleep and better weight gain for your baby. The message they want to convey is that they are there for you and that they care, that you are enough, that they won't judge you and that you should prioritise your mental health – the implication being that switching to infant formula makes life easier and somehow saves your mental health. Many of these companies even provide care lines and online support to offer a 'helping hand' to mothers with breastfeeding difficulties or mental health issues. Formula is a necessary product for many parents. It is not the enemy. But manipulative advertising, whose goal is to make you doubt your ability to breastfeed, is.

It's not just infant formula companies who are trying to convince you to buy their products. You will see ads for lots of other products, such as bottles, pumps, breast massagers, silicone milk collectors, sleep monitoring devices, white noise machines, expensive cribs, supplements, silver cups, nipple creams, sleep training programs, lactation cookies and anti-colic drops. The list is endless. But their goal is the same; to convince you that buying their product will make your life easier – more sleep, less night-time waking, more 'hands-free' time, lower risk of Sudden Infant Death Syndrome (SIDS), more energy, more milk, balanced hormones, and fewer problems. Some companies even claim that their products are 'a life saver' or 'a game changer.'

So, beware of predatory marketing and the way in which it is targeting YOU. Constant exposure to advertising can make you feel unfulfilled, anxious and inadequate, and can put you at risk of buying stuff you don't need.

To Post or Not to Post?

> On average, children have 1,300 photos of themselves circulating on social media platforms before the age of 13, before they are even allowed to have an account.
>
> François Macron

One of the most natural responses to having a new baby is to want to share the joyful news with friends and family. And with oxytocin flowing in abundance, you may even feel like sharing your news with the world. But have you given much thought to whether or not you really want to share your baby's image on social media? Sharing intimate images of birth, breastfeeding and babies on social media has become normalised. There are certainly positives to that, in raising awareness about the reality of birth and breastfeeding. But, it is worth considering how you may be compromising your baby's privacy by posting their image online. The European Union Charter of Fundamental Rights mandates that 'everyone has the right to respect for his or her private and family life, home and communications.' (article 7) and 'everyone has the right to the protection of personal data concerning him or her' (article 8). This charter applies to everyone, including babies, who are unable to consent to having their images shared. In addition to compromising your baby's privacy, there are also some potential risks to posting their images on social media:

- *Digital kidnapping* – this is where people take images of infants from the internet or social media and repost them as their own (yes, weird, but it can happen!)

- *Identity theft* – This is another worst-case scenario, but there is a risk that someone will pick up on details you share about your baby and use them to steal their identity and commit fraud. Barclay's Bank has predicted that *sharenting* (documenting your children's lives on social media) will account for two-thirds of identity fraud against young people by 2030

- We cannot assume that what we regard as normal or acceptable now, will be regarded as such a decade or two for now. While we may regard 'sharing' (ie, publishing) our babies' images on social media as harmless, our babies may question our actions when they are older, and feel angry that their privacy was violated. This may cause them to question your judgement. One American teenager called Sonia Bokhari reported feeling 'utterly embarrassed and deeply betrayed' when she discovered that her mother and sister has been sharing images of her on Facebook for years.

There are ways to post on social media while still protecting your baby's privacy. You could post a photograph in which your baby's face is hidden or you could redact their face (using a little heart emoji!).

Finally, if you are asked by someone, for example, a healthcare professional, if they can post your or your baby's image on social media, ask for some time to think it over. Consider why they want to post your image. Do they have something to gain? Are they promoting a product or a service? Who may see the image? You may ultimately say yes, but a little bit like the BRAIN technique that was discussed in Chapter 4, pause and consider all aspects of the request and its implications for you and for your baby.

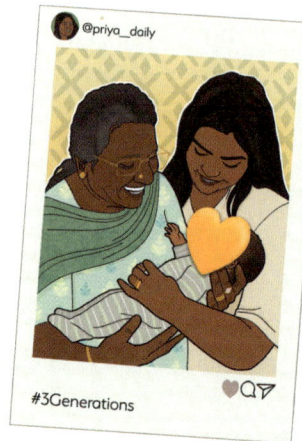

> *Everyone has a right to NOT be a commodity. To not be data. To not have their privacy compromised or traded in exchange for likes or follows.*
>
> Keats-Citron, 2022

Social Media is Addictive

Social media platforms want as much of your attention as they can get and as such, they are designed to be addictive. Their goal is to make money through advertising. The more you scroll and like and share, the more time you spend on the platform, and the more advertising you see. This is due to algorithms that the platforms use to determine what content you see. It is worth giving some consideration to how much of your attention (regarded as the most valuable commodity in the world today) you want to give to social media platforms. Are you in control of your social media use, or are their clever algorithms keeping you scrolling for longer than you want? Is your social media use affecting you in any way? If you've seen the Barbie movie you may remember America Ferrera's character Gloria, who worked for Mattel and came up with an idea for a *Sad Barbie* who spent 'six hours a day scrolling Instagram.' You probably don't want to be Sad Barbie, so take ownership of your use of social media.

CHAPTER 8

Sore Nipples and Tricky Nipples

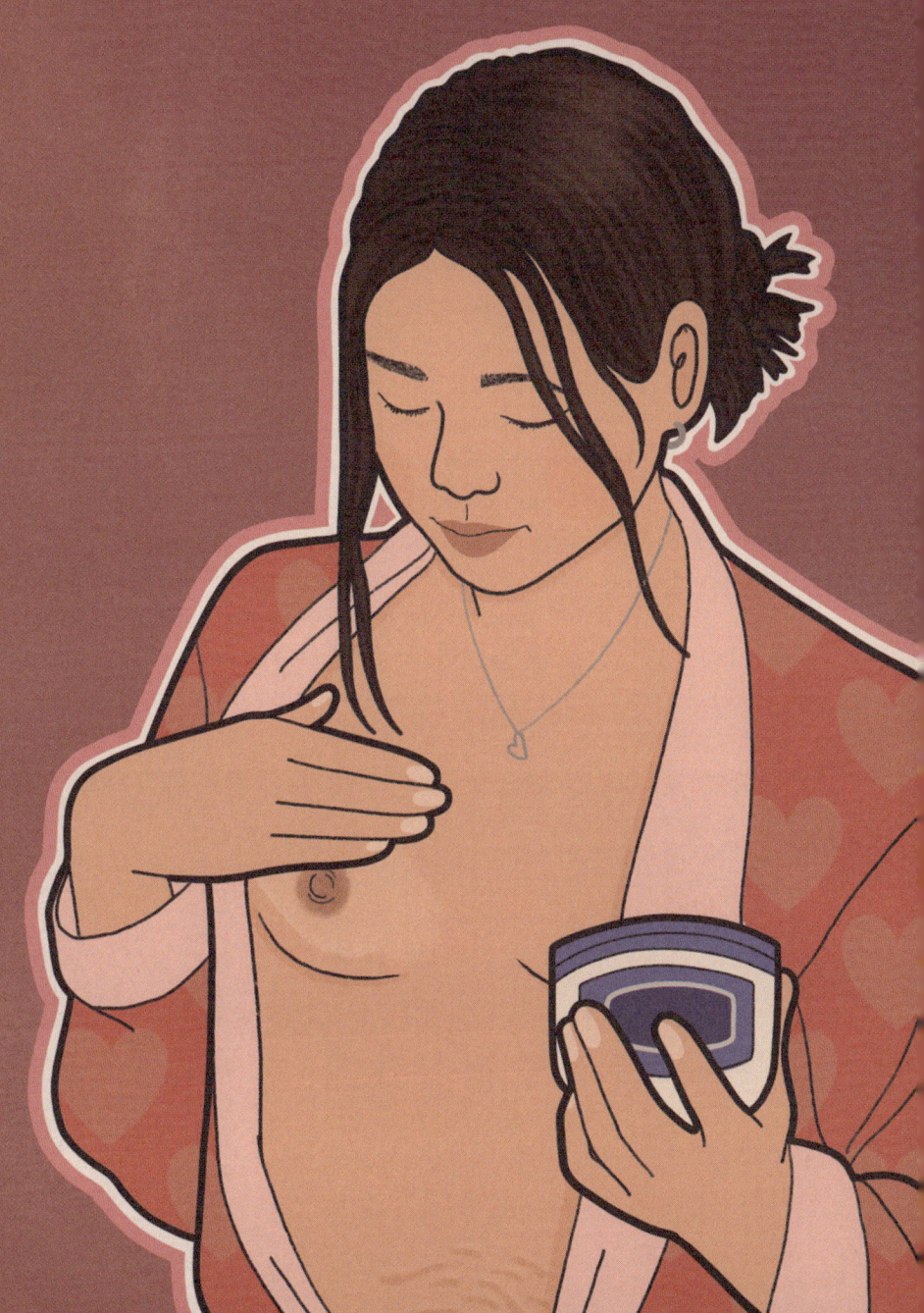

Most nipples are the perfect size and shape for breastfeeding, and for most people breastfeeding will be pain-free. However, some mothers will experience nipple pain or find that their nipples (due to their shape or size) are a little bit trickier than the average nipple. Whatever the case may be, the important thing to know is that with skilled support there is usually a way to continue breastfeeding or providing milk for your baby.

Sore Nipples

Sore nipples are the most common problem reported by breastfeeding parents in the first few weeks postpartum. If you have sore nipples, it is important to identify the cause, figure out the most appropriate solution, and determine how to treat your nipples if they are damaged. Working with a skilled breastfeeding supporter or IBCLC to help you in that process is really important. While some nipple tenderness and sensitivity are normal in the first week or two (due in part to higher levels of prolactin), consistently sore or damaged nipples are not.

Sore nipples are usually related to your baby's latch. Often small changes to your position or your baby's position can make a significant difference to how your baby latches and the level of pain you experience. Some general tips that can help optimise your baby's latch, get a little bit more breast tissue into their mouth and get your nipple into a *safe space* (beyond your baby's gums and in towards their palate) where it is not going to be compressed are

- Drop your baby's hips a little lower
- Gently pull you baby in a little closer to your body by applying pressure to their back
- Ensure your baby's chin is touching the underside of your areola and that their neck can extend (this enables them to open wide)
- Check if there is anything else you could do make you and your baby comfortable

Sometimes nipple pain when your baby is feeding can be due to damage sustained by a shallow latch when your milk was coming in – so the pain may not indicate a current latch issue. Look at the shape of your nipple after the feed. If it is a normal rounded shape, the pain is probably not latch-related. If the nipple is flattened or lipstick-shaped, there most likely is a latch issue.

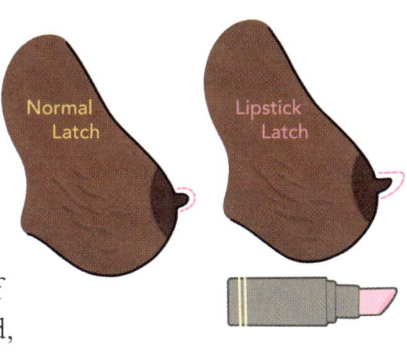

If you feel pain when your baby first latches, don't unlatch them immediately. Wait for a few moments or until your milk lets down. Sometimes babies will shimmy their way into a good latch and adjust themselves once the milk starts flowing. So, pause, breathe, see if the pain subsides.

If changes to latch and positioning don't help, there may be some other underlying cause of pain. These causes include vasospasm, tongue tie or something to do with your baby's oral anatomy, baby clamping due to muscle tension in their jaw, and thrush.

Vasospasm

Vasospasm is when blood vessels in the nipples constrict and reduce blood flow to the area. It can cause a throbbing/burning pain during or after breastfeeding or between feeds. Cold makes the pain worse.

Vasospasm can result from your nipple being compressed when your baby has a bad or suboptimal latch. If this is the case, the nipple is likely to be flattened or misshapen after feeding. Or you may experience vasospasm if you suffer from Raynaud's phenomenon (decreased blood flow to the extremities in response to cold or stress – do the tips of your fingers turn white when you're cold?). Vasospasm is also a possible side effect of Labetelol, a medication for high blood pressure.

How do you know if you have vasospasm? Your nipples will probably turn white after feeding due to the withdrawal of circulation. They may then turn purple, before eventually returning to their normal colour. This is called a *triphasic* colour change. You will probably experience pain in your nipples (which can radiate into your breasts) as the circulation returns to the blood vessels.

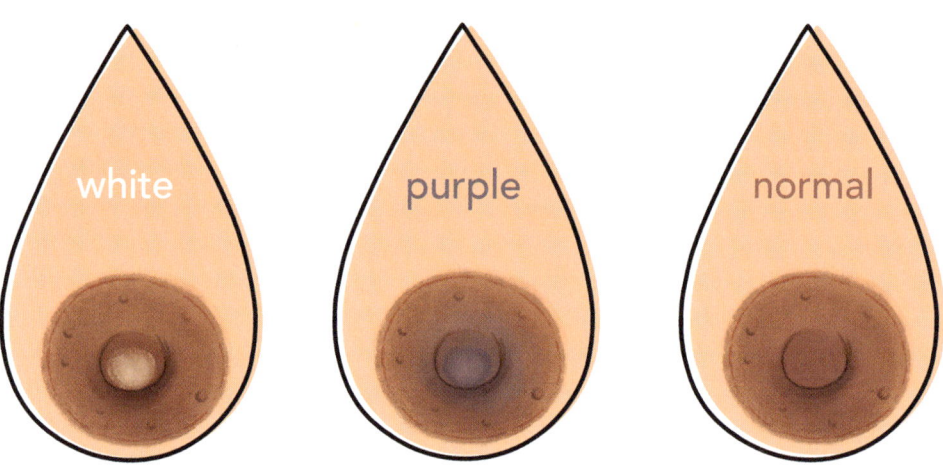

Managing Vasospasm

- Ensure that your baby is latching as well as they can – ask a breastfeeding supporter for help. If improvements to latch and positioning don't help, there may be something else at play. Eg. tongue tie.

- Apply dry heat to your nipples after breastfeeding (for example, a dry facecloth or muslin warmed on a radiator).

- Don't expose your nipples to the cold.

- Ensure you stay warm – an extra layer of clothing may help, or woollen breast warmers (yes, here is such a thing).

- Massaging your nipples gently between your thumbs and forefingers after feeding can encourage circulation

- Caffeine can make vasospasm worse, so reduce your intake of caffeinated tea and coffee (or drink decaf).

- Vitamin B6, Magnesium, Calcium, fish oil and evening primrose oil supplements (3mg twice a day) are thought to lessen the effects of vasospasm.

- Very occasionally a drug called Nifedipine can be prescribed to relieve the symptoms of vasospasm. If you have tried other measures and nothing's working, talk to your GP about Nifedipine and seek guidance from an IBCLC. Like all other medications, there are side effects to consider, and it is possible that Nifedipine's side effects could outweigh the benefits.

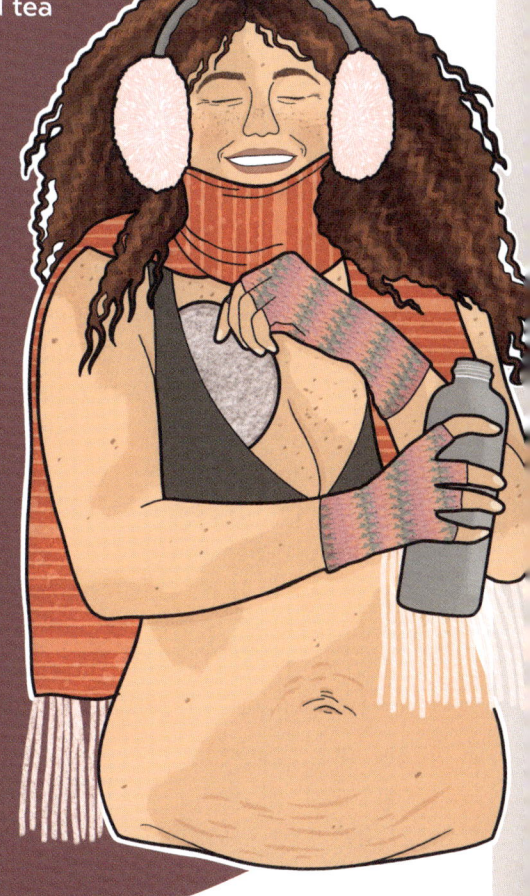

Vasospasm is often misdiagnosed as thrush because the symptoms are similar. It's important to have skilled support to try and determine the true cause of the pain you are experiencing.

Tongue tie

A tongue tie (the medical term is ankyloglossia) is when the frenulum, the small piece of tissue that anchors the tongue to the floor of the mouth, is so tight or short that it significantly restricts tongue mobility. Sometimes this limited tongue mobility can result in difficulties breastfeeding, such as a shallow latch and sore nipples, a baby that is unable to latch or effectively transfer sufficient milk when they are breastfeeding. If your baby has a tongue tie you will probably be able to see it when they cry and feel it if you sweep your finger under their tongue. But the visual appearance of a frenulum does not always mean that your baby is tongue-tied.

Quite often when a baby has a tongue tie, the mother's nipple will be flattened after breastfeeding.

When a tongue tie has been identified as the cause of breastfeeding difficulties, a frenotomy (tongue-tie release) — a procedure in which the frenulum is cut or released using scissors or a laser — is usually recommended. The goal of the frenotomy is to give the baby greater tongue mobility and improve breastfeeding. It is a very quick procedure and you can feed your baby immediately afterwards.

Between 4 and 10% of babies have a tongue tie (depending on what study you look at), but not all of them will require a frenotomy.

These are things you should consider if someone has identified a tongue tie and referred your baby for a frenotomy:

- Are you clear about what problem will be fixed by the frenotomy?
- Has the person who recommended the frenotomy done a thorough breastfeeding assessment?

- Have all other possible causes of breastfeeding problems been ruled out?
- Have you tried different positions to help improve your baby's latch?
- Will the person referring you be able to support you *after* the frenotomy has been done?
- Will the frenotomy be performed in a clinical setting?
- Have the risks of performing the procedure been explained to you?
- How do you feel about consenting to your baby having a frenotomy? If you are unsure, could you get a second opinion?

Sometimes a frenotomy is a no-brainer and is absolutely the solution to breastfeeding problems. But in the past decade tongue tie has been increasingly over-diagnosed. In my own private practice I see a large number of babies who have had a frenotomy performed with little or no apparent improvement in breastfeeding. Often, we discover that there is more going on, for example, the baby may have a significantly recessed chin and/or a high bubble palate – both of these anatomical variations can affect breastfeeding. Or we may discover that the mother has low milk supply. I also see a lot of parents who have been told that their baby has a *mild tongue tie* or that they *might* have a tongue tie, when in fact their baby's oral anatomy is perfectly normal. So, it is very important to have a thorough consultation and breastfeeding assessment with an IBCLC before a decision is made to refer your baby for a frenotomy.

Is wound massage necessary after a tongue tie release?
There is no evidence that doing wound massage after a tongue tie release is necessary. In fact, it could be painful and distressing for a baby (and parent) and contribute to them developing a feeding aversion. Sometimes gentle suck training exercises will be recommended for babies following a tongue tie release. So long as your baby does not object to them, these exercises may help your baby learn to breastfeed more effectively.

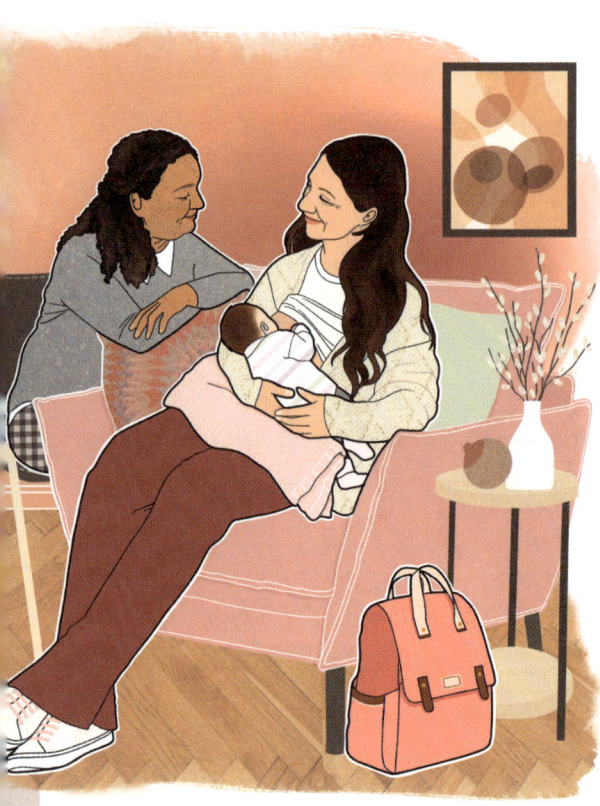

What about Posterior Tongue Ties?

A posterior tongue tie is one which is further back along the underside of the baby's tongue. It is not as obvious as classic or anterior tongue tie which attaches close to the tip of the tongue. While posterior tongue ties can affect breastfeeding, there is currently not enough evidence to support their release. Often other interventions such as adjustments to positioning can help, coupled with time and growth. Babies grow very fast and this means continual changes to their oral anatomy and their jaw, particularly in the first few months. Sometimes improvements in latch and feeding can be seen over time. There isn't always a quick fix for a breastfeeding problem.

Do lip ties and buccal ties affect breastfeeding?

There is insufficient evidence to support releasing either lip ties or buccal ties and these procedures are not commonly performed in the UK and Ireland. If you have been advised that your baby has lip or buccal ties, try to get a second opinion. A baby's upper lip does not have to flange out in order for them to have a good latch. In fact, many babies' upper lip will be in a neutral position when feeding.

Thrush

The cause of your nipple pain *might* be thrush – but it probably isn't. Thrush, or *candida*, is a fungal infection that can occur on your nipples or in your breasts, as well as other places in the body. Women who have a history of vaginal thrush or who have recently taken antibiotics are more susceptible to nipple thrush.

However, thrush is very often incorrectly diagnosed when mothers report sore nipples. Typically, they are advised to use a topical cream to treat the 'thrush' and then subsequently realise it isn't thrush when it they are still experiencing pain after a few days of use.

> **IF IT'S NOT THRUSH, THEN WHAT ELSE COULD IT BE?**
> It could be vasospasm, dermatitis, a bacterial infection or nipple irritation caused by pumping. Working with a GP and/or an IBCLC will help determine the cause of the pain.

Signs and symptoms of thrush include

- An itching or burning pain around the nipples and areola that can radiate into the breasts. Some women describe it as feeling like 'shards of broken glass' in their breasts.

- Nipples are very sensitive to touch – so much so that you don't want to have anything in contact with them.

- It's on both breasts.

- Nipples sometimes look pink and shiny or red and flaky.

- Your baby may have thrush in their mouth – thick white plaques on the insides of their cheeks, tongue, or palate or in the corners of their mouth. They may also have thrush on their bum – a bright red nappy rash.

- Sometimes with thrush, babies become fussier when they breastfeed.

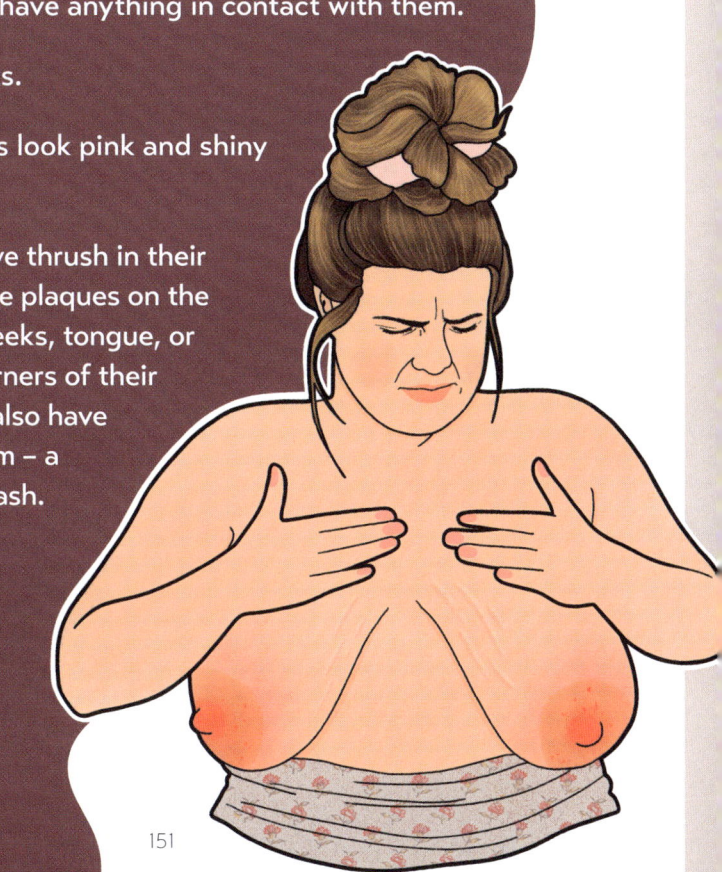

If you think you have thrush, see your GP. If they agree that it's thrush, they will advise on the most appropriate treatment – usually an anti-fungal cream (Miconazole) for your nipples and anti-fungal oral gel (Miconazole) or drops (Mystatin) for your baby. In severe cases, you will also be advised to take Fluconazole tablets (Please note: Fluconazole should not be taken in combination with Domperidone or Erythromycin).

Can you continue to breastfeed while you and your baby are being treated for thrush? Yes! Can you give your baby frozen breastmilk that you expressed while you had thrush? Yes! Don't throw it out!'

The following measures are recommended to prevent the thrush infection spreading:

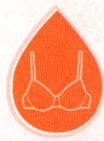
Wash bras, towels and anything else that comes into contact with your breasts in hot water.

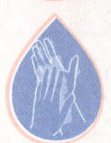
Wash your hands before and after feeding, after applying creams and after nappy changes.

Sterilise any feeding bottles, teats or soothers after use.

Also, take care to keep your nipples dry – thrush loves moist environments.

Blebs (Milk Blisters)

A bleb, or milk blister, occurs when skin grows over a nipple pore and milk gets backed up behind it. It looks like a little white dot on the face of your nipple and can feel sore when your baby feeds. Most of the time, a bleb will resolve spontaneously with continued responsive feeding (or pumping). However, occasionally blebs can be stubborn and difficult to clear. These are some measures that may help you clear a stubborn bleb:

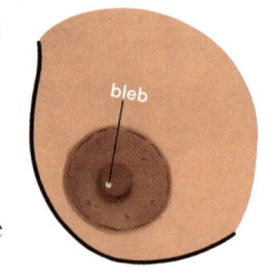

- Soften the skin by applying a warm, moist compress before breastfeeding.

- Placing a cotton pad with some olive oil on it into your bra between feeds can also help to soften the skin and clear the bleb.

- If the above measures don't work, you could try applying a mild steroid cream (eg 1% hydrocortisone) to the affected area three times a day after feeding. Gently wipe off any residual steroid cream with a damp cotton pad before breastfeeding.

Couldn't you just stick a needle in the bleb to clear it? This is not recommended, but if the usual measures are not working, it's something you could ask your GP to *unroof* the bleb. It's a little bit like removing a splinter – the skin is lifted up rather than pierced.

A lecithin (a fat emulsifier) supplement is sometimes recommended for mothers who experience recurrent blocked ducts or blebs. However, there is no evidence that it works. Anecdotally some parents report that lecithin helps, while others report no effect.

Treating Damaged Nipples

If your nipples are cracked or abraded (ie, skin is broken and nipple looks raw), you need to figure out how to heal them and keep breastfeeding or providing milk for your baby. It's important that you determine the cause of the damage. Usually it's latch-related friction or compression of the nipple, but damage can

BUT WHAT ABOUT AIR-DRYING NIPPLES?

The advice to air-dry sore or cracked nipples is outdated. Research has found that moist wound healing results in wounds healing 50% faster than air-drying.

also result from pumping – a poor fitting flange or very high suction.

The recommended treatment for cracked or abraded nipples is *moist wound healing*. This involves keeping the area moist by covering it with some kind of barrier. Doing so facilitates faster healing and promotes the growth of new skin cells. It also helps to prevent a scab forming. The kinds of barriers you could use to promote moist wound healing include breast milk, Vaseline and nipple creams. There is no evidence that nipple creams (which tend to be quite expensive!) are any more effective in promoting moist wound healing than either breastmilk or Vaseline. Many nipple creams contain lanolin, which some people may be allergic to.

Other products that can be used to help heal nipples include:

Compresses – Compresses contain lanolin or a plant-based oil. You put them on after feeding and they help to keep the nipples moist. Some women find them soothing, but they are probably not going to help with deeper wounds. Don't leave a compress on for longer than 30 minutes.

Hydrogel Pads – These pads also promote moist wound healing. One pad can be used for 24 hours – you just remove it when feeding. If you keep them in the fridge they can feel lovely and cooling when you put them on.

Polymem dressings – These dressings promote moist wound healing but unlike Multimam compresses and hydrogel pads, they absorb exudate from a wound. So, they would be a good option if you have an oozy crack on your nipple. Polymem dressings help to reduce inflammation and keep a wound clean.

Medihoney products – These products contain medical-grade sterilised Manuka honey and include creams, gels, and dressings. Medihoney has anti-bacterial properties and can help promote moist wound healing. It can help to heal quite deep nipple wounds that have not responded to other treatments. Healing could take up to three weeks.

Silver cups – these are little silver cups that can be placed on nipples between feeds. They are purported to help with moist wound healing, and some women find them helpful. However, use with caution. Leaving these cups on your nipples for too long can result in them sitting in milk, and this can cause the skin to become macerated. If you are using silver cups, I would suggest leaving them on your nipples after feeds for 15 – 20 minutes max.

Aloe Vera Gel – It's not commonly used on nipples but there is some evidence that it can help relieve the pain of nipple trauma and help with healing.

Working with an IBCLC will help you choose the most appropriate treatment for your nipples, if indeed a product is needed. Breastmilk plus time may be the answer.

What if a crack is infected? – Oozy yellow pus or a yellow crust on your nipple suggests that there could be a bacterial infection present. If this is the case, washing your nipples in warm soapy water will help to clear the biofilm. It is important to see your GP as nipples with a bacterial infection may require treatment with an antibiotic ointment. It is safe to continue breastfeeding or give your baby your milk when you have a bacterial nipple infection.

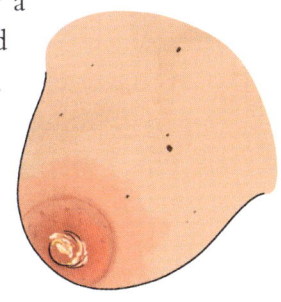

Can you continue directly feeding your baby at the breast?
It depends on the level of pain you are experiencing and whether breastfeeding will get in the way of nipple healing. Getting support

with latch and positioning and continuing to feed your baby directly at the breast is certainly easier. But there may be situations where taking a break from direct breastfeeding and pumping instead is advisable (while your nipples are healing and the cause of the damage is being addressed). For example, if you are waiting for your baby to have a tongue tie release, you may prefer to pump and bottle feed.

Please note: There are other less common causes of nipple pain and/or itching such as eczema, psoriasis and herpes simplex, which I have not covered here. If you are concerned, it is important that you reach out for breastfeeding support and/or medical help.

Idiopathic Nipple Pain

Idiopathic pain is pain for which a cause cannot be identified. It's not common, but idiopathic nipple and breast pain can occur in some breastfeeding mothers. Talk to your GP about options to help you manage the pain and seek support to continue breastfeeding. Some breastfeeding medicine doctors in the US recommend a low-dose SSRI antidepressant medication to treat idiopathic pain so that's something you could discuss with your GP.

Large, Flat, Short and Inverted Nipples

Nipples come in all shapes and sizes and most of them are perfect for breastfeeding. However, a small percentage of nipples can make breastfeeding more challenging – I call them *tricky nipples*.

In theory, flat or short nipples should not make latching and breastfeeding difficult – because babies *breast*feed, rather than nipple feed. But sometimes flat/short nipples can make it harder for a baby to get the nipple far back enough into their mouth to trigger a suck reflex. Often

large

small adjustments to positioning or nipple shaping can help.

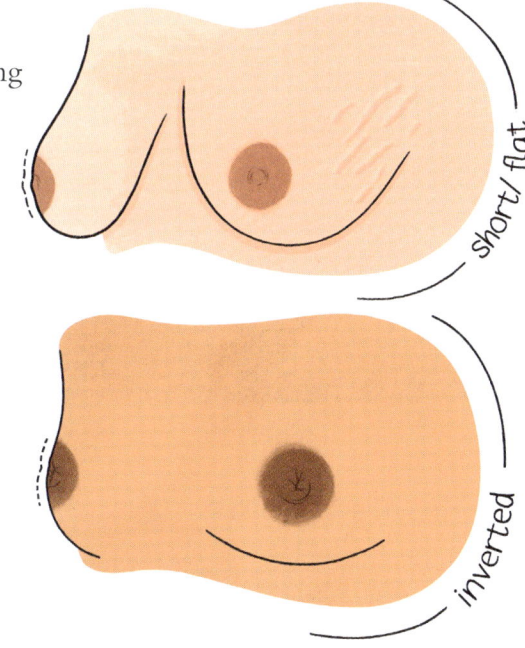

Inverted nipples can be a little bit more challenging, particularly if they invert when they are stimulated. These are referred to as *true* inverted nipples. Some nipples look inverted, but they will pop out when stimulated. Breastfeeding is possible with these *inverted-appearing* nipples. Adjustments to positioning and/or nipple stimulation, for example, rolling the nipple between your thumb and forefingers or even using ice on it, can make latching much more manageable.

With true inverted nipples, latching and breastfeeding can be very challenging, but that's not to say impossible! Much depends on your breast shape and whether you can easily make a *breast sandwich* with your areolar tissue. I have seen some cases where despite trying absolutely everything, mothers with true inverted nipples were unable to directly breastfeed, and also some where mothers were able to breastfeed their babies.

A lot can change over the course of a couple of months: areolar tissue can become more protractile and babies' jaws grow and enable them to open their mouths wider. Both of these factors can make latching on to tricky nipples easier.

There are a few products that some mothers find help to get their babies latched and breastfeeding well:

Nipple shields – not recommended as the first port of call for latching issues, but sometimes using nipples shields can be a game-changer.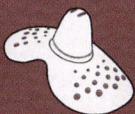

Nipple everter (latch assist) – this little device can be used before breastfeeding to pull nipples out.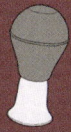

Supple Cups - These are little silicone cups that you put on your nipples for a short time before breastfeeding in order to draw them out.

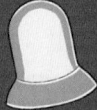

Breast Shells – they can be used to protect sore nipples from contact with clothing but some mothers find that wearing them before feeding gently draws nipples out.

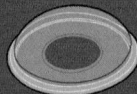

Nipple Shields

These are thin silicone covers that are placed over your nipple when breastfeeding. In some circumstances, using a nipple shield can help a baby latch and transfer milk effectively. Ideally, you should get help with latching and positioning before you try a nipple shield, and only use it once your milk has come in.

When can a nipple shield help?

Using a nipple shield may help to support direct breastfeeding where

- a mother has flat or inverted nipples

- a baby is struggling to latch or maintain a latch because of their oral anatomy (high palate or tongue tie) or a recessed chin

- a baby needs some extra intraoral stimulation (eg, a preterm baby) to get them sucking

- a mother is transitioning her baby from bottle to breast feeds

- a mother's nipples are damaged and direct breastfeeding is painful

What type of shield to use?
Nipple shields come in different brands, shapes and sizes. An IBCLC can help you choose the most suitable one for your nipple. Sometimes you may have to try a couple of different types before you find the shield that works best for you.

How to put a nipple shield on?
Stretch the edges of the shield out before placing it over your nipple. The shield should draw your nipple into it and stay in place with a little bit of suction. Putting the shield on properly can take some practice. It is advisable to have an IBCLC or midwife observe a feed with a nipple shield to ensure your baby is transferring milk effectively. Can you hear swallows? Is your baby drinking? Is your breast softer after the feed? Can you see milk in the shield after your baby has fed? If your baby is transferring milk well, the answer to all of these questions will be yes.

How to clean shields?
Wash nipple shields in warm soapy water and then rinse well.

How long to use the nipple shield for?
This depends on your baby and on the reasons you needed to use it in the first place. Some babies will need to use a shield for the duration of their breastfeeding journey. Other babies will transition to being able to breastfeed without them after a few weeks or months. Try not to put pressure on yourself to stop using the shields. Very often it is the baby who decides at some point in time that they no longer need them.

Tips for weaning from nipple shields:
Try removing the shield towards the end of a feed to see if your baby will latch without it. Also, try doing skin-to-skin when you can so that your baby gets plenty of opportunities to latch without the shield. It can also be helpful to offer your breast without the shield while your baby is half asleep.

Nipple shields often get a bad rap. Mothers are frequently told that they should stop using them. But the reality is that sometimes using a nipple shield is the difference between being able to breastfeed and not being able to breastfeed. So hooray for nipple shields.

Pierced Nipples

Most women with nipple piercings can breastfeed without any difficulty. It is recommended that you remove your jewellery prior to starting breastfeeding. The piercings will probably close-up but you can always get them done again after you have finished breastfeeding. You can opt to remove and replace your nipple jewellery before and after each feed, but it may just be more hassle than it's worth. If you do this, be careful about hand hygiene.

There is a small risk that piercings could obstruct milk flow or cause low milk supply. This is because they can damage the ducts and/or nerves in the nipple. There is no way to know in advance if your piercings will affect breastfeeding so you just have to wait and see.

CHAPTER 9

Mastitis, Blocked Ducts and Breast Pain

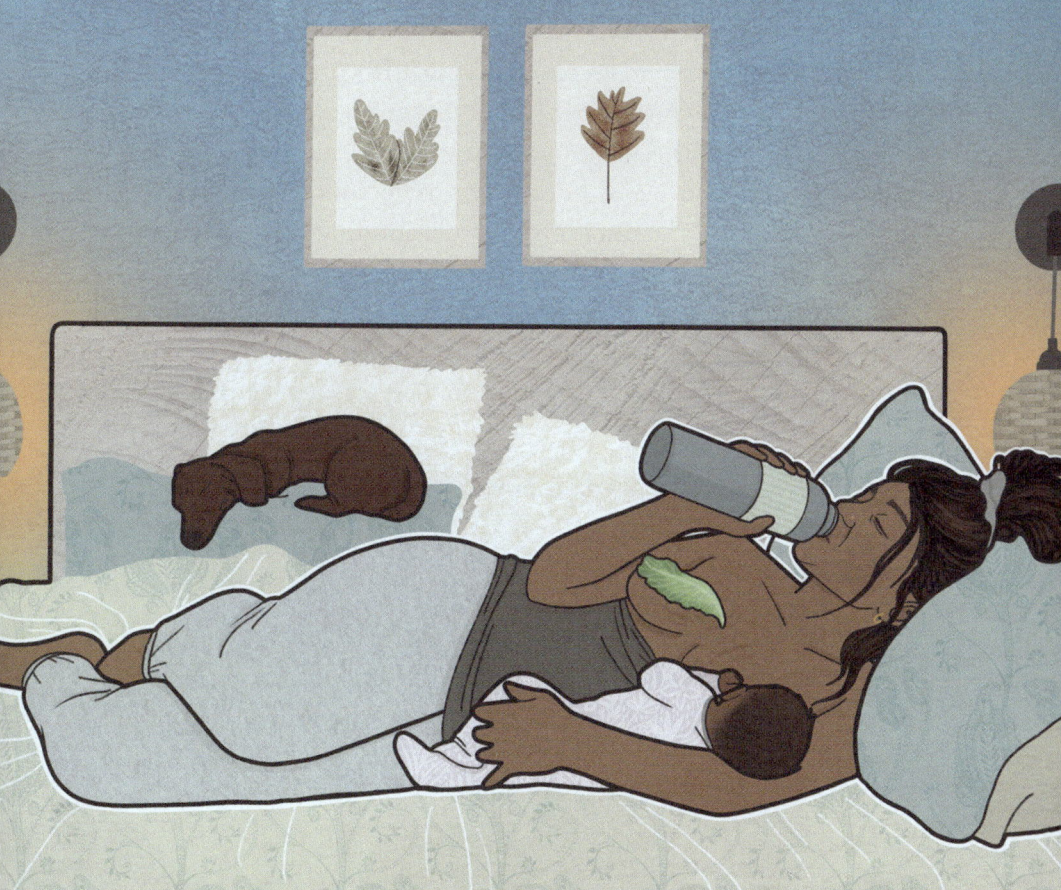

Blocked Ducts

A blocked duct occurs when an area of the breast around a duct (or ducts) becomes inflamed, and blocks the flow of milk towards the nipple. As a result, milk can get trapped in the lobules behind the affected duct. The area may feel tender to touch and hard and lumpy, even after breastfeeding. It may also look red.

Blocked ducts have several possible causes, including longer gaps between breastfeeds, baby sleeping longer at night, shorter than usual breastfeeds (for example, if you're busy), a baby that is not removing milk efficiently, or overproduction of milk. They could also be caused by pressure from a tight-fitting bra. Most mothers who breastfeed will experience blocked ducts at some time. If you get blocked ducts, avoid applying firm pressure or kneading the area behind the duct – there is often a temptation to do this with the goal of forcing the milk to move towards the nipple. However, applying firm pressure and kneading can be counterproductive as it can push milk from the duct into the surrounding tissue and increase the risk of mastitis, a common inflammation of the breast tissue.

Blocked ducts often resolve themselves with continued breastfeeding, but if you have a persistent blocked duct you could try the following measures (in conjunction with continued responsive feeding):

- Ensure you make time for breastfeeding and try to relax (this will help your milk to flow)

- Do a little gentle massage of your breast before feeding – light circular movements and gentle tapping, and gentle sweeping movements towards your armpit.

- Apply a warm compress to your breast before feeding.

- Ensure your baby is well positioned and latched – go back to basics!

- After breastfeeding, apply a cold compress or an ice pack to the affected area (to reduce inflammation).

- Rest. And make sure you're drinking plenty of fluids.

- If your breast still feels sore after feeding, you could consider taking Ibuprofen.

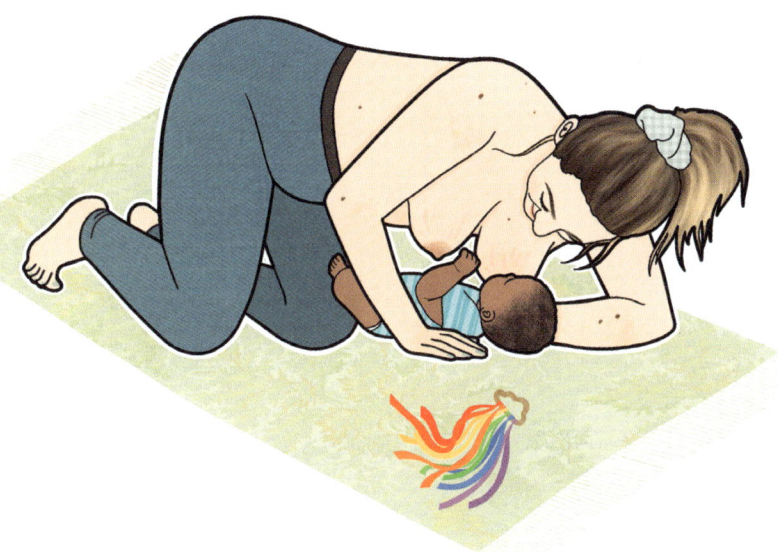

Some women find dangle feeding helps to clear blocked ducts. If the blocked ducts do not resolve within a few days, if the area becomes red and inflamed and/or you develop a fever, contact your GP as it could be mastitis.

Mastitis

Mastitis, inflammation of the breast tissue, occurs most commonly in the first four weeks postpartum (10-20% of mothers experience it). It is usually caused by suboptimal milk removal – the breast becomes very full of milk and this leads to inflammation and swelling. Mastitis can also result from nipple damage, oversupply or pressure on the breast (wearing a very tight bra or applying too much pressure during massage).

Mastitis can be non-infective or infective. Infective mastitis must be treated with antibiotics.

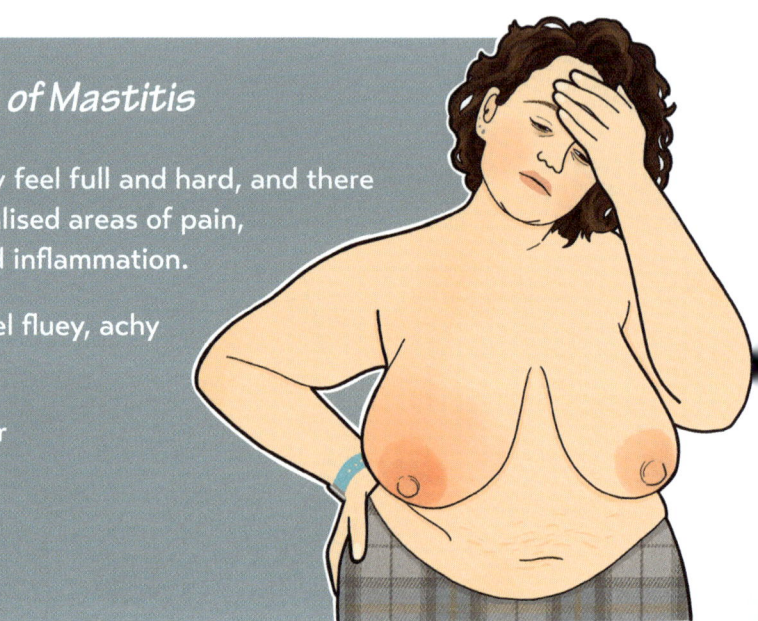

Symptoms of Mastitis

- Breasts may feel full and hard, and there may be localised areas of pain, redness and inflammation.

- You may feel fluey, achy and tired.

- A high fever

- Nausea

- Chills

So, what should you do if you experience any of the above symptoms? These are things that can help:

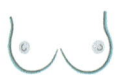 Don't panic! Continue breastfeeding your baby responsively (or pumping and feeding your baby your milk). You cannot pass mastitis on to your baby through your milk.

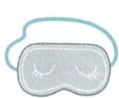 Try to get as much rest as you can – mastitis may be your body's way of telling you to slow down.

 Avoid emptying your breasts with pumping – this could trigger increased milk production, which isn't going to help. After a breastfeed or a pump, your breasts should feel softer, but they don't have to be completely emptied.

Apply a warm compress before feeding (this can help milk to flow).

 Apply ice/cold compress or cabbage leaves (from the freezer) to your breasts after feeding to reduce inflammation.

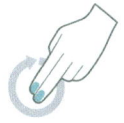 Avoid forceful or deep massage. Instead, if your breast is very full try gentle lymphatic drainage before feeding/pumping. It helps to move lymph fluid away from the breasts.

- *Get comfortable and lean back*
- *Warm your hands*
- *Make circular massage movements just above your collarbones and in your armpits*
- *Gently massage from your nipple radially outwards towards your armpit and upwards towards your neck.*

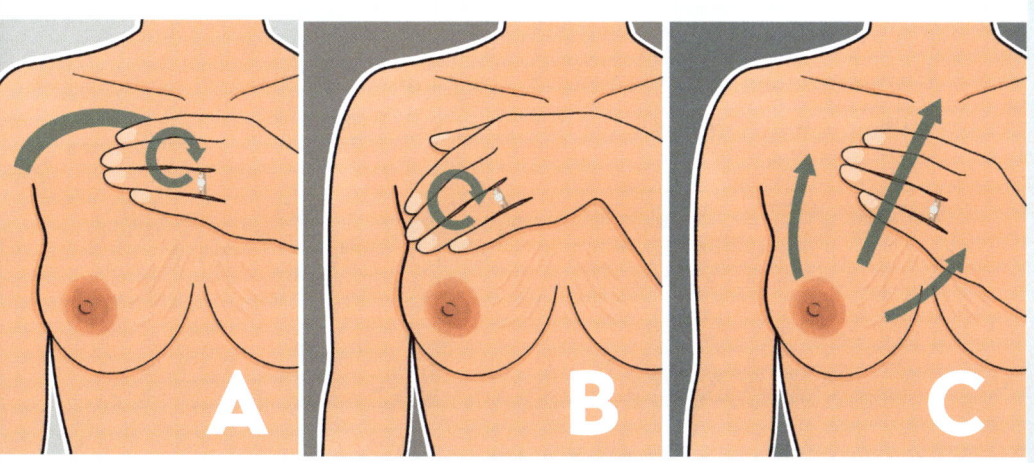

 Wear a supportive bra that fits well.

 Take Ibuprofen and/or paracetamol for pain relief (both are safe to take when you're breastfeeding)

 Ensure you drink plenty of fluids

IF YOUR SYMPTOMS DO NOT RESOLVE WITHIN 24 HOURS, OR IF YOU START TO FEEL WORSE, CONTACT YOUR GP. YOU MAY NEED ANTIBIOTICS.

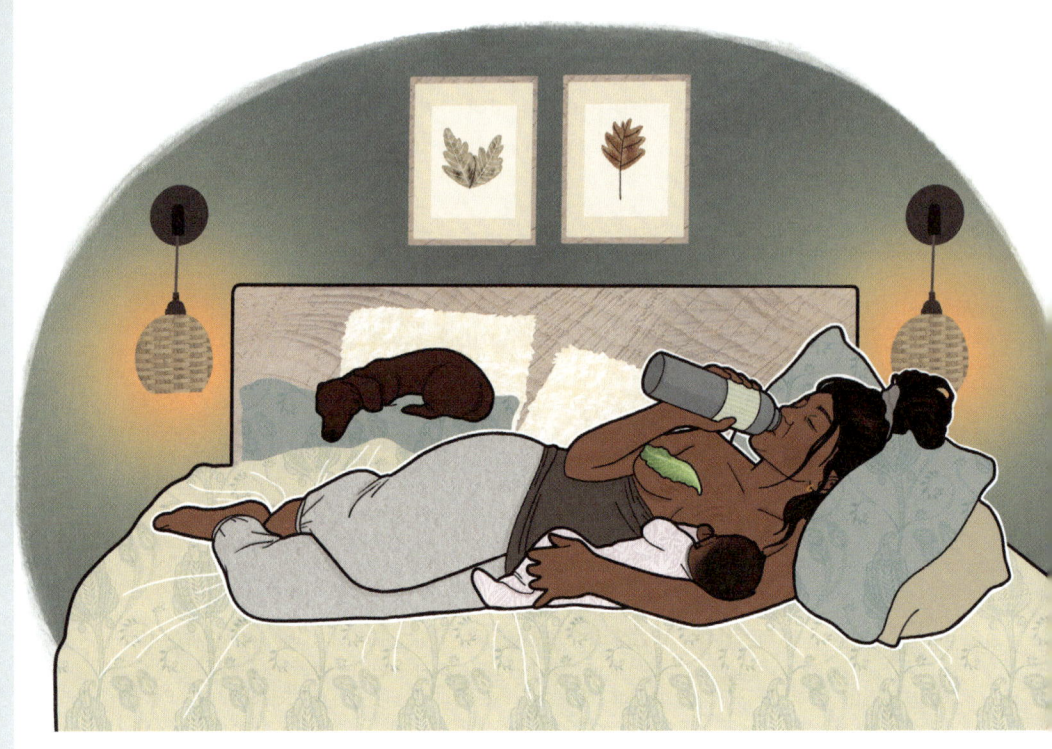

If you are diagnosed with mastitis, it is important that you keep the milk flowing. Don't stop breastfeeding or pumping!

> *Milk production can temporarily drop when you have mastitis, but it should be possible to bring it back up again*

Antibiotics are safe to take when breastfeeding and will not adversely affect your baby. Most GPs will prescribe Flucloxacillin (penicillin) 500mg four times a day for a course of seven to 14 days. If you are allergic to penicillin, alternatives such as Clindamycin or Cephalexin can be prescribed. Occasionally, women with mastitis will need to be readmitted to hospital to get IV antibiotics. If you are readmitted to hospital, you should be able to bring your baby with you and continue breastfeeding.

A mastitis infection might make your milk taste salty — this may cause your baby to fuss a little bit when feeding.

If you get repeated bouts of mastitis or if you continue to experience pain in your breasts or if the antibiotics you have been prescribed don't resolve your symptoms, there may be an underlying cause that needs to be addressed. See an IBCLC and your GP. In these situations, doing a breastmilk culture is advisable. This involves taking a small sample of your breastmilk and sending it to a laboratory which will investigate what specific bacteria are present.

Abscess

An abscess is a localised, walled-off collection of pus in the breast. It develops in approximately three percent of women who get mastitis and requires surgical drainage to get the pus out. Sometimes an abscess can be felt in the breast, as a round, smooth mass, a bit like a small egg. The area may also be tender. The presence of an abscess can be confirmed by diagnostic ultrasound.

Opinions differ among breast surgeons about how best to remove the pus from an abscess. Some will remove the pus using a needle and syringe (aspiration) while others will opt to put a drain in (incision and drainage). Continuing to breastfeed from the affected breast may be possible while the abscess is being treated – it depends on the location of the abscess. If it is very close to the nipple, direct breastfeeding could be difficult. Either way, you should continue to regularly remove milk from the breast, if not by direct breastfeeding, then by pumping. Sometimes mothers choose to stop feeding from the affected breast altogether, and just feed from the unaffected side.

Having an abscess can be very upsetting and women sometimes worry about being left with scarring. Whatever concerns you have, talk to your breast surgeon and let them know that you wish to continue breastfeeding (if that is what you want to do). Sometimes people who don't have much breastfeeding training or experience lack an understanding of the strong, embodied feelings mothers can have about this topic.

Breast Lumps and Bumps

When your breasts start producing milk, it is normal that they will sometimes feel lumpy or bumpy. But if you ever feel a lump that you think is not normal or a lump that does not go away, speak to a healthcare professional. These are some examples lumps that can present when you're lactating:

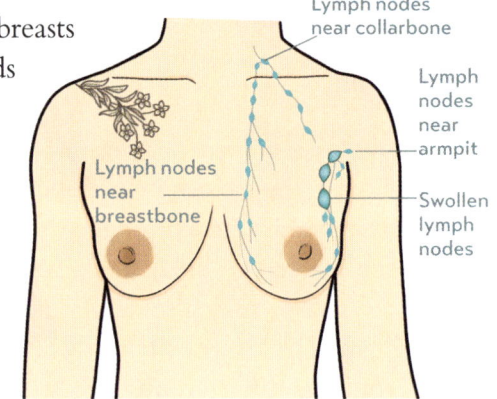

Swollen Lymph Nodes: When breasts start to lactate, the lymph glands produce more lymph fluid. This fluid removes the waste products of milk synthesis and bacteria from the breasts and absorbs excess blood from tissue spaces. Most of this lymph fluid flows into the lymph nodes in the armpits. When a mother's milk comes in and is increasing in volume, large volumes of lymph fluid can sometimes accumulate in the lymph nodes, causing lumps in the armpits. Usually, these lumps resolve within a week or two. Keep breastfeeding responsively and stay hydrated. You could also try cold compresses to reduce inflammation around the lymph node area. If the lumps become painful or don't resolve, speak to a healthcare professional.

Galactocele: This is a benign milk-filled cyst and is not very common. It can range in size from 1cm to 10cm and its presence can be confirmed with an ultrasound. Galactoceles can be aspirated or drained but they may refill with milk, so several aspirations may be necessary. Small galactoceles do not need to be drained.

Fibrocystic Breast Tissue: Some women have fibrocystic or lumpy breasts. The lumps are caused by little cysts and collections of fibrous tissue in the breast. This is a non-cancerous condition. Women who have fibrocystic breast tissue can breastfeed. However, their breasts may feel a little bit more tender and ropey at times, especially when their breasts are quite full.

Referred Breast Pain

Referred breast pain is also known as Mammary Constriction Syndrome (MCS). It is deep pain in the breasts that results from tension in your shoulders and upper back. If other causes of breast pain have been explored and ruled out, it is possible that you are experiencing MCS. The following measures can help to alleviate the pain associated with MCS:

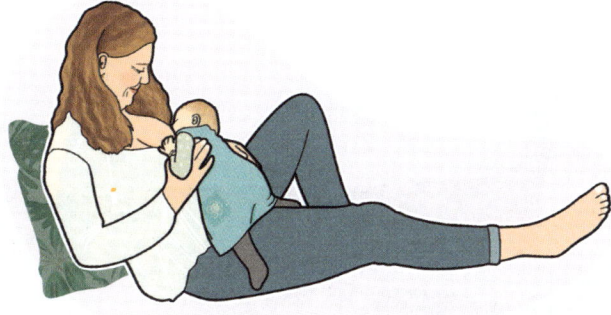

Consider the position of your body when you are breastfeeding – Are you hunching over? Are your shoulders tight? Are you taking your baby's weight in your arms or shoulders rather than supporting them with your body? Think about how you may make yourself more comfortable and use gravity to support your body and your baby's weight. Lean back, shimmy your hips forward, drop your shoulders.

Breathe into tight areas of your body – If you can identify where you are holding tension, closing your eyes and consciously moving your breath in and out of that area could help release tension. Just three long, slow inbreaths and outbreaths could make a difference. Another way to use your breath would be to scrunch up your shoulders on an in-breath and then release them as fully as you can on a long, slow out-breath.

Pectoral Muscle Massage – Your pectoral muscles are located just above your breasts. Gently massaging the pectoral area before breastfeeding is thought to reduce MCS pain. Using your fingers or the palm of your hand, make circular movements to the area, using only as much pressure as feels comfortable.

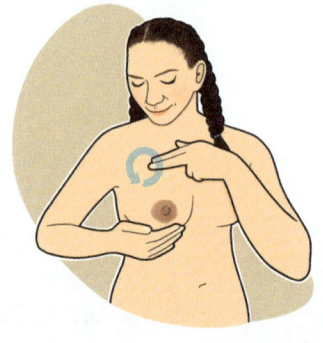

Take a few minutes to relax and *gently stretch the muscles in your upper back* by lying on the floor with a rolled-up towel or semi-inflated pilates ball between your shoulder blades.

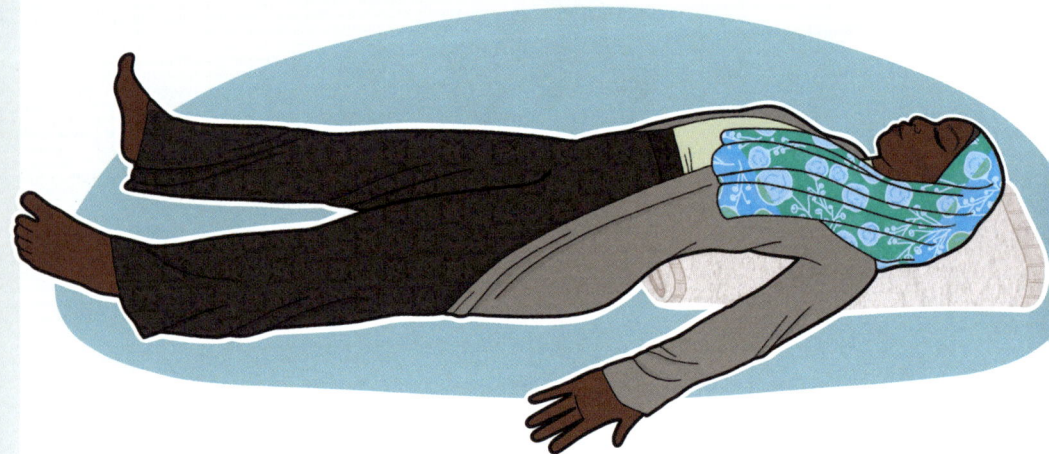

Oversupply

Oversupply is when you produce significantly more milk than your baby needs. It can make breastfeeding very stressful for both you and your baby. Mothers who have oversupply are likely to experience uncomfortable breast fullness, breast pain, recurrent mastitis and blocked ducts and leaking/spraying that can make breastfeeding in public difficult. Babies of mothers with oversupply often experience fussiness when feeding, spitting up, wind, digestive discomfort and mucousy or explosive poos. These babies are also likely to gain weight very rapidly, often at twice the rate of other babies.

Sometimes oversupply can be triggered by too much pumping in the first few weeks post-partum, but there isn't always an obvious cause. I have found in my experience supporting parents with oversupply, that milk production tends to regulate from around 12 weeks post-partum. But to help you manage oversupply and dampen down milk production before this, these are some measures that you could try:

If you are pumping, gradually decrease it – with fewer pumping sessions, and removing slightly less milk each time you pump. Aim to remove only as much milk as you need to feel comfortable, rather than emptying your breasts. Over time, this will give your body the message to make less milk.

Recline when breastfeeding – this can make it easier for your baby to manage a forceful flow of milk. Side-lying can also help to make feeds less fraught.

When your milk lets down at the beginning of a feed – You could unlatch your baby and allow the flow to subside before relatching them. Or you could try to reduce the flow of milk by cupping your breast and applying pressure back towards your chest, away from your nipple. You can gradually release this hold once your baby settles into the feed.

Feed your Baby from just One Breast per Breastfeed – Doing this can help to reduce milk production by leaving the opposite breast full for a longer period. You may need to hand-express a small amount of milk for comfort though – it's a fine line between keeping your breasts fuller for longer and staying comfortable.

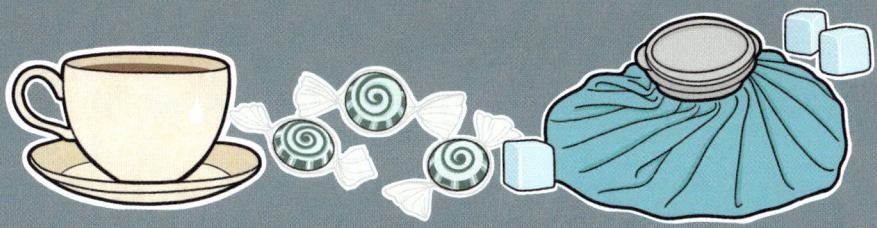

Use Cold Compresses or Ice packs on your Breasts after Feeding – Cold or ice packs can provide pain relief, reduce inflammation and bring down milk production.

Jiggle your Breasts Before Feeding – There isn't a whole lot of evidence that doing this helps, but the idea is that if you gently jiggle and shake your breasts before feeding, there will be more fat in your milk at the beginning of the feed. This is thought to reduce the large volume of lower-fat milk that your baby drinks and, in turn, reduce gassiness and the explosiveness of their nappies. It's worth a try.

Herbs that reduce Milk Production – Peppermint, Sage and Parsley are said to reduce milk production. You could drink peppermint tea, suck peppermint sweets, throw more parsley into your stuffing and take sage in capsule format.

If the above measures do not work, seek out support from an IBCLC. They may be able to talk to you about other measures that could help, or medications that reduce milk production with pseudoephedrine or an oestrogen-containing contraceptive pill. And of course, seek advice from your GP if you are considering taking any medication.

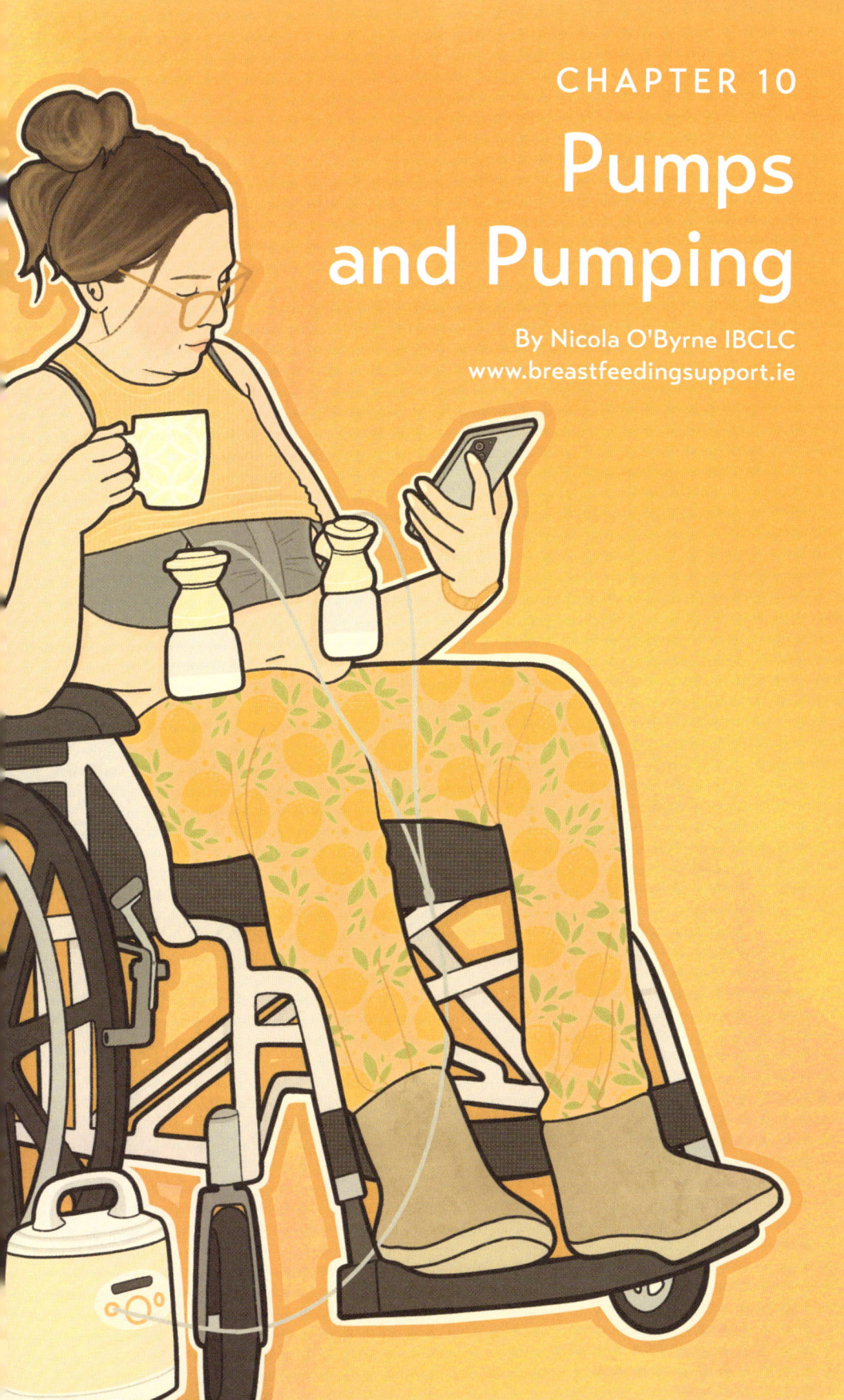

Introduction

It's important to know that you can breastfeed your baby for six months or longer without ever using a bottle or a breast pump. However, many mothers today are very busy and using a breast pump can help them to continue breastfeeding while getting on with their lives.

In this chapter I'm going to discuss the reasons why you may be advised to use a breast pump in the early weeks after your baby is born and how to start pumping milk so that you can give your baby expressed breastmilk should you need to leave your baby or if you choose to use some expressed breastmilk by bottle every day.

Exclusive Pumping

Some mothers pump all their breast milk and don't feed their babies directly at the breast. This is called exclusive pumping. Some people will choose to pump exclusively, while others may have no choice if direct breastfeeding hasn't worked out or their baby is struggling to latch and they still want their baby to have breast milk. Mothers of preterm babies often start out on their feeding journey with exclusive pumping. This enables them to provide milk for their baby until such time that their baby is developmentally ready to do some or all feeds at the breast.

To start exclusively pumping, you need to

1. Hand express colostrum every two-three hours for the first 36 – 48 hours after your baby is born. Please note: the Medela Symphony pump has a setting for hand expression.

2. Towards the end of day two or beginning of day three, start using a multiuser pump (also referred to as a *hospital-grade pump*) on both breasts eight to ten times in 24 hours. Volumes will increase daily, and you will be aiming to get at least 750mls by day 10 postpartum. It is normal to get more milk from one breast and have higher amounts in the mornings and during the night.

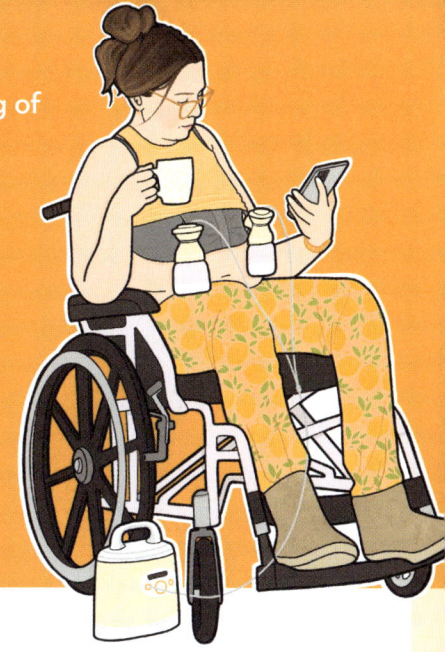

Using a strong multiuser breast pump is essential to obtain a good supply. Parents usually rent these pumps – examples include the Medela Symphony and the Ardo Carum. Once the supply is established, many mothers find they can pump less frequently and still get the same volume.

Occasional Pumping

Many breastfeeding mothers choose to do some pumping – it could be once a day or a couple of times a week, or whenever needed. Mothers may pump because they:

- have to be away from their baby for short periods of time
- want to have some expressed milk stored in their freezer for use at a later date
- want to give their baby some milk in a bottle in the evening
- want to give their milk to an older infant

You can use an app to keep track of how much milk you are pumping. Or alternatively, you can download a free pumping log sheet from the internet.

Many mothers find that the easier time of the day to pump is after a morning breastfeed. Remember to have realistic expectations around the volume of milk you can pump *after* your baby has breastfed. You may get approximately 20-60ml. If you wait 30-60 minutes after breastfeeding to pump, you may get a little bit more milk.

Triple Feeding

Triple feeding is the term used when a mother is asked to breastfeed her baby on both sides, pump breast milk, and feed her baby pumped milk after every breastfeed.

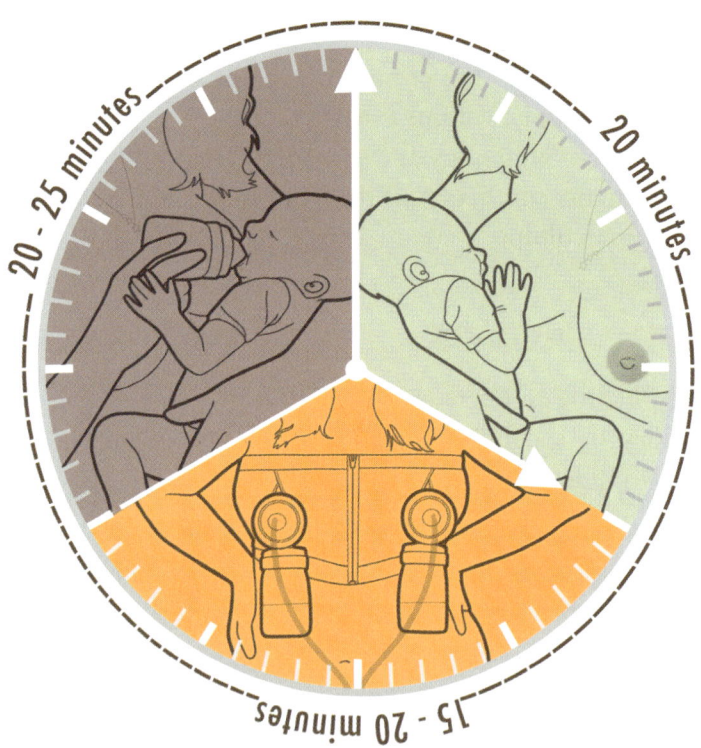

- 20 minutes breastfeeding (both breasts)
- 5-20 minutes double-pumping
- feed the milk obtained to the baby by bottle

This may be suggested in the early days after discharge from the hospital if your baby has lost more than 10% of their birth weight or if you have risk factors for low milk supply.

Triple feeding is very difficult to keep up for long and the strain may eventually affect a mother's mental health. So ideally each feed should take about one hour:

- 20 minutes breastfeeding (both breasts)
- 5- 20 minutes double-pumping
- feed the milk obtained to the baby by bottle

Unfortunately, triple feeding tends to take much longer than that, especially as new parents struggle with putting pumping parts together, sterilizing pump parts and bottles, changing the baby's nappy and feeding the baby expressed milk. Ideally, triple feeding should last no longer than three to five days, after which a professional should readjust the plan to make things easier for the parents.

Some tips that can make triple feeding easier:

There may be *no need to sterilise* each *time* you use your breast pump. If your baby is term and healthy you need to sterilise your pump parts only once in 24 hours. After using the pump, you can wash the bottles in warm soapy water and rinse and leave them to dry before the next pump.

Warm the flanges (the parts of the pump that go on your breasts) before pumping by placing them in a bowl of hot water and then drying them with a kitchen towel. This helps to increase the volume of milk you can pump.

Hands-on pumping – gently massage your breasts before pumping, use your hands to gently compress while you are pumping and do some hand expression after your pump. All of this can help to increase the volume of milk you pump.

You will get more milk *using heat on your breasts* during pumping has been proven in the research to remove the milk faster.

Using a *pumping bra* or cutting holes in an old bra can help so that you don't have to hold the bottles in place all the time.

In temperatures under 25°C you can pump back into milk that's been previously expressed up to six hours.

It may be possible to reduce pumping times from eight in 24 hours or perhaps cluster a few pumping times together two-hourly so that you can have a longer break to sleep.

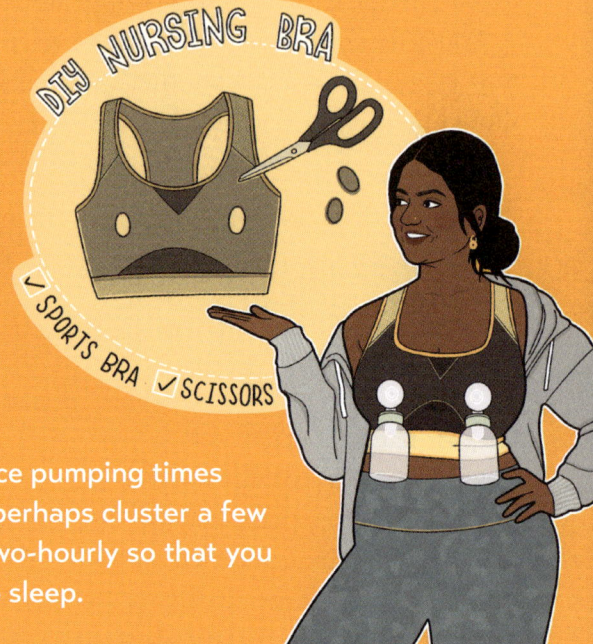

Pumping for a Preterm Baby

If your baby is born before 36 weeks (and hence is called preterm), it's quite likely you will need to express some breastmilk. Preterm babies that are under 32 weeks have not developed their suck, swallow and breathing coordination and will need expressed milk by tube until they mature. Some points about expressing for a preterm baby:

- Skin-to-skin with your baby (kangaroo care) is wonderful for helping build milk supply.
- Sterilising all pumping parts and handwashing is vital as your baby does not have a strong immune system.
- Your midwife will help you start hand expressing colostrum for the first 24-48 hours, then you will need to use a multiuser pump to double pump 8 times per 24 hours.

- Volumes will rise each day and sometimes one breast will give more than the other. You may get more milk in the morning and less in the evening.

- Keeping a log of milk volumes is useful.

- Hopefully by day 10 post birth you'll be getting around 800mls in 24 hours.

- Store your milk in containers the NICU nurses give you, carefully labelling them with your name, date and time of expressing.

- Generally, the NICU uses all the milk for the first 14 days then freshly expressed from the previous 24 hours. This means your baby gets the highest level of immunity possible.

Transferring to breastfeeding

Once your baby is stable and able to suckle you will start doing some small breastfeeds – they may only take a few sucks at first or just attach to the breast and do nothing – it's all good and every few days they will improve. The IBCLC in the NICU will help you work out a plan to drop pumping and switch to full-time breastfeeding.

Silicone Milk Removers and Collectors

Silicone milk removers are not breast pumps. There are different types of silicone milk removers – some use suction and drain from your breast (usually while you're breastfeeding on the other breast), while others just collect dripped milk.

Milk removers that use suction to remove milk while you're feeding on one side should be used with caution, especially in the early weeks of breastfeeding. To ensure your baby gets enough milk, feed them on both breasts before using a silicone milk collector. This enables them to get the easily available milk in your breasts and helps to reduce the risk of oversupply.

Breastmilk removers or collectors such as breast shells and other devices which sit into your bra while you are feeding don't use suction. They passively collect dripped milk. These are generally a safer option. However, the milk should not be sitting against your skin for longer than two hours as it's more likely to have a higher bacterial growth. Generally, silicone milk removers do not need to be sterilised. They just need to be kept clean. It's not unusual for mothers to find that they can collect small amounts of milk in the early weeks of breastfeeding but once their babies are six weeks-plus they may not get effective milk removal with silicone milk removers.

Types of Breast Pumps

Breast pumps have improved immensely over the last twenty years. Parents have a huge choice now about what type of pump they use. But, if you are exclusively or predominantly pumping, it's important to know that using a strong pump from the beginning is essential if you want to optimise your milk supply.

Hand pumps: These are mechanical devices that require you to create a vacuum and extracting milk by alternately squeezing and releasing your hand around the handle on the pump. Some mothers prefer using a hand pump and find that they can get higher volumes of milk than using an electric pump, while others find the hand action tiring.

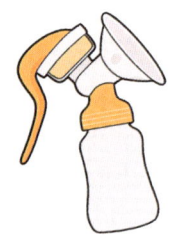

Wearable pumps: Wearable pumps are worn directly over the breast, inside your bra, and the milk is collected in the bottom of the pump. Sometimes they are connected to a smartphone app where you can increase and decrease the vacuum and turn the pump on and off. The big benefit of these pumps is that they enable you to be hands-free and to move around and do other things. For example, you could pump while preparing a meal or playing with your baby or older infant.

Most of these wearable pumps are quiet and the more expensive ones tend to be quite discreet. It is important to make sure that you have fitted the flange correctly to your nipple size. In my experience, mothers who have longer, softer breasts may struggle a little bit with positioning wearable pumps.

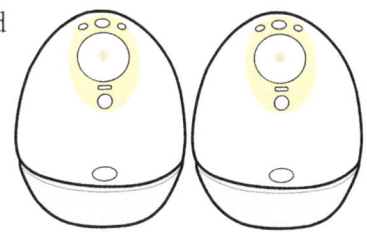

Semi Wearables: These pumps are a bit cheaper than wearable pumps. They collect milk directly at the breast in cups and they have a small motor which generally sits in the mother's pocket or on her waistband. They're discreet and quiet and usually more efficient than the wearables. These pumps can also be linked to a smartphone app which will record pumping times and volumes.

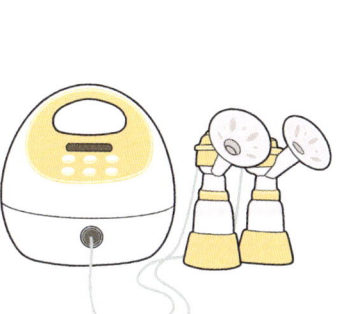

Electric pumps: These are standard single and double pumps. That must be plugged in to power outlet. Some have rechargeable batteries that can be used anywhere once they are charged. These pumps vary massively with the amount of vacuum they can exert and with their rate of cycles (speed). It is important that you know how to use your electric pump properly so that milk removal is optimised. Take the time to read the instruction manual and seek help if you need it.

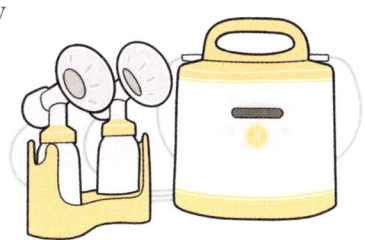

Multiuser (Hospital) Pumps: I like to say these are the Rolls Royce of Pumps. They have very robust, powerful motors. They are suitable for use between mothers once the tubing and membranes have been changed. These pumps are used in hospitals and can be rented once mothers go home, if needed.

They are very effective in removing milk. So, somebody who has a very strong milk supply would need to be very careful to ensure they don't trigger too much milk production. However, for a mother with low milk supply, these pumps give the best chance of stimulating as much breastmilk production as possible.

Flange Sizing – Does it Matter?

The flange (also sometimes called a *breast shield*) is the piece of hard plastic that sits over your breast when you pump. The vacuum draws your nipple into the neck of the flange. Traditionally, the standard size of flanges is around 24 millimetres. Most women have much smaller nipples than 24 millimetres. So, it's a good idea to know the diameter of your nipple so that you can choose an appropriately sized flange. I would advise if it is less than 22 millimetres in diameter that you purchase an accessory such as an insert or a new flange in the correct diameter. In my experience, using a smaller flange feels more comfortable, prevents pain when pumping and results in increased breastmilk output.

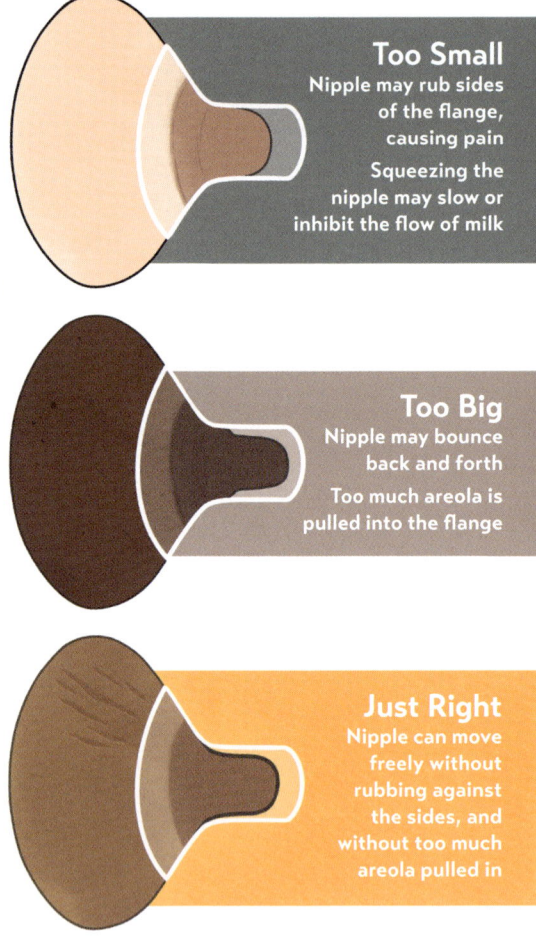

Too Small
Nipple may rub sides of the flange, causing pain
Squeezing the nipple may slow or inhibit the flow of milk

Too Big
Nipple may bounce back and forth
Too much areola is pulled into the flange

Just Right
Nipple can move freely without rubbing against the sides, and without too much areola pulled in

Flanges come in a range of different sizes, from as small as 12mm to as large as 32mm. You may need to try a couple of different flanges before you decide on the one that will work best for you. Ultimately, be guided by how pumping feels with a particular flange, rather than the size you think you should be using.

Choosing a Bottle and Paced Feeding

There are so many bottles and teats on the market, it can be very hard to see past all the marketing telling you that they are anti-colic and that they mimic breastfeeding. The truth is that no bottle behaves like the breast. A bottle cannot work like the breast. *It is the person giving the bottle to the baby who can adjust the flow.* And it is more common for a baby to have *flow confusion* rather than the classic *nipple confusion* that we hear about. Flow confusion or preference is where a baby struggles to switch between the slow, steady flow of milk when they breastfeed and a faster flow of milk when bottle-feeding. Lactation consultants prefer a bottle teat that has a curved edge and is not very long. This enables the baby to open their mouth wider when they latch on to the teat. The caregiver adjusts the flow of milk by tilting the bottle up or down depending on how fast the baby is swallowing. This is called *paced bottle feeding* and is a technique worth knowing It is used especially for younger babies who may be at risk of flow confusion. It really does work. Giving a bottle this way enables the baby to swallow slowly and coordinate their suck, swallow and breathe rhythm. They don't gulp down the milk and are less likely to take in lots of air. Generally, when the baby takes a rest from sucking, the caregiver drops the bottle down a little bit so that there is no milk leaking out of the teat while the baby is not sucking. When the baby starts to suck again, raise the bottle up to allow milk into the teat.

Amounts in volumes that babies take very massively. Over the first few weeks, I'm frequently asked how much milk should I give in a bottle? That depends on whether you were giving a baby some extra milk after breastfeeding or whether you were replacing a breastfeed. Most babies take anything from 60 to 90mls in the early weeks, increasing to 120mls after four to six weeks. The key thing is to watch your baby. Watch for cues that they are full and don't keep trying to finish the feed.

Using Your Pump

If everything is going well with breastfeeding, it's best to stick with exclusive breastfeeding for the first few weeks so that your baby learns how to suck and establishes your milk supply. From three to four weeks, many mothers start to feel more confident about breastfeeding and may consider pumping. Some prefer to wait until six weeks, and some parents don't ever use a pump or a bottle.

Most people find that they can pump higher volumes of milk in the mornings.

Most modern pumps now have two phases:

- *The first phase is the Initiate or Stimulation phase* when you turn the pump on. It stimulates the milk to start flowing (the letdown reflex) and mimics babies' sucking behaviour when they first latch (fast sucks and low suction).

- *The second type of pumping phase is the Expression phase.* It mimics how babies suck once milk has started to flow. Most pumps will automatically change to this phase after two minutes of the stimulation phase. The expression phase is slower and has a higher vacuum than the initiate phase.

You will be able to hear and feel the change in rhythm when your pump switches from the stimulation phase to the expression phase.

You can increase the vacuum of your pump. Once your milk is flowing and the pump is operating on the expression phase, you can turn the vacuum up as high as is comfortable for you. But don't turn it up too high as this could cause you pain and/or nipple damage.

When the milk flow slows down after the letdown, many mothers find that if they go back to the stimulation phase again on their pump they may be able to get a second let down.

How long should pumping sessions be? I would always advise not pumping for more than 15 or 20 minutes at a time. And pump every two to three hours rather than four-hourly.

Bottle Refusal and Reluctance

Newborn babies up to about six weeks will always accept a bottle in their mouth. Their sucking reflex is involuntary at this stage. When you put anything in their mouth, they will suck it. After six to eight weeks, this becomes a voluntary thing where they can decide whether they're going to accept it or not. And even sometimes if a baby has accepted a bottle in the early days, when the parents go back after six weeks, sometimes the baby won't take it. The baby is not being stubborn or fussy. It's that they are confused, they don't know what to do. It is a completely different set of oral muscles that are used to extract milk from a bottle than those that are used to breastfeed. So, gentle, patient and kind attempts to introduce the baby back to the bottle by the mother (because that's who they trust most) usually work best. And here are some other ideas which I have found to have helped over the years:

◊ Warming your breastmilk

◊ Distracting your baby by singing or praising them

◊ Swaying or rocking your baby while attempting the bottlefeed

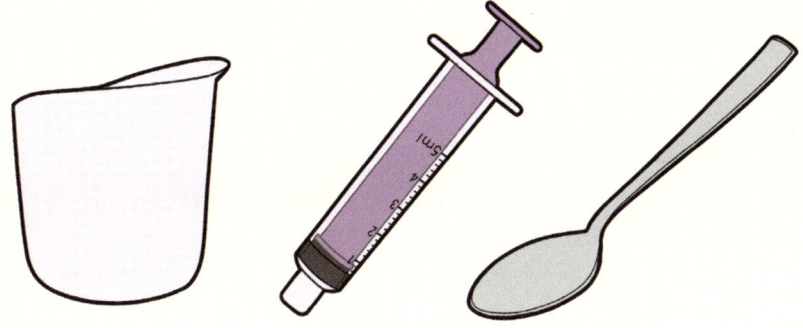

Sometimes, however, a baby won't take the bottle and that can be traumatic for everybody. To keep trying, in that case, I suggest using another way to give the baby fluids if the mother is apart from her baby. It does mean that the person who is minding the baby has a full-time job, but it may be possible to give the baby breast milk from a cup. Or a syringe. Or a dropper. Sometimes trying a feeding cup with a spout instead of a bottle can work. It's best to use one that is free-flowing (the baby doesn't have to suck to open a valve). You'll find one in the supermarket on the lowest shelf as they are not the fancy ones.

Storing Expressed Breastmilk

Breast milk is a live substance. The more recently the milk has been expressed, the more antibodies and antibacterial agents it has. As the days go by, the bacterial counts in breast milk drops because the antibodies in the breast milk are consuming them. However, after about five days the bacterial count starts to increase. Here is a chart which tells you how long breast milk can be stored:

Breastmilk storage Chart

	Freshly Expressed Milk	Thawed Milk
Room Temp	Up to 4 hours – 6 hours under 25 degrees	Up to 2 hours
Cooler Pack	Up to 24 hours	Up to 24 hours
Fridge	5 to 7 days (at the back on the fridge, not in the door)	Up to 24 hours
Freezer compartment inside a fridge	2 weeks	Do not refreeze
Fridge Freezer (with separate door)	3 to 6 months	Do not refreeze

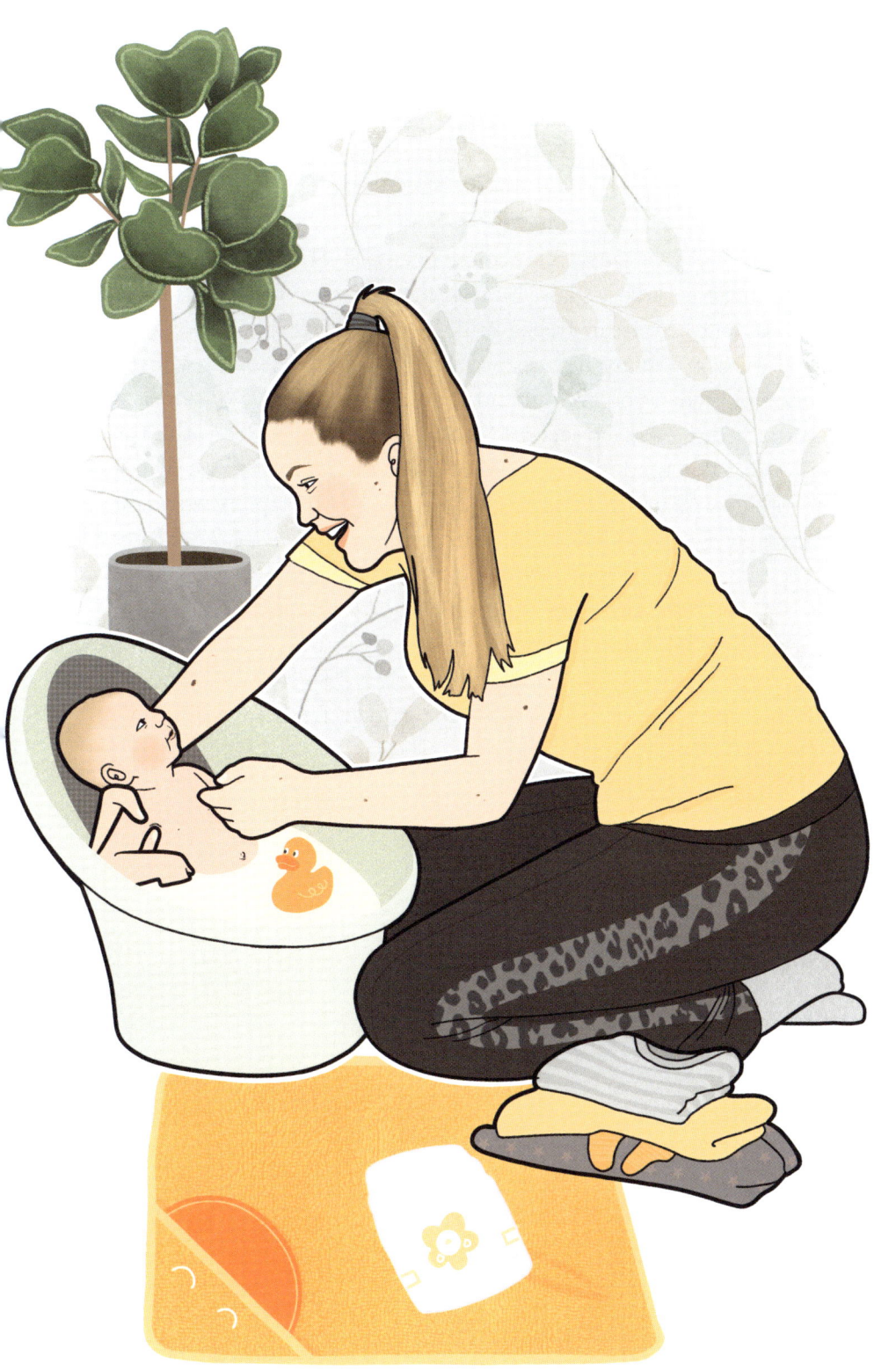

THE MOST COMMON QUESTIONS I'M ASKED ABOUT STORAGE OF BREAST MILK ARE

Can I mix milk that's freshly expressed with milk from the fridge into the same bottle and feed it to the baby? Yes, you can.

What's the best way to store my breast milk? The optimal storage container for milk is glass. Next is hard plastic. And then breastmilk storage bags. You can freeze milk in ice cube trays or in containers. And there are many devices available online for keeping your breast milk cold when you are out and about, or for storing your breast milk in the fridge or the freezer. Once milk is removed from the freezer, it needs to be used within 24 hours. You can defrost it fast by putting it into warm water or running under a warm tap. *Never microwave breastmilk as you will kill off all the goodness and risk making the milk too hot.*

What can I do with milk that has expired or can't be given to the baby? You can use it for sticky eyes. You can use it to bathe the baby, put it into their bathwater as a moisturiser. Never, ever throw it out! Even if you put it on the plants in the garden, it'll help them!

CHAPTER 11

Postpartum Mental Health and Breastfeeding

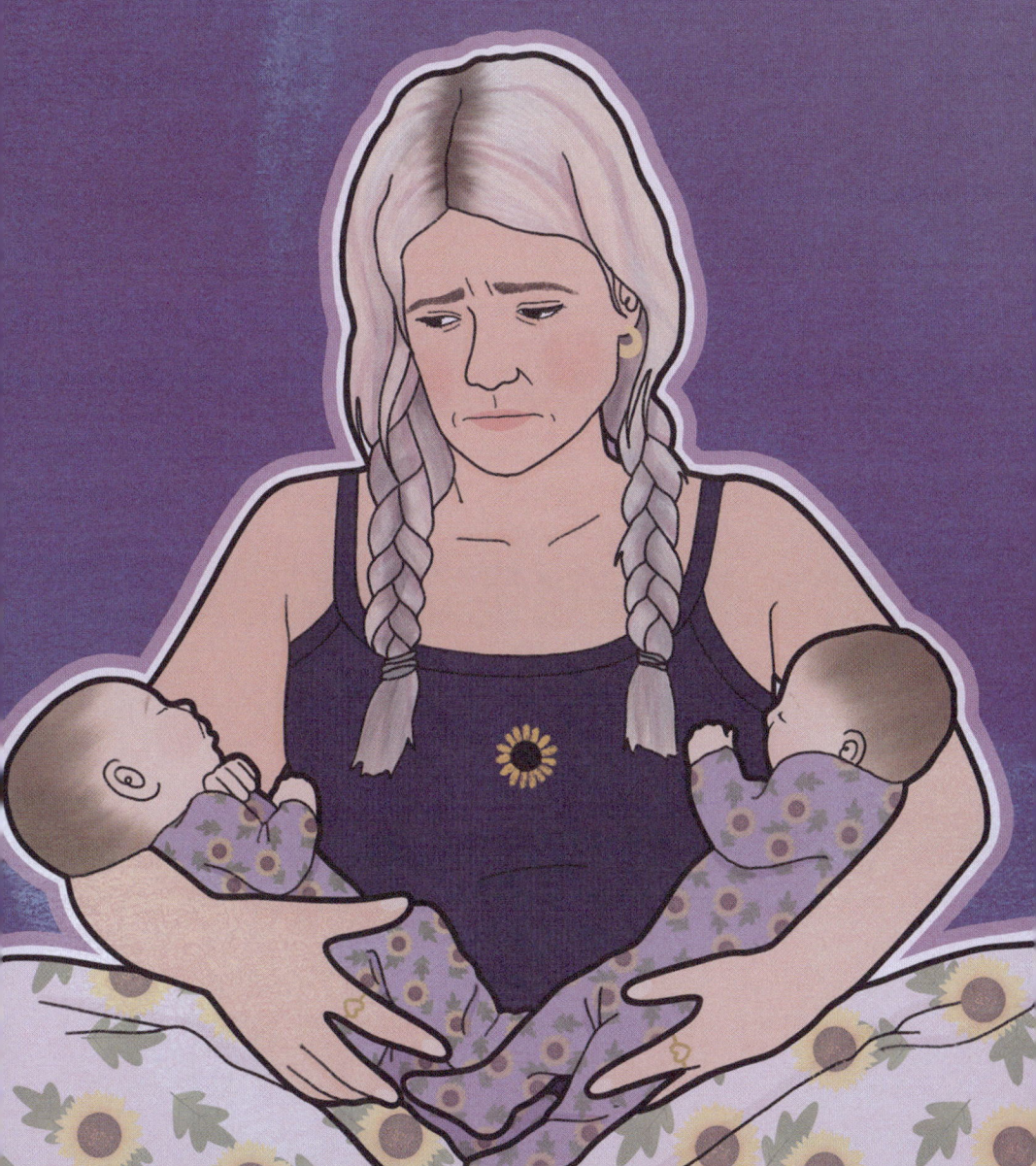

We tend to think of the postpartum period as a time of great joy and happiness for mothers as they bond with and get to know their new baby. While it is all of those things, it's also a time when new mothers can feel quite vulnerable, overwhelmed and unsure of themselves as they navigate what will probably be the biggest and most profound change they will ever experience – becoming a parent.

> *When Meghan Markle Duchess of Sussex was a few months postpartum she was asked by a journalist how she was. She replied that her experience of being a new mom was 'a very real thing to be going through' and that it had been a struggle for her. Meghan didn't provide any further explanation of the nature of her struggle, but reading between the lines, I think we can assume that she had postnatal mental health challenges. The interview shone a light on what a difficult time new motherhood can be and how important it is to support new mothers, see their struggles and ask them how they are.*

Emotions tend to be quite raw and heightened after you've had a baby, which means that you will probably be more sensitive and react more strongly to events and things people say. This is completely normal. Oxytocin, the feel-good hormone, is flowing in abundance and your heart is more open – this is a good thing. It facilitates love, connection, bonding and attachment. But this openness and vulnerability and the demands of being a new mother put you at an increased risk of a mental health condition such as depression and anxiety. The postpartum period is also a time when past traumas – even things that happened decades ago – can surface in a surprising and unwelcome way. It is important to be mindful of this and to know the difference between normal postpartum feelings and thoughts, and feelings and thoughts that may be symptoms of a mental health condition.

Often when breastfeeding mothers experience mental health challenges, the finger of blame is pointed at breastfeeding. The rationale is that breastfeeding must be too demanding for the mother and that switching to formula feeding would make life easier and improve mental health. But the reality is that for many mothers who have mental health challenges, breastfeeding can actually help them feel better about themselves. Of course, that is not always the case. Some mothers may choose to stop breastfeeding or to reduce the amount of breastfeeding. There is no one-size-fits-all when it comes to how you do motherhood, mental health and feeding your baby. The important thing is that you decide what you want, what is right for you, and find the right support to help you with that. Also, remember that having a mental health challenge is not your fault. Approximately one in five mothers will experience a mental health challenge in the postpartum period. Seeking help when you need it does not make you a bad parent and does not risk you losing custody of your baby.

I hope that this chapter will help you to better understand postpartum emotions and mental health, so that you can be accepting of your new sensitive self and know when to seek mental health supports.

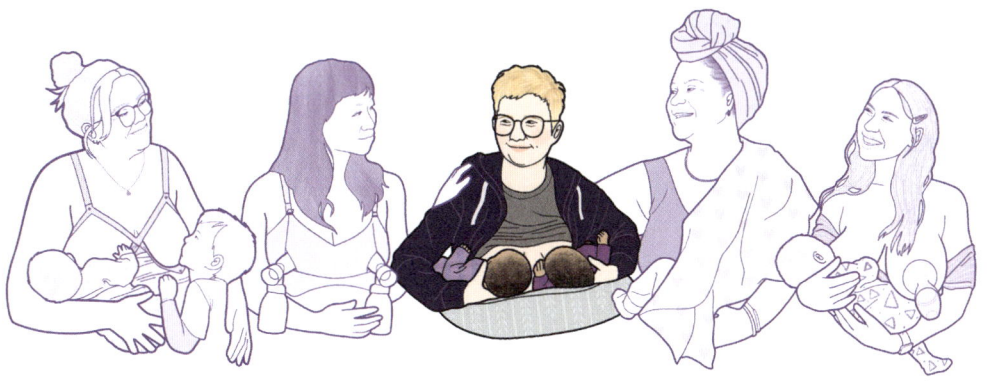

The Baby Blues

With all the hormonal changes you go through after you have had your baby and the lack of sleep, it is normal to experience mood changes. You will probably feel overwhelmed and have days when you feel sad and tearful. This is normal. Often these feelings come around three days postpartum, but they usually don't last beyond the first week. These sad feelings in the first week are called *the baby blues*. If your sad feelings last for longer than a week, it is possible that you are depressed. Talk to someone. The sooner you get help and support, the better.

> On day three, I had THE BIGGEST and longest sob I have ever had, and I can still feel it in my chest when I think about it now. I just couldn't stop crying all day – and it's only because I had a lovely student midwife friend (Zelle) who checked in on me that morning and warned me that it might happen, that I knew I was OK and didn't panic! I hadn't heard about this day three thing before, or how profoundly it would hit.
> The next day I felt back to myself!
>
> Lauren, Illustrator

Postnatal Depression (PND)

Approximately 13% of mothers are affected by postnatal depression (PND) in the first three weeks postpartum. While breastfeeding can help to protect against PND, breastfeeding difficulties put you at greater risk for it. This is just one of the reasons why support is so crucial in the early days, particularly if you are finding breastfeeding hard.

Other factors that put new mothers at an even greater risk of PND (and other mental health difficulties) include

- a history of depression or other mental health problems
- preterm delivery
- having a multiple birth
- birth trauma or caesarean section birth
- lack of family and social support, isolation
- stressful life events such as a recent bereavement
- a pregnancy that was unplanned
- depression during pregnancy
- being neurodivergent
- the death of a parent before the age of 11

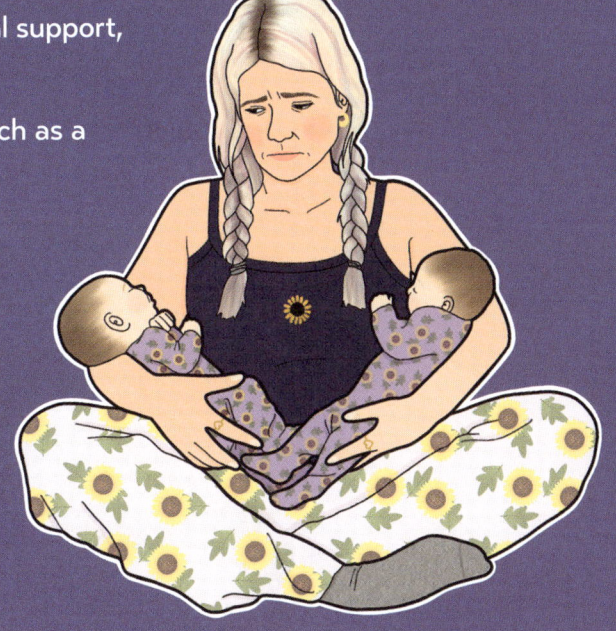

But PND can also occur in the absence of any of the above risk factors. It could be triggered by hormonal changes, or there may not be an obvious cause. The important thing is that you recognise it for what it is and reach out for help. So how do you know if you have PND, and that it's not just the baby blues?

Baby blues tend to be transient, meaning you could feel very down for a few hours or a day, and then bounce back the next day and feel more like yourself again. With PND, however, you are likely to feel very down most of the time. Other symptoms include

Breastfeeding for longer than one month is associated with a 37% lower risk of postnatal depression.

- Feeling a sense of hopelessness, or like you've lost yourself. Some mothers report having PND as feeling like they are in a black hole.

- Feeling reluctant to go out and see people or to do much of anything.

- Difficulty enjoying your baby or feeling like you're not bonding with them.

- Having a sense that you're not as good a mother as you should be.

- Difficulty making decisions or concentrating.

- Lack of energy and motivation, or a persistent sluggish feeling.

- Changes in eating and sleeping patterns.

- Persistent anxiety, not being able to relax.

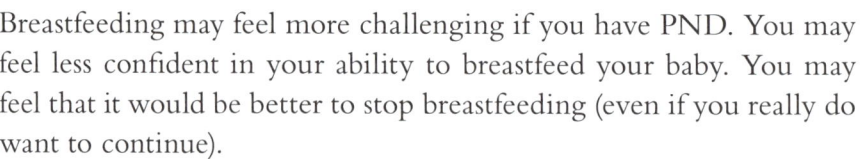

Breastfeeding may feel more challenging if you have PND. You may feel less confident in your ability to breastfeed your baby. You may feel that it would be better to stop breastfeeding (even if you really do want to continue).

So, what to do if you think you are ticking a lot of the above boxes? Contact your GP or other primary healthcare provider so that you can get the help and support you need. They may suggest psychological and/or social supports, or cognitive behavioural therapy (CBT). You may also be prescribed an anti-depressant. Most anti-depressants, particularly the Selective Serotonin Reuptake Inhibitors (SSRIs) that are commonly prescribed for PND, are safe to take when breastfeeding.

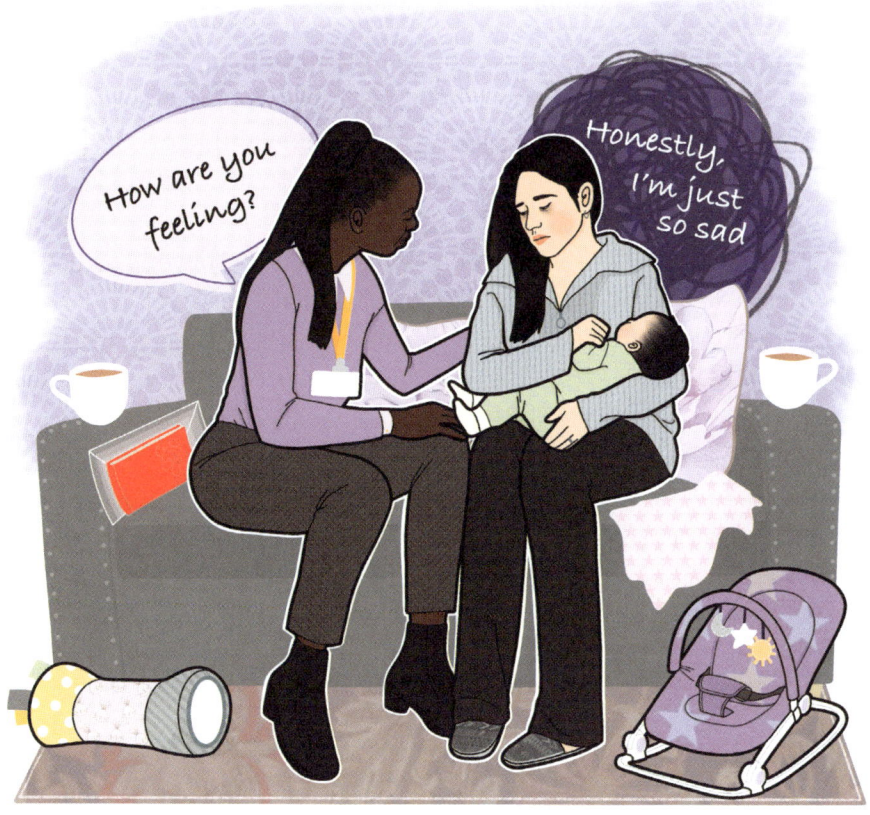

Postnatal Anxiety

Mothers are more likely to experience postnatal anxiety than postnatal depression, yet anxiety tends to be under-recognised by healthcare professionals and as a result is under-treated. Factors that can contribute to postnatal anxiety include a lack of family support, having had a difficult birth experience, a history of mental health issues and breastfeeding difficulties. Some degree of anxiety as you transition to motherhood and get to grips with caring for your new baby is normal. It is the most important job you will ever do, and the stakes are high! It is normal to wonder if you're doing it right, to worry about your baby's weight gain and to check their breathing when they are sleeping. An easing of this anxiety is usually a matter of time and a process of learning to trust in your abilities as a mother. In addition to worrying about your capacity to parent, you may also feel anxious about losing your sense of self-identity and worry that you'll never get back to feeling *normal* again. You may fear that you'll struggle to be the competent person in the workplace you were before you had your baby or that you will never be able to enjoy having sex again, or that your body will never be your own again. These feelings are normal and usually subside as your confidence gradually increases.

Sometimes though, levels of anxiety can go beyond what is considered *normal* and have a detrimental effect on your wellbeing and on your experience of being a mother. If you are constantly worrying, feeling on edge, feeling a sense of dread, unable to relax, and/or experiencing physical symptoms such as tightness in your chest or a fast heartbeat, it is important to seek support because these symptoms suggest that you have postnatal anxiety (as opposed to the normal levels of anxiety that new parents experience).

If you are concerned about postnatal anxiety, contact your GP, health visitor or public health nurse. They will help you to find the support you need – whether it is mindfulness, talk therapy, gentle exercise, cognitive behavioural therapy and/or medication. Also talk to a partner or a close friend or family member about what you are experiencing. Sometimes just opening-up and feeling heard can be a significant first step towards managing your symptoms.

What about breastfeeding? Are there aspects of breastfeeding or feeding your baby that are causing you anxiety or that you are finding difficult? Talking things through with an IBCLC or a breastfeeding volunteer could help you figure out ways to make things easier. The goal of a breastfeeding professional or volunteer is never to convince you to exclusively breastfeed. It is to meet you where you are at and help you find a way to feed your baby that works for you and that supports your mental health.

Postnatal Obsessive-Compulsive Disorder (OCD)

Obsessive Compulsive Disorder is a type of anxiety that involves recurrent unwelcome thoughts or ideas which result in distress and urges to respond with excessive behavioural compulsions, for example, repeated washing or sterilising bottles. New mothers are five times more likely to develop OCD than other women. There are a number of reasons for this – the immense changes you're experiencing, the demands of caring for your baby, the realisation that you can't control everything, adjusting to a routine that is baby-led, the stress of keeping your baby safe and hormonal changes. Another factor could be a gulf between your expectations of how motherhood was going to be for you and the messy, chaotic reality. Symptoms of OCD include

- A fear of your baby coming to harm
- Concerns about germs and infection
- An intense focus on the volume of milk you are producing and/or pumping (particularly if you have low milk supply)
- Intrusive or scary thoughts – for example, of harming your baby or of doing something wrong, overfeeding them or not feeding them enough
- Constantly checking on the baby
- Anxiety about inappropriate sexual arousal when breastfeeding
- Obsessively following routines related to feeding, winding baby and getting them to sleep

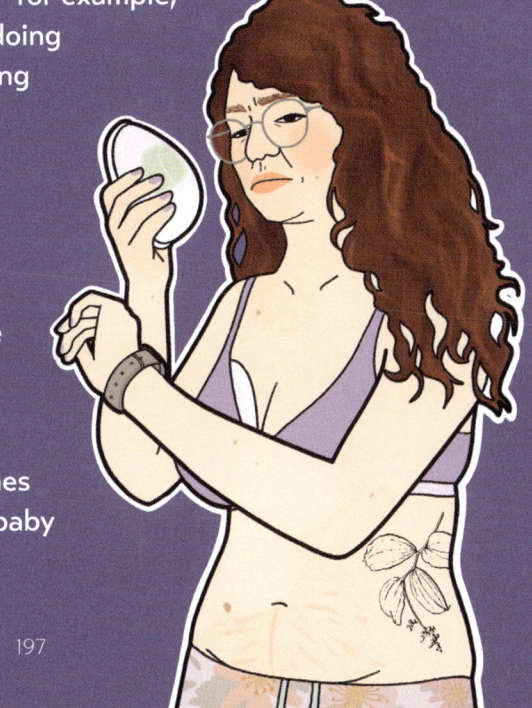

These symptoms can get in the way of you being able to relax and enjoy early motherhood. They do not mean you are a bad mother. Talking to a mental health professional and getting treatment will help. If you feel overwhelmed or feel that you tick some of the boxes for postnatal OCD contact your GP or the appropriate postnatal mental health services. They will be able to discuss treatment options. Your GP may also talk to you about taking medication that is compatible with breastfeeding. The fact that you are breastfeeding should not get in the way of taking appropriate medication. There is almost always a safe option.

Attending a face-to-face breastfeeding or new mothers' support groups can also help alleviate the symptoms of postnatal OCD. Being in a shared space with other mothers gives you an opportunity to see normal newborn behaviour, learn about breastfeeding and engage socially with others.

Postpartum Psychosis

Postpartum psychosis is a rare but very serious mental illness that can develop in the postpartum period. It can manifest within days of giving birth or after a few months. Women who have been diagnosed with bipolar disorder or who had postpartum psychosis before are at a greater risk of it occurring. The symptoms of postpartum psychosis can begin suddenly and include

- Extreme mood swings – from feeling elated to feeling tearful
- Racing thoughts, restlessness
- Feelings of paranoia
- Having irrational or delusional thoughts
- Difficulty sleeping, staying awake for days
- Hallucinations – seeing or hearing things that are not there
- Being more chatty and excitable than usual

- ☁ Not making sense when speaking and rapid speech
- ☁ Behaving in ways that are out of character
- ☁ Feeling detached from people around you, and perhaps disconnected from yourself
- ☁ Thinking of harming yourself or your baby

If you experience any of these symptoms, contact your GP or mental health services as soon as possible.

Treatment for postpartum psychosis requires hospitalisation, mood stabilising medication and psychological supports. It can be a difficult and distressing time. Whether or not a mother can be supported to continue breastfeeding or providing milk for her baby depends on many different factors, such as the medications she has been prescribed and whether she can be admitted to an inpatient unit with her baby. If a mother must be apart from her baby for a time, it is important that she be supported to pump and that she have access to a hospital-grade pump. Sudden weaning (the term used to describe stopping breastfeeding or lactation very quickly) can put a mother at risk of mastitis and/or abscess.

There are several Mother and Baby Units throughout the UK but unfortunately none in Ireland.

Birth Trauma

Birth trauma is a birthing experience that is characterised by unwelcome or unpleasant experiences that have negative psychological and/or physical consequences for the mother, and which in some cases can result in serious injury to the mother or her baby. Many factors can contribute to birth trauma: complications, obstetric violence, invasive procedures/exams, unwanted physical touch, emergency c-section, admission of a baby to the NICU and mother-baby separation, having a general anaesthetic, and the resurfacing of past traumatic life events. Trauma can also result from a mismatch between a woman's expectation of how a birth will be and the reality of her experience or a perception

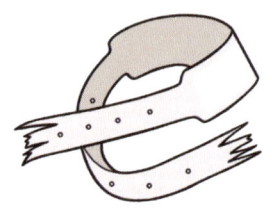 of a lack of caring by labour and delivery staff. Birth trauma is complicated. And it's subjective. So, people who have similar experiences can internalise them in different ways. Whatever feelings you have around your birth experience are valid and should be respected.

No matter how you birth your baby, the experience stays with you and becomes part of your story with your baby. My 92-year-old mother-in-law, May, can recall the details of the births of each of her four children. She can recount in vivid detail not only the events of each of the births but how she was treated, things healthcare professionals said to her and how these experiences made her feel. It's as if the memories of the birth experiences are retained in a different, more embodied way than those of other life experiences. Good, bad or indifferent, your birth experiences stay with you.

If you have experienced birth trauma, you may find yourself having flashbacks to the birth and reliving the fear, the sense of helplessness or the feeling of being violated. You may also experience enduring physical pain or feel detached from your baby or family members. Birth trauma and its effects can lessen as the months and years pass, but it doesn't go away easily. It is important that you get help to process the experience, whenever you feel ready to do so. That may be weeks, months or years after you have given birth. Some options you could consider are psychotherapy, speaking with a birth trauma resolution therapist, cognitive behavioural therapy and/or speaking with hospital staff to gain a better understanding of what happened and why.

Having a traumatic birth can affect breastfeeding in different ways:

- The stress and trauma can result in a delay in your milk coming in
- Mother-baby separation can also delay milk coming in and potentially interfere with breastfeeding – the baby's first feed may not be at the breast

- ☁ Birth trauma can lessen a mother's sense of breastfeeding self-efficacy (the feeling of 'I can do this')

- ☁ A physical injury, for example, a perineal tear, could make finding a comfortable position to breastfeed in more challenging

- ☁ Birth trauma can affect how a mother feels about her body and her breasts – some mothers may not want to breastfeed after a traumatic birth while others will be more determined to breastfeed

Sometimes, when a mother has experienced a traumatic birth, breastfeeding and providing milk for her baby become more of an imperative for her, even if she hadn't intended to breastfeed. She may have a sense of wanting to do something *right* after perceiving that she has *failed* to have the birth experience she had hoped for. The mother may have a sense of wanting to prove herself and feel very determined to make breastfeeding work. She could also have an instinctive sense that breastfeeding will be healing for her and her baby, or a way of making peace with her body.

On the other hand, birth trauma can result in some women choosing not to breastfeed. A mother may feel too physically traumatised to breastfeed her baby or that she is 'not in the right headspace' to do it (this is an expression I have heard from women I have worked with). If you experience birth trauma and you choose not to breastfeed, you should do so without feeling any guilt or shame and you should be supported in that decision.

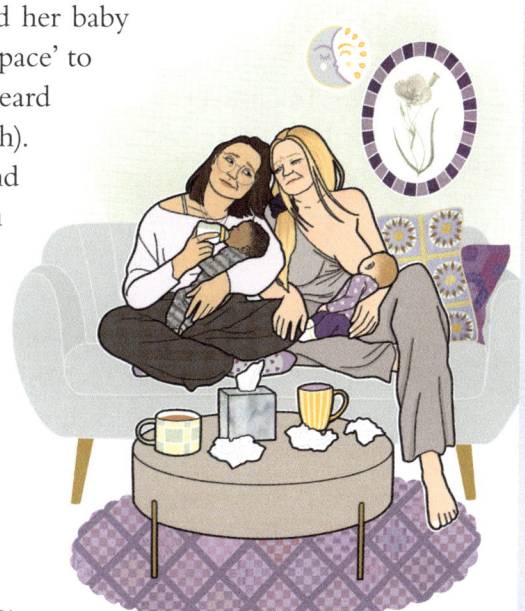

All women should be given respectful, sensitive and caring support irrespective of how they choose to feed their babies.

If you are breastfeeding following birth trauma, it is important to have skilled and individualised support as early as possible. Do tell a midwife or lactation consultant that you are feeling fragile and that you had a difficult birth, and that you really want to breastfeed. Also let those helping you know if you are feeling physical pain or if you don't want to be touched. Communicating your needs and your feelings makes it easier for staff to provide you with sensitive support. Try to be gentle with yourself. See how you feel about breastfeeding and remember it can take time to build your confidence and recover from the trauma you experienced.

Note: After a traumatic birth, breastfeeding can be triggering for some mothers and cause flashbacks to the birth. If this is the case for you, seek help. Talk to someone (a therapist or IBCLC) who can help you to figure out how best to feed your baby, whether it's direct breastfeeding, exclusive pumping or stopping breastfeeding altogether.

Dysphoric Milk Ejection Reflex (D-MER)

Dysphoric Milk Ejection Reflex is a condition that some breastfeeding mothers have whereby they experience a sudden, intense rush of negative feelings at the beginning of a breastfeed or a pumping session, just before their milk starts to flow. The types of feelings that women who have D-MER describe include sadness, anger, dread, irritability, detachment, anxiety, hopelessness, and despair. They may use expressions like 'being hit by a wave of doom' or 'going into a very dark place' to describe the experience. The bad feelings can last for a few seconds or for a few minutes. But usually by three to four months postpartum, women with D-MER find that they no longer experience symptoms.

It can be shocking to experience D-MER, especially when you have had an expectation that you're going to feel a rush of oxytocin when your milk lets down. It can feel like you are the only person who is having this experience. But you're not. D-MER is real, it's not in your head and it may be caused by a sudden drop in the hormone dopamine.

If you think you have D-MER, talk it through with someone – a volunteer or peer breastfeeding supporter, or a lactation consultant. Or perhaps ask in an online or face-to-face support group about the condition. You may find there is someone else who has had a similar experience to you.

When the wave of bad feelings hits you, these are some things that may help:

- Distract yourself – watch TV, scroll on Instagram, listen to music, or play a game on your phone

- Focus on your breath – in-breath, pause, out-breath, pause......

- Focus on your baby

- A few drops of rescue remedy or a homeopathic treatment (while not evidence-based, some mothers report that it helps!)

- Have a drink of water

- Repeat a little mantra to yourself, something like 'This a D-MER. These thoughts and feelings will pass.'

- For more information about D-MER go to www.D-MER.org.

Breastfeeding Aversion Response (BAR)

BAR is like D-MER, but differs in that mothers who have it experience very strong negative feelings – aversion, revulsion and wanting to unlatch their baby – for the *duration* of feeds, rather than just when the milk lets down. BAR can be experienced by mothers for the duration of a breastfeeding relationship, but for some it can start when their infants are older. BAR can be difficult for mothers and emotionally upsetting, especially when a mother has a strong desire to continue breastfeeding. Some mothers who have BAR may decide to stop breastfeeding, but many others find a way to continue. Some techniques and strategies that can help if you are breastfeeding and you have BAR are

1.

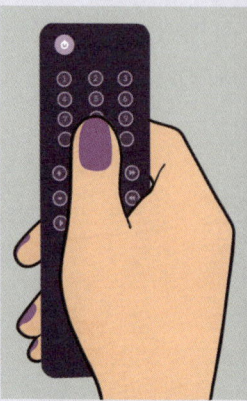

Distraction while breastfeeding, for example watching television or scrolling on Instagram

2.

Using some kind of **guided meditation** like *Yoga Nidra* while breastfeeding (yoga nidra apps can be downloaded on the Google Play Store or iTunes)

3.

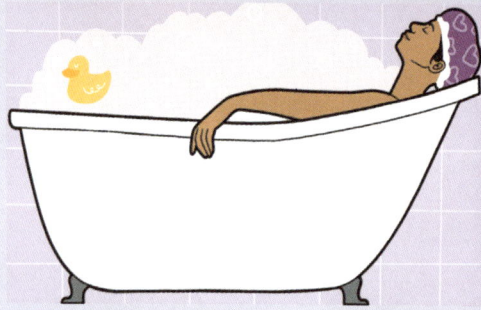

Selfcare – acknowledge that you are having a challenging time breastfeeding, and find some way to care for and nurture yourself. What helps you to feel good and to relax? Going for a walk on your own? Having a relaxing bath?

4.

Breathing Exercises – there are lots of yoga-based breathing exercises that can help you to get through breastfeeds when you have BAR. Focusing on your breath can help take you away from the internal dialogue in your mind around the BAR and from the physical sensations of BAR. You could just follow your inbreath and outbreath or try square breathing – follow your inbreath, pause, outbreath, pause – and visualise these four stages of each breath as a square.

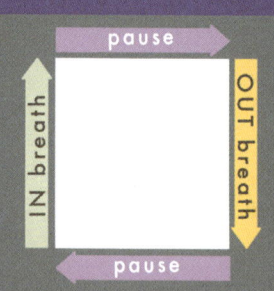

5.

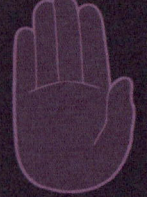

Establish some **Boundaries** – For example, to limit the time your baby spends at the breast or limit the number of feeds you do per 24 hours*. Or you may decide to limit the duration of your breastfeeding journey.

6.

Seek out Support – you may find support online or in face-to-face breastfeeding support groups. There are some BAR support groups on Facebook. The one run by Zainab Yate (author of 'When Breastfeeding Sucks') is called *Aversion Sucks – Peer to Peer Breastfeeding Support*.

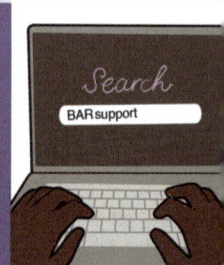

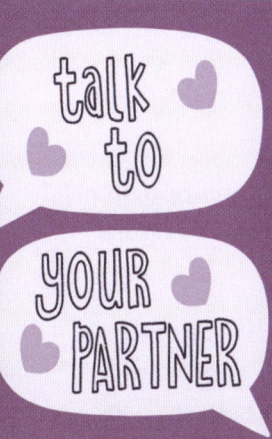

7.

Talk to your Partner and help them to understand what you are feeling. When they understand more about what having BAR is like, they are better able to support you.

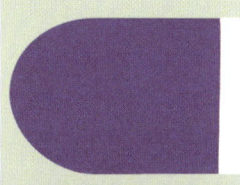

8.

Magnesium Supplement – Some mothers find that taking a magnesium supplement can help to lessen the intensity of BAR sensations.

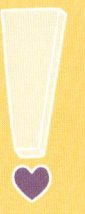 **9.** Remind yourself that having BAR is not your fault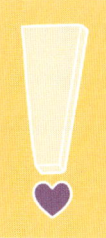

*If you decide to limit feeds or time your baby spends at the breast, you may need to consider supplementation with expressed breastmilk or infant formula, especially if your baby is quite young. Chatting to a breastfeeding supporter or IBCLC could help you determine if your baby is going to need supplementation.

IN SUMMARY

Exclusive breastfeeding protects maternal mental health, but mothers experiencing breastfeeding difficulties are more likely to suffer from postnatal depression or anxiety. This is why **breastfeeding support is so crucial in the early days postpartum.**

The quality of the support you receive matters. It is vital that you are working with professionals who understand and respect your feeding goals and have an appreciation for the nuanced nature of breastfeeding.

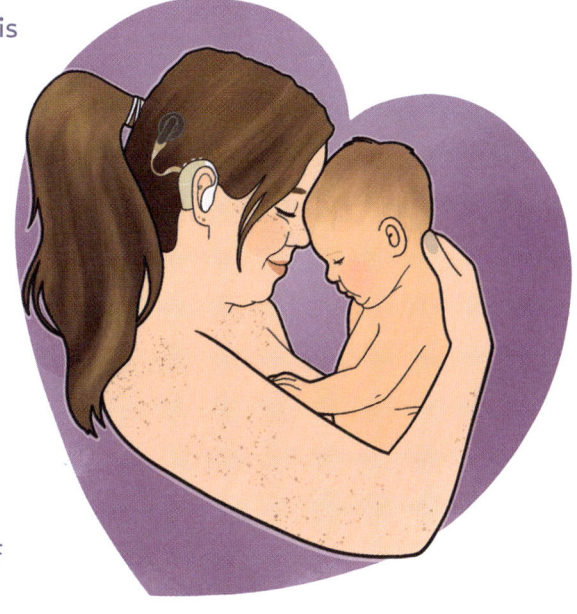

Good mental health and a positive breastfeeding experience are not mutually exclusive.

There is no one-size-fits-all solution when it comes to supporting a mother's mental health. Give yourself space and time to figure out what is going to work for you and your baby.

Sometimes mental health difficulties can affect mother-infant bonding, but remember that *bonding is an ongoing, continually unfolding process.* If it is derailed at any stage, you can get back on track later.

Mental health difficulties are not your fault. They do not mean you are a bad mother.

No matter what you are going through, you are not alone. There are professionals who can help and there are other mothers having similar experiences.

CHAPTER 12

Breastfeeding and Sleep

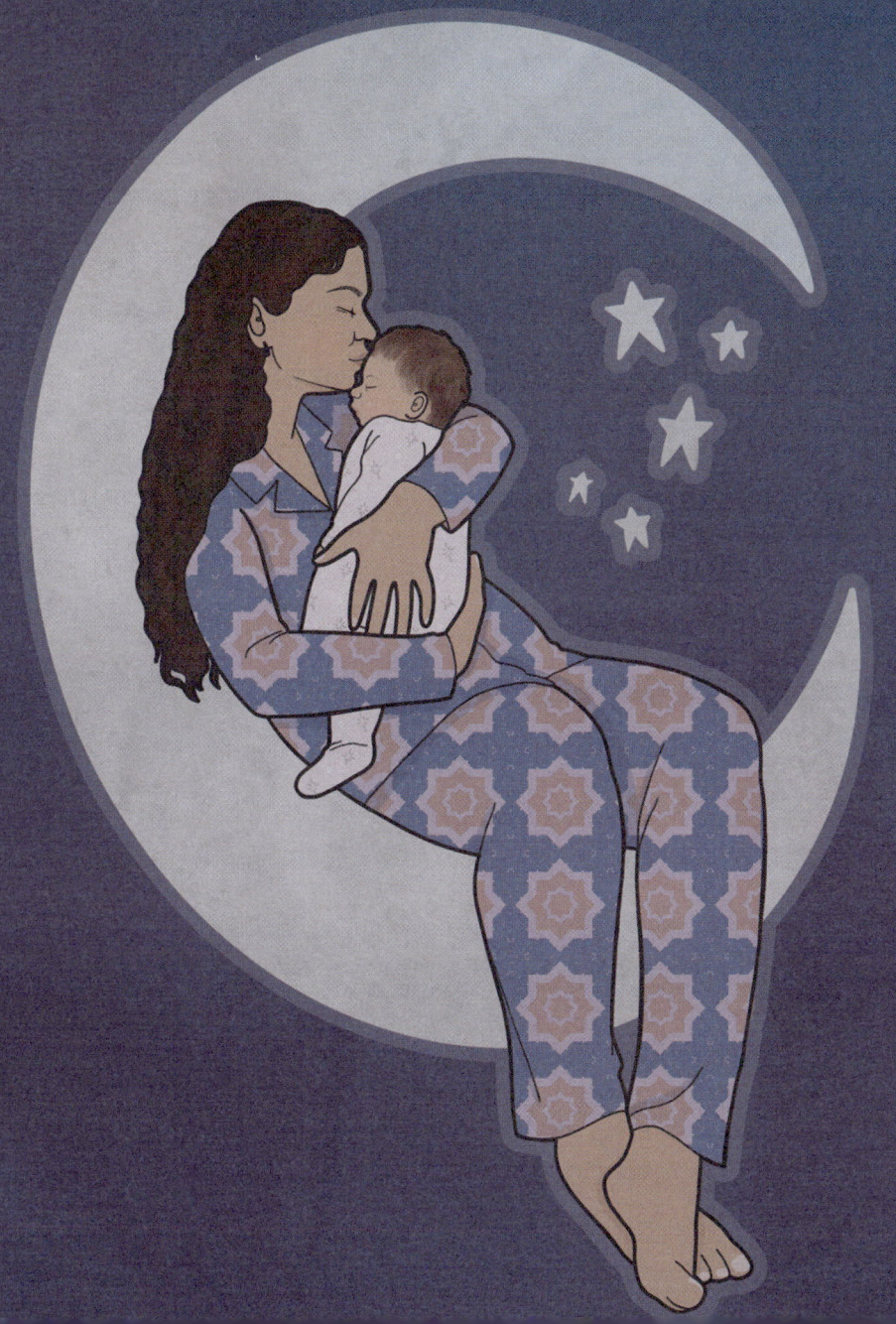

I hardly even know where to start with this chapter. So much has been written on the topic of infant sleep already. Look at the shelves in the parenting section of your local bookshop and you're likely to find at least a few books on the topic. They will all be promising a *solution* or some kind of *fix* to the *problem* of your baby waking during the night. Sleep deprivation is an age-old challenge that parents of small babies have always had to contend with. In this chapter I don't offer solutions, but I explain what normal is, why babies wake, and common myths around infant sleep. I also offer some ideas for optimising your own sleep and surviving the early months. So many of the challenges parents face when it comes to how their babies sleep, have to do with trying to reconcile their expectations of how their babies *should* sleep with the reality of their baby waking several times a night.

Your Expectations

What expectations do you have for your baby's sleep? What have you heard? What have you read? And what have you subconsciously picked up about how babies should sleep? Perhaps you've heard that babies start sleeping through the night from 12 weeks. Or that babies should be sleep-trained early on to get them into a good routine. Or that babies need to sleep during *sleep windows* and be awake during *wake windows*. Maybe you've heard about the *cry-it-out* method of sleep training. Or you may have heard that it's important to do *parent-led* parenting from the beginning, or that co-sleeping is dangerous? Maybe you have a sense that if you do everything right, your baby will be on board with whatever sleep schedule you implement? Do you think that babies should be able to *self-soothe* themselves to sleep? You probably have more perceptions about how babies sleep than you realise! Unfortunately, some of these ideas can get in the way of you being able to accept the reality of how *your* baby sleeps. So, let's look at normal infant sleep.

Normal Infant Sleep

Small babies need to wake frequently during the night. This is not some kind of cruel design flaw to punish you, but a clever evolutionary adaptation that keeps babies alive and facilitates optimal growth and development. Babies have small tummies and a very fast gut transit time (compared to that of adults), so filling them up for the night just isn't going to work (if only!). Babies need to breastfeed frequently at night. This is normal. In the early days babies can wake three to four times to feed. And for other reasons too. Remember the fourth trimester? Babies are in the process of adapting to being in the world and to not being in your body, and having their circadian rhythms controlled by you. When they are born, they don't produce melatonin – one of the main hormones involved in controlling circadian rhythms. So, they are simply not capable of knowing when they are tired and getting themselves off to sleep. And they don't know the difference between day and night. Babies start to secrete melatonin from around one month of age and by four to six months of age they are producing as much as they need and start to develop their own circadian rhythms. This does not mean that they will magically start sleeping through the night at this stage, but that they will *begin* the process of adapting to their own circadian rhythms – by having some longer stretches at night, and becoming tired in the evening time.

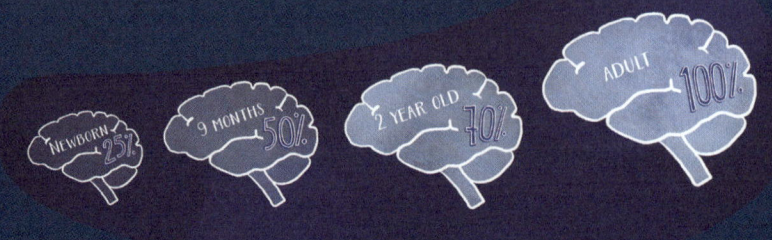

Your Baby's Brain Development: At birth, a baby's brain is 25% of its adult brain size. At nine months it is 50% of its adult brain size and by two years it is 70% of its adult brain size. To support this rapid brain growth, babies need lots of frequent feeding (especially at night), cuddles, caring touch, communication and responsive care.

Another reason why babies wake frequently at night is brain development. Most of your baby's brain growth and development happens during the night, especially during light sleep phases – which babies have more of than adults. Babies encode memories during this light sleep, cells grow, neural pathways develop, and connections are made. Babies can wake easily from these light sleep phases, but they are important for brain growth and development.

Spending a large part of the night in light sleep phases and waking frequently helps to protect babies against SIDS (Sudden Infant Death Syndrome). Even partially breastfeeding helps to reduce your baby's risk of SIDS.

Please note: Even if your baby is formula-fed, the risk of SIDS is still very low, especially if you follow safe sleeping guidelines such as putting your baby on their back to sleep, placing them on a firm sleep surface such as a mattress, and ensuring there are no soft toys or cot bumpers in their cot.

Babies can also wake during the night just for reassurance and cuddles. It's their way of communicating with you and of building their confidence. Think about it – night times are dark, and maybe even scary to a baby. On a primal level they may feel a greater need for physical contact and a feeling of safety during the night.

> *A human infant is biologically designed to sleep next to its mother's body and to breastfeed intermittently throughout the night, at least for the first year of its life.*
>
> McKenna and Gettler, 2017

Co-Sleeping with Your Baby

Co-sleeping describes the practice of sleeping on a flat surface with your baby. In most cultures around the world co-sleeping is the accepted norm. But our Western perspectives on where babies should sleep at night-time are a little bit different. The received wisdom is that babies should sleep in a cot and be apart from their parents, and that this fosters independence and an ability to self-soothe. But where do these ideas come from? They can be traced back to Victorian notions about child-rearing practices which enshrined discipline and order, and which were guided by the belief that children should be reared along scientific lines. Parents were advised not to spoil babies and that crying was natural and a way for a baby to exercise their lungs. Sticking to a rigid routine, as little handling as possible, and avoiding spoiling a baby were recommended. And in regard to sleeping arrangements, co-sleeping was deemed unhygienic and was generally associated with poverty. In contrast, having a baby sleep in a cot, preferably in their own bedroom, became the middle class ideal. These ideas grew in popularity for most of the 20th Century and were reinforced by maternity hospital practices in the 1950s which were based around formula feeding babies on four-hourly schedules.

Attitudes to co-sleeping have been changing over the last few decades and there has been a growing acceptance that co-sleeping is a normal practice and that it can be done safely (see the next section for safe co-sleeping guidelines). Whether or not you co-sleep is a personal decision. As with parenting, there is no one right way to do family sleep arrangements. Only you can know what feels right for you and your baby and what is going to work best for your family. But for mothers who are breastfeeding there are some benefits to co-sleeping that you may like to consider:

- You don't have to get out of bed to feed your baby at night-time! This can mean more sleep for everyone.

- You are less likely to wake fully when breastfeeding, and it may be easier for you to get back to sleep.

- It can be enjoyable – that feeling of having your baby close at nighttime.

- Many babies settle more easily when they are in close physical proximity to their mother.

- There is some evidence that co-sleeping helps protect babies against SIDS because they spend more time in light sleep phases.

- Frequent breastfeeding ensures your baby gets the milk they need to grow and optimises your milk supply.

- There is a kind of physiological co-regulation between a mother and her baby when they co-sleep – the mother's breathing, heart rate and temperature will influence those of her baby, and vice versa.

- Fathers can benefit from co-sleeping. One study found that when fathers sleep close to their babies, their testosterone levels drop. Lower testosterone levels enable fathers to engage in more sensitive and responsive parenting.

- A couple of studies have found that adults who co-slept with their parents as infants have higher self-esteem than adults who did not co-sleep as infants.

In my work seeing breastfeeding families over the years, one of the things I have come to learn is that sleeping arrangements are not a one-size-fits-all. Some parents will fully co-sleep, some will have their baby in a cot or bassinet, and some will sleep in separate bedrooms for a time (mother and baby in one room and the partner in the other). It's up to you to determine what is best for your family.

Safe Co-Sleeping Guidelines

Whatever sleep arrangements you intend to have in place, the reality is that most breastfeeding families will do some amount of co-sleeping. So, it's important that you are aware of the safe co-sleeping guidelines.

The following criteria should be met in order to co-sleep safely with your baby:

You/Your Partner	Your Baby
Are exclusively breastfeeding and feeding responsively	Is healthy and full-term
	Is on their back
Are sober	Is lightly dressed so they don't overheat
Don't smoke	
Sleep on a flat surface (your bed) with your baby and not on a sofa or armchair.	Is not swaddled
	There are no pillows or covers around their face

- Don't leave your baby on their own in your bed.
- Bear in mind that giving your baby infant compromises the safety of co-sleeping. If your baby is having significant volumes of infant formula, it may be safer for them to sleep in a crib or a cot.
- If you are taking medication that affects your sleep (makes you drowsy or makes you sleep more deeply), it may be safer to have your baby sleep in a crib or cot.

Sleeping with your baby on a sofa is not safe.

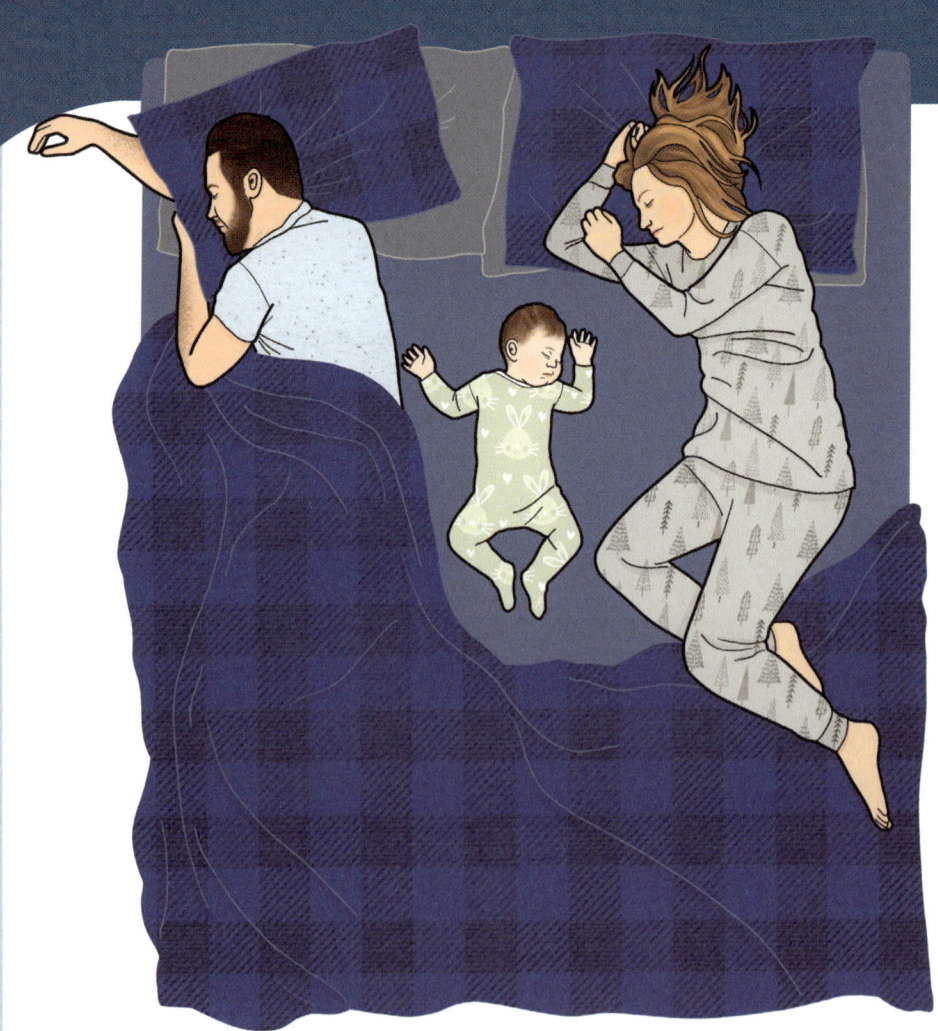

Breastsleeping

Breastsleeping is a relatively new term that was coined by American anthropologists to describe the practice of bedsharing and breastfeeding. It suggests that these activities are so intertwined that you can't really talk about one without talking about the other. Breastsleeping recognises that close physical proximity between a mother and her baby, especially during the night, is an important aspect of establishing breastfeeding. It also acknowledges the uniqueness of the connection between the mother and her baby, regarding them as one physiologic entity – *a dyad*.

Another way to think about the concept of breastsleeping, is that there is often overlap during the night between breastfeeding and sleeping. They don't always occur as stand-alone behaviours – babies can breastfeed when they are half asleep, as can mothers. You don't have to be fully awake to breastfeed. This can be a helpful way of understanding night-time feeding and sleeping with your baby.

Night-time Parenting

Awareness of night-time parenting as a concept can help in coming to terms with the intensity and exhaustion of night-time breastfeeding. Basically, babies and infants have needs during the night, not just during the day. Before I had my first baby I never gave any thought to the notion that your responsibilities as a parent don't end at 8pm at night when your baby goes to sleep (if indeed they go to sleep at 8pm). But the reality is that babies, especially those that can't yet tell day from night, need you as much during the night as they do during the day. They need to feed, they need reassurance when they wake, they need connection and security, and they need you to keep them warm. As your baby gets older their needs are not quite as intense during the night, but there will be times when they need hugs and soothing after waking from a bad dream or if they are sick. There are no rigid rules about how you should do night-time parenting. It will vary from family to family. But try to give yourself the space to explore the idea.

Sometimes it's a matter of reorienting your expectations. Having parenting responsibilities through the night is normal. When you respond to your baby during the night, you are doing what mothers have done for millennia. You are not doing anything wrong and you are not *failing* to get your baby into a routine.

Sleep Training

There has been a proliferation of *paediatric sleep consultants* over the last decade offering a range of different solutions to your baby's sleep *problems*. This speaks to the difficulty parents have coping with how their babies sleep and a societal lack of knowledge about infant sleep and normal newborn behaviour. Sometimes it's really hard and can feel like you're in the trenches when you're surviving on very little sleep. But many sleep consultants are perpetuating the idea that normal infant sleep is an illness that needs to be cured. Having said that, some people do benefit from the support of someone trained to assist families with their infant's sleep. If you do decide to use the services of a sleep consultant, these are a few things I suggest you consider:

PLEASE NOTE:
Sleep training your baby has the potential to undermine breastfeeding as it may lead to fewer breastfeeds during the night. This can affect your baby's weight gain and cause a drop in your milk supply.

- **Is there actually a problem that needs to be fixed?** Often parents perceive that their baby has a problem with sleep when in fact they are behaving as they should do. Talking things through with a voluntary breastfeeding counsellor first could help to determine whether or not there is a problem. What you perceive as a problem may be a developmentally normal sleep pattern for your baby.

- What **qualifications** does the sleep consultant you are planning to work with have? There is no standardised qualification for sleep consultants – courses are online and last between six weeks and six months.

- Is the sleep consultant answerable to an accredited **governing body**?

- Does the sleep consultant have training in or **knowledge of breastfeeding?** Ideally you want to find someone who understands breastfeeding and can factor your wish to continue into the methods they recommend for you.

- What **methods** does the sleep consultant advocate? Cry-it-out? Some sleep consultants use more gentle and holistic approaches to supporting families with their infant's sleep than others.

Myths about Breastfeeding and Sleep

Giving your baby a dreamfeed will make them sleep for longer:
The idea with *dreamfeeding* is that you feed your baby at around 10.30 or 11pm without fully waking them, in the hope that their big full tummy will make them sleep for a longer stretch. It's generally associated more with formula feeding than breastfeeding. So, could you give your breastfed baby a dreamfeed? You could certainly try but there is no guarantee it will work. And there is also the risk that you will actually fully wake your baby. Another thing to consider is that encouraging your baby to take a dreamfeed, could interfere with the process of establishing your milk supply. And if your baby did sleep for a longer than usual stretch, you may end up with very full or engorged breasts as a result.

Introducing infant formula will result in your baby sleeping for longer stretches:

This is often suggested to breastfeeding parents who may be struggling with nighttime wakings. But there isn't actually evidence that introducing a bottle of infant formula will result in your baby sleeping for longer stretches at nighttime. Milk is only one of the reasons why babies wake at night-time. And as per the above point, introducing the bottle of formula could interfere with your supply and put you at risk of engorgement or blocked ducts.

Babies need to learn how to self-soothe:

Babies are not able to calm themselves down when they cry or settle themselves when they are upset. Their brains just don't yet have what it takes to perform these functions. What babies need is responsive parenting, irrespective of how they are fed. When you respond by holding, touching or feeding your baby you *co-regulate* them. Responding in this way helps your baby to develop the skills to be able to self-regulate when they are ready. It gives them the message 'I am here for you' and helps to build a foundation for secure attachment and good emotional health later in life. Your baby learns to trust you and this is the basis for being able to form healthy relationships in adult life. Being responsive fosters independence, when your baby is ready for it.

Feeding your Baby to sleep is a bad habit:

Being able to feed your baby to sleep is one of the greatest things about breastfeeding! It is *not* a bad habit. Breastmilk contains hormones such as tryptophan and melatonin which induce feelings of drowsiness in babies, so drifting off to sleep with a bellyful of warm milk is to be expected. Furthermore, a baby's levels of the hormone cholycystokinin (CCK) rise immediately after breastfeeding and this also contributes to their feeling relaxed and sleepy.

It's OK to leave your baby to cry it out. They are just protesting a big change:
No, it's really not. Babies are unable to soothe or calm themselves when they are upset. They need you to help them regulate their emotions and to reassure them that you're there and that everything is OK. It's not aways possible to know what your baby is trying to tell you when they cry – they could be hungry, cold, afraid, or have a dirty nappy. But the important thing is that you let them know you're there for them.

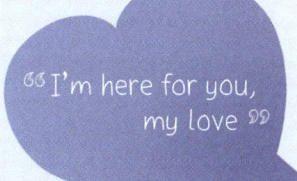
"I'm here for you, my love"

When will your baby start sleeping through the night?

Good question, but unfortunately the answer isn't that simple. All babies are different. Some will sleep for five and six hour stretches from early on while others will still be waking for breastfeeds (or for other reasons) several times a night up to the age of one, or even beyond that. Even the concept of *sleeping through the night* is subjective – is it six hours? Eight hours? Ten hours? Babies do start to sleep more according to their own circadian rhythm from around 12 weeks, but that does not necessarily mean sleeping for extended periods during the night without needing to feed. Talk to other parents at a support group about what night-times look like in their households and they will all tell something slightly different. Try to let go of the idea that your baby *sleeping through the night* is a box that has to be ticked, or that successful parenting means having a baby who is a good sleeper. Can you be patient with your baby? Can you trust that they will sleep for longer stretches when they are developmentally ready?

Survival Tips

Lack of sleep and broken sleep during the night is one of the hardest things to cope with as a new parent. As a new mother, you will also be recovering from the birth of your baby (no matter what kind of birth you had, it is a big deal for your body and you need time to recover), learning how breastfeeding works and trying to figure out your newborn baby's needs. There is no secret formula for making your baby sleep through the night, but here are some ideas that may help you survive the early months:

Take a Nap during the Day

So many of the mothers I see are hesitant about the idea of taking daytime naps. It's not surprising really. Our culture doesn't support napping during the day – we get up, keep going all day and then go to bed at whatever time we go to bed. People often equate napping during the day with laziness or with being unproductive, which is ridiculous really when you think of the way in which afternoon siestas are the norm in many other countries. Sometimes napping during the day can take a little getting used to, but it is very necessary during the early days of parenting so that you can catch up on broken sleep during the night. Even a 20 – 30 minute nap could help you get through the day and make everything a bit easier.

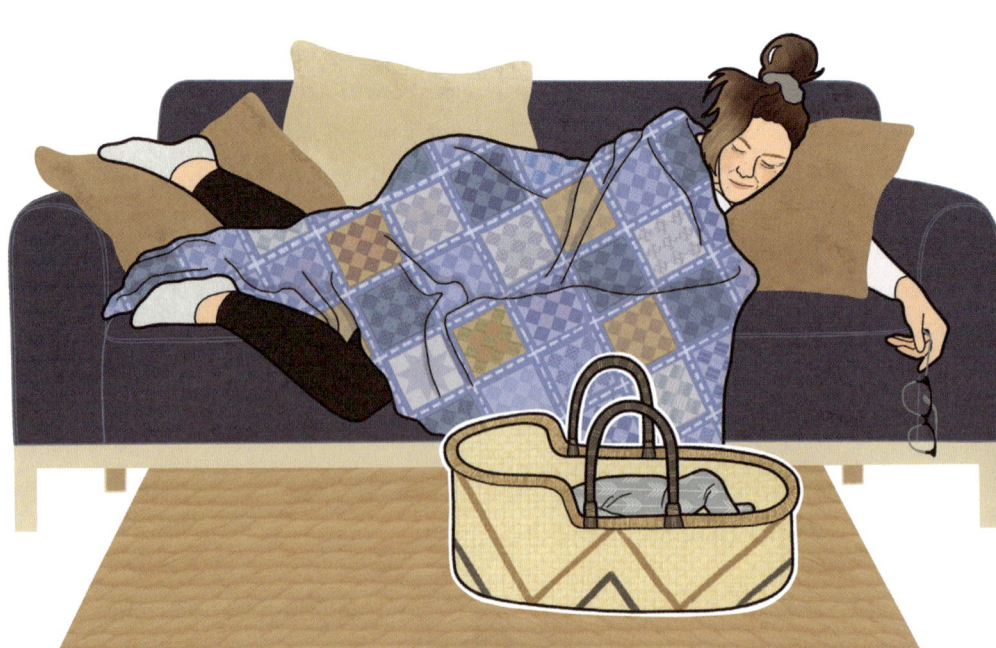

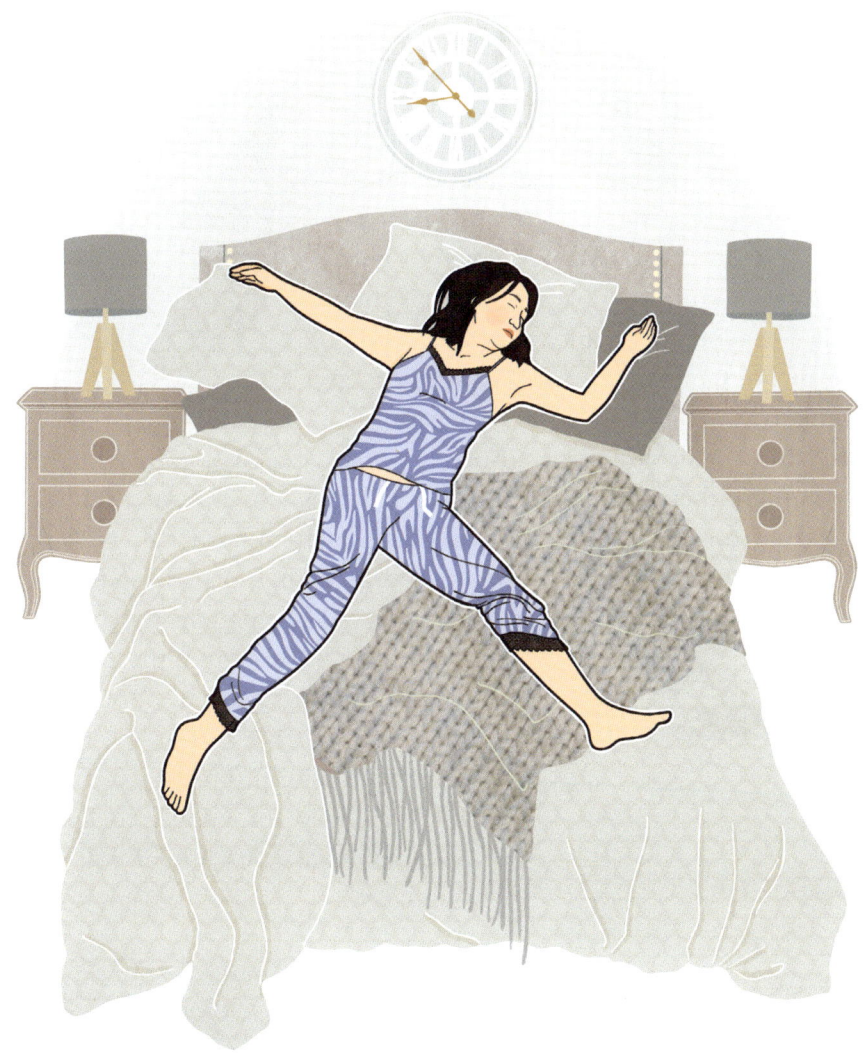

Go to Bed Earlier

Again, this seems like a no brainer, but when you're sleep deprived and struggling to survive the early weeks of parenting it may not seem that obvious. Feed your baby in the evening – they may want to cluster feed for an hour or two – and when you feel they are done hand them over to your partner so they can sleep on their chest. Go to bed yourself and your partner can bring your baby to you when they next wake for a feed. Even if you only get one or two solid hours of sleep, it's a head start on the accumulated hours of sleep you get during the rest of the night. Mothers often find they will go into a very deep sleep for a couple of hours if they go to bed at 8:30/9:00pm.

Accept all Offers of Help and Ask for Help

If you're feeling exhausted and on the verge of not coping, is there anyone you could ask for help? Is there anyone who could give you a couple of hours of their time – maybe they could take your baby out for an hour or two in their stroller or carrier while you go to bed or have a bath? It's OK to need help. Our Western culture is not particularly good at caring for new mothers, unlike some other cultures which have a tradition of caring for the mother up to six weeks after she has given birth. I've seen this in action with Indian friends when they have a baby. Their parents will come to stay for two or three months and cook nutritious meals and care for the baby when the mother sleeps. So don't be shy about asking for what you need. It's very easy for people to assume you're managing just fine if you don't say otherwise.

Talk to a Voluntary Breastfeeding Counsellor or Peer Supporter

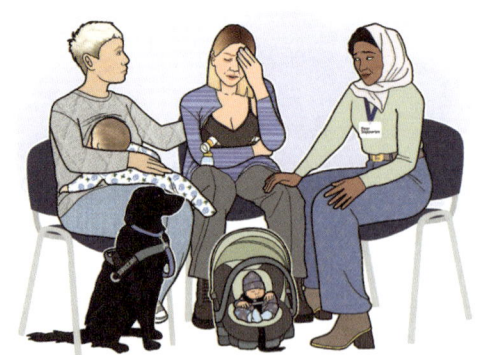

When you're exhausted or feel like you are at your wits end, talking to someone who understands breastfeeding and gets how hard the night-times can be, can really help. Having a chat with someone who is trained to listen gives you space to get it all off your chest and often can result in your getting some clarity on your situation. In addition, a voluntary supporter may have some little nugget of wisdom to offer you or a different perspective.

Attend a Breastfeeding Support Group

Breastfeeding support groups are about connection and being in a shared space with people who are having similar experiences to yourself. They are mothers who are breastfeeding and may also be struggling with exhaustion and broken sleep. So attending a friendly group gives you the opportunity to be heard, to hear what helps other people cope and to be reminded of the fact that you are not alone.

Try to See Things from Your Baby's Perspective

This doesn't give you more sleep at night, but understanding what is going on for your baby or what they are trying to tell you when they wake at night may help you accept where you're at with your baby. Maybe your baby needs lots of reassurance at nighttime. Maybe your baby needs to feed a lot. Maybe your baby's brain is growing very fast and needs lots of nighttime feeding to fuel that growth. Remember, your baby is only ever responding to instinct. They are not being intentionally difficult!

Do a Reset

What does this mean? When you are exhausted, sometimes having a decent stretch of sleep can make you feel refreshed and better able to cope. Could you arrange with your partner to get a solid four-hour stretch of sleep? This might mean pumping or hand expressing some milk for your partner to give your baby if they wake. Feed your baby before you sleep and give them a feed when they wake. Please note: The length of time you give yourself to sleep will depend on the age of your baby. As your baby gets older, you may be able to get a five- or six-hour stretch. But in the first couple of months, four (maybe four and half) hours is probably as long as you would want to go without feeding.

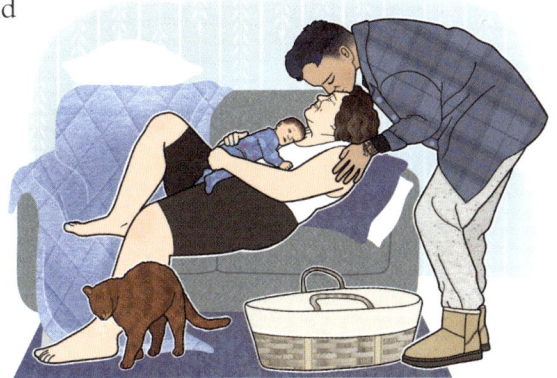

Make a Change to your Family's Sleep Arrangements

Lots of families do this when a new baby arrives. Think about what will get you all the most possible sleep. That may be you, your partner and your baby in the bed. Or it may mean your partner sleeping in a spare room while you and your baby bedshare. Or it could mean your baby in a cot beside your bed. Try and keep yourself in the moment and remind yourself that changes to sleeping arrangements are temporary.

Try to Get Some Time Outside During the Day

A good brisk walk and some fresh air can get some endorphins flowing if you're feeling exhausted or low. Even when you don't feel like it, it can shake up your energy and clear the head.

Follow the Path of Least Resistance

Many parents I see are convinced that they have to get their baby down at a certain time of the day and this can often lead to angst and stress when the baby protests and decides they don't want to be apart from their parents. So, instead it may be easier to just keep your baby with you in the evenings, either sleeping on you or in a bassinet. What's the easiest thing? Just do that. It won't be forever.

CHAPTER 13
When Breastfeeding is Hard

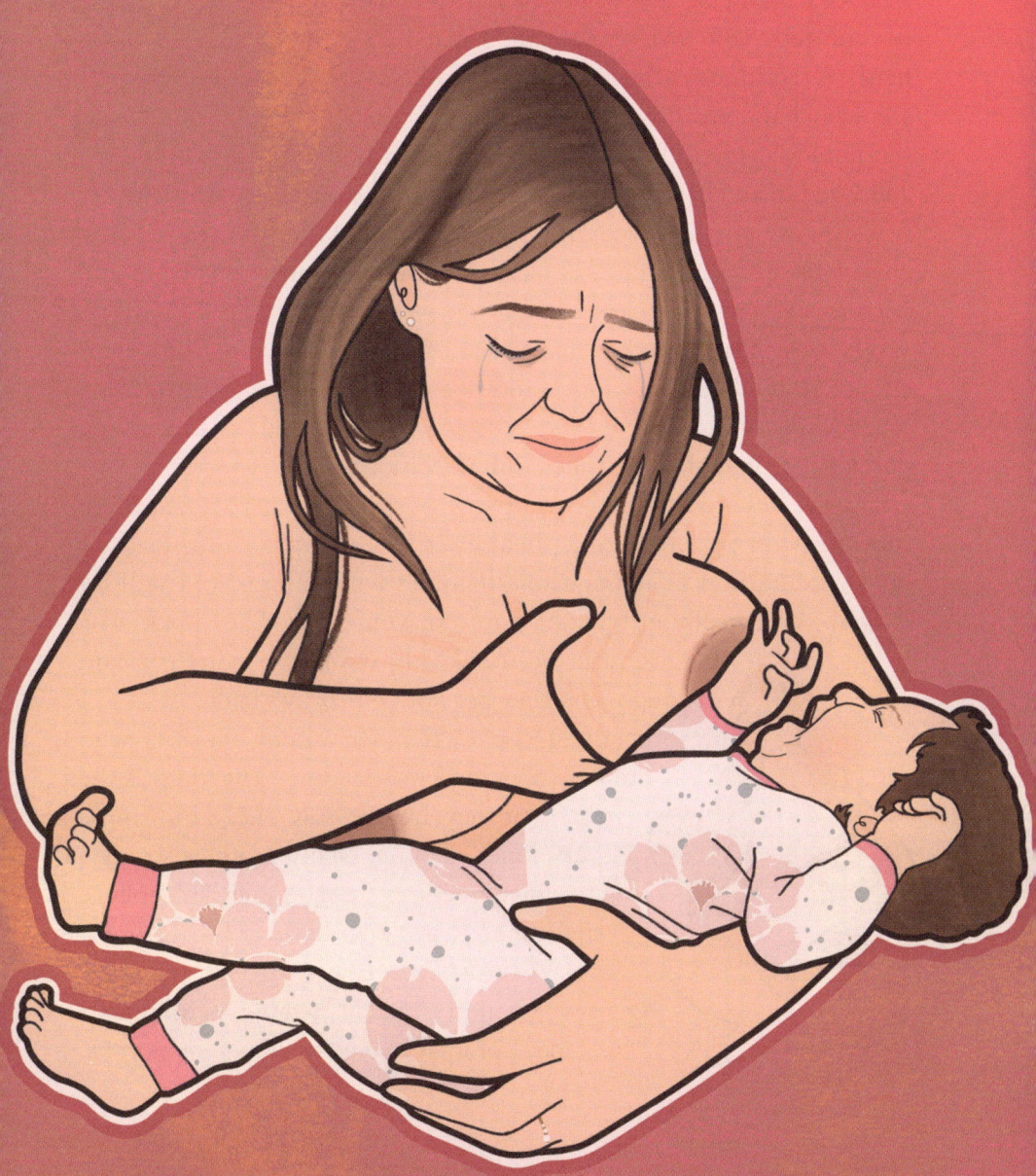

Sometimes breastfeeding is really hard and mothers are unable to breastfeed in the way they had hoped they would. The emotional fallout from these kinds of situations can be really devastating.

As a lactation consultant I know this better than anyone because I see the difficult cases – the non-latching babies, the low milk supply, the recurrent mastitis, the high-needs babies and the persistent nipple pain. I see how the mothers are affected: grief, upset, anger, loneliness, sadness, shame, disappointment. And confusion, because when you're pregnant no one tells you that breastfeeding can be so hard. A common grievance from mothers I see who have breastfeeding difficulties is that the potential for difficulties they face were not addressed in antenatal breastfeeding classes. The purpose of this chapter is to discuss in a balanced and honest way the types of breastfeeding challenges that some mothers face, the resultant impact on them, and ways to navigate these situations.

The first thing I want to make clear, is that breastfeeding difficulties are not your fault. There are a multitude of reasons why a breastfeeding journey can be derailed. The causes can be related to underlying physical or physiological issues, infant sensory issues, genetic factors, circumstances around the birth or lack of timely skilled breastfeeding support. Mothers often blame themselves when breastfeeding does not go according to plan and equate difficulties with failure. So, I will say it again, breastfeeding difficulties are not your fault. They don't arise because you did something wrong or didn't try hard enough, and they are not your baby's fault.

Something else I often see among mothers who are experiencing breastfeeding difficulties is the belief that they are the only one. This can be a very lonely feeling. Many mothers struggle with breastfeeding and some experience challenges that don't have a simple quick fix. If breastfeeding was easy for everyone, we wouldn't need lactation consultants and voluntary breastfeeding supporters.

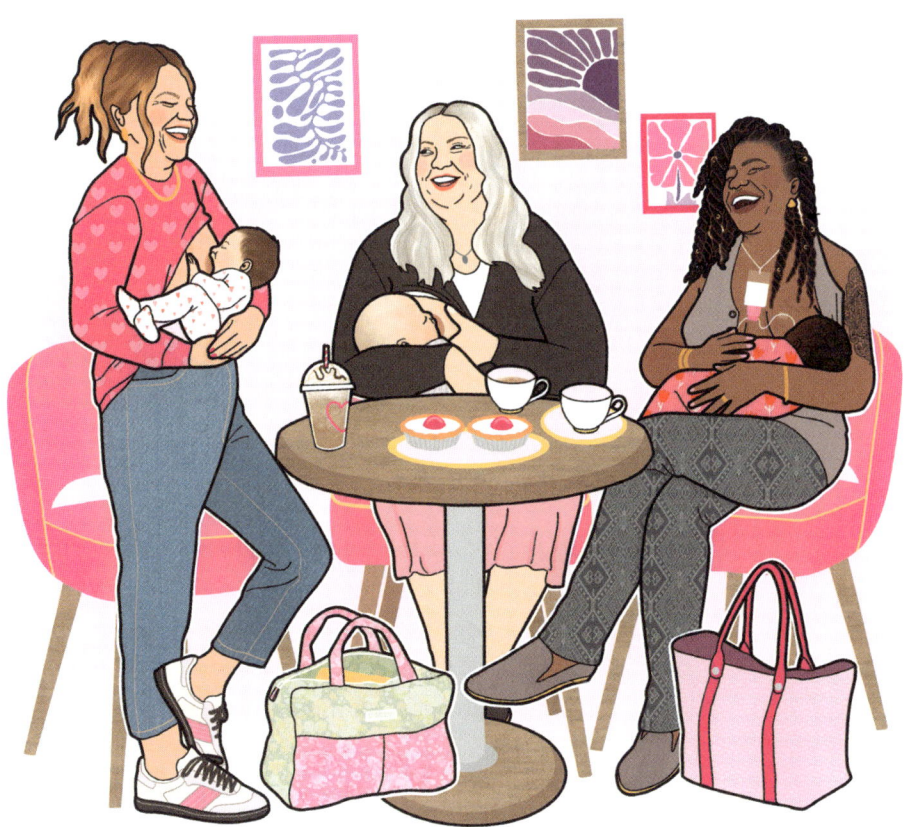

Organisations like La Leche League were founded because of a recognition that breastfeeding can be difficult and that mothers need support. If you experience breastfeeding difficulties, please know that you are not alone and that support is available.

Breastfeeding difficulties are real and their emotional impact on parents can be huge.

Causes of Breastfeeding Difficulties

These are the most common causes of significant breastfeeding difficulties that I encounter in my work as a lactation consultant. They all have the potential to cause stress, anxiety, depression, anger and trauma. Breastfeeding difficulties can also result in a mother or parent experiencing social isolation (because sometimes they avoid breastfeeding support groups) and a profound sense of disappointment that their breastfeeding journey is not as they had hoped it would be.

Low Milk Supply

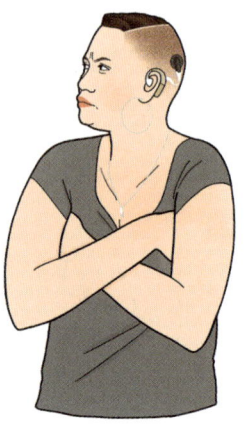

This is the most common cause of breastfeeding difficulties that I see. It can result in mother feeling inadequate, feeling like they have failed their babies and feeling self-conscious emotions such as shame and guilt. Low milk supply is discussed in detail in Chapter 14.

A non-latching baby

Most babies will be able to latch and feed directly at the breast. But, for a small cohort of babies, this may not be possible, despite the best efforts of the mother and support from a lactation consultant. Sometimes the road towards getting a baby to latch can be a long one. When a baby is unable to latch and a mother wants to provide them with their milk, they will exclusively pump and feed them their milk in a bottle. This can work well for some mothers, indeed some mothers choose to exclusively pump. But if exclusive pumping is not how you envisioned your breastfeeding journey, it can be very difficult, both practically and emotionally.

These are some of the situations in which feeding a baby directly at the breast may not be possible:

A preterm baby that has been bottled-fed pumped milk – Most babies who have been tube or bottled-fed from birth can transition to full breastfeeding. But sometimes that transition can be challenging. It could be that the baby finds switching from one way of feeding to another too overwhelming, or that the mother struggles with switching from scheduled pumping and feeding to the more unpredictable routine of direct breastfeeding. Transitioning from bottle to breast can take time, growth and patience. It may not always happen according to the timeline that you want. So, whether it's a case that it's a long road for you and your baby to get to where you want to be with breastfeeding or it's that you just can't arrive there, it's hard. It's exhausting and emotional, and you will need support.

A baby that has anatomical variations that make direct breastfeeding difficult – Some babies are born with anatomical variations that make it difficult or impossible for them to latch and feed directly at the breast. For example, a baby with a cleft palate, may not be able to breastfeed. Or a baby may be born with a congenital condition that makes direct breastfeeding difficult (for example low tone or issues coordinating sucking, swallowing and breathing).

Childhood/sexual Trauma – A mother's past traumas may be triggered when their baby latches directly to their breast and as a result they may choose to exclusively pump. It can be traumatising to be confronted with unexpected memories of past events that may have been buried. And upsetting to feel that you are unable to breastfeed your baby directly.

Inverted Nipples – It may not always be possible to directly breastfeed if you have truly inverted nipples. This can be difficult to accept, particularly if you've absorbed the narrative that there is always a solution to breastfeeding problems. You may not perceive exclusive pumping and bottle feeding as a solution, or at least not a solution that you want.

Forceful Hands-on Assistance with Latching – It is possible that some babies will develop an aversion to latching or being at their mother's breast due to rough or forceful hands-on assistance from a healthcare professional (HCP) in the early days postpartum. Sometimes HCPs (with good intentions) will end up forcefully pushing a baby's head to their mother's breast in an attempt to get them latched. This kind of approach is counterproductive as it can result in the baby developing an aversion to latching. Usually, with a great deal of patience and sensitive support, these babies will come round and breastfeed. But getting to that point can be difficult.

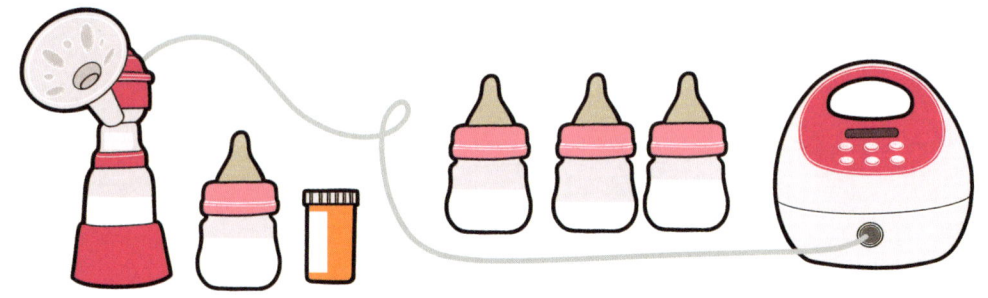

Oversupply and Recurrent Mastitis

These are among the most difficult cases I support parents with. There isn't a quick fix and mothers are very often given conflicting advice and advised to stop breastfeeding, despite wishing to continue. It can be difficult for partners too, and I have seen situations where a partner wants the mother to stop breastfeeding because they don't want to see them have to go through another mastitis infection. If you have oversupply and/or recurrent mastitis it is very important that you get skilled and individualised support from a GP (or other healthcare professional who understands lactation and can prescribe antibiotics) and from an IBCLC. Most cases that I have seen where a mother experiences oversupply and repeated bouts of mastitis resolve around the 12-week mark, but reaching that point can be difficult. It can feel unfair that you are having such an awful time with breastfeeding and frustrating if you can't seem to reduce your milk production (despite doing all the things you've been advised to do). See Chapter 9 for more information on oversupply and mastitis.

Ongoing Nipple Pain

Usually when a mother experiences persistent nipple pain, we can find a cause and do something about it. But occasionally there will be no apparent cause for nipple pain. It's possible that the underlying cause of pain could be psychosomatic (that is, some kind of mental stress or traumatic memory which manifests as physical pain). Or it could be that a parent has very sensitive nipples. Or both. But in these kinds of situations, it can be hard to say definitively why the mother is experiencing pain. Sometimes mindfulness practices can help, or if the mother has a sense that there is some kind of emotional pain at the root of her physical pain, she could consider talk therapy. Talking things through with an IBCLC or an experienced voluntary breastfeeding supporter will also help the mother figure out how to keep breastfeeding or providing milk for her baby.

Feeding Aversion

Over the years I've seen a handful of babies with what appears to be feeding aversion – not a breastfeeding issue as such, but an apparent aversion to any kind of oral feeding, including bottle feeding. In most cases, the feeding aversion became apparent when the baby was two to three months old. It is immensely stressful for parents when this happens.

Babies who are feeding-averse may exhibit the following behaviours

- Show feeding cues less frequently than other babies.

- Feed for a very short time and then become upset and refuse to take any more milk. They may turn their head away from the breast or bottle, cry or arch their back.

- Breastfeed or bottle-feed only when they are very sleepy. Sometimes they will feed better during the night than during the day.

- Cry or show signs of distress when the parent holds them in a feeding position.

- Gain weight slowly. Or stop gaining weight. They may fall through centile lines on growth charts.

It's not always possible to say why a baby has developed a feeding aversion. But it could be related to

- A negative association with feeding – perhaps related to something that happened when they were very small, for example, being pushed to feed when they didn't want to, being intubated, or choking on milk.
- Some kind of physical pain or discomfort the baby is experiencing.
- A sensory issue which only becomes apparent when the baby is older.

The normal parental response when a baby is not gaining well is to try to get more milk into them – offering more breastfeeds, trying to make the baby feed longer than they want to and also giving extra milk in bottles. The response of the baby, who picks up on all of this increased effort to get them to feed more, may be to become even more feeding averse! It can be a vicious and stressful cycle. When you are in a situation like this, it can be difficult to find appropriate support. I suggest you work with an IBCLC who has some experience working with feeding aversion and also work closely with a paediatrician or your GP. Parents that I have worked with whose baby had a feeding aversion report that they found the book 'Your Baby's Bottle-feeding Aversion: Reasons and Solutions' by Rowena Bennett immensely helpful. Buying the book enabled them to join a Facebook support group for parents experiencing similar issues. The parents found it validating and helpful to be able to connect with other parents who understood what they were going through.

You Don't Enjoy Breastfeeding

Many mothers are surprised to discover just how much they love breastfeeding. But some mothers discover that they just don't like it.

And that's OK. However, it can be difficult when you want to provide your baby with your milk. You may choose to pump, or you may keep going for a specific length of time. The feelings you have about not enjoying breastfeeding can make you feel alone, and as if there's something wrong with you (there isn't!), particularly when you have a lot of friends who are breastfeeding. Try to accept all that comes up for you regarding breastfeeding. Honour your inner voice and see if you can let it guide you, whether it guides you to keep going or to stop breastfeeding altogether.

As we've previously mentioned, some mothers experience a phenomenon when breastfeeding called breastfeeding aversion response (BAR) whereby they feel very strong negative feelings during breastfeeding and an urge to unlatch their baby, even when they want to breastfeed. See Chapter 11 for more information on BAR.

Breastfeeding an Unsettled Baby with Allergies or GORD

Breastfeeding a baby who has been diagnosed with an allergy or with gastroesophageal reflux disease (GORD) can be very challenging. Often breastfeeding can be fraught – babies may not settle easily after feeds and may need to be kept upright, or may need more frequent feeding. The other big challenge is trying to access skilled support to breastfeed. Mothers are often given conflicting advice or are advised to switch to expensive hypoallergenic formulas. There is no one size fits all when it comes to these types of issues, so it is important that you work with professionals who can meet you where you're at and support you to continue breastfeeding. It can also be helpful to connect with mothers having similar issues.

Suboptimal Breastfeeding Support

There are lots of IBCLCs, midwives, health visitors, nurses and GPs who provide excellent, sensitive and evidence-based breastfeeding support to parents. But, unfortunately there are also a small number of healthcare professionals who perhaps don't have sufficient or up-to-date training, or who may not have adequate interpersonal skills to be able to provide the kind of breastfeeding and lactation care needed by some parents. It can be immensely frustrating if you can't seem to find the help you need, when you need it. Because breastfeeding and lactation support is time sensitive. Not being able to access appropriate care when you need can result in significant and ongoing issues with breastfeeding. And the experience can contribute to feelings of anger.

The Emotional Fallout

It's a big deal when breastfeeding is hard or doesn't work out as you had hoped. You may have had a vision of yourself as a breastfeeding mother or have had an expectation that if you encountered difficulties, that you'd simply address them by accessing skilled help and support. However, we know that the reality isn't always that straightforward. There has been a growing awareness over the last decade of how difficult breastfeeding experiences impact mothers and parents emotionally. Breastfeeding difficulties can contribute to mental health challenges such as postpartum depression and anxiety, and that psychological well-being is linked to whether a mother perceives her breastfeeding journey as a *success* or a *failure*. If breastfeeding is hard, if it falls short of how you imagined it would be, you may experience some of the following emotions:

Devastation: This is a big, dramatic word, but devastated is how many mothers feel when breastfeeding is hard or when it has been derailed. Breastfeeding doesn't exist in a vacuum – it is intertwined with how you feel about yourself as a mother and how you see yourself in the world. It is about self-identity. So, when breastfeeding is hard it can feel like you have lost an expected vision of yourself as a breastfeeding

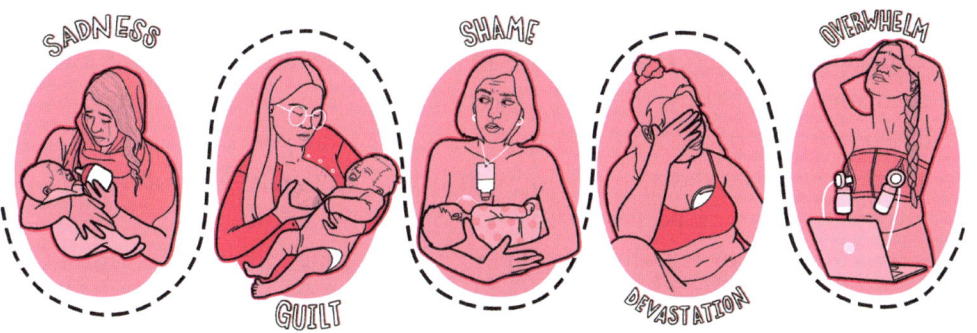

mother, being in shared spaces with other breastfeeding mothers. This loss can be very difficult to come to terms with. It can take time to grieve the loss, make peace with your experience and find a new motherhood self-identity that is not contingent upon having a perfect or easy breastfeeding journey.

Guilt and Self-Blame: One of the reasons parents choose to breastfeed is because it supports optimal infant health. Parents want to do *the best* for their babies by exclusively breastfeeding. If exclusive breastfeeding is not possible and parents have to supplement with infant formula, they may feel guilty that they haven't done enough or that they're letting their baby down (even when they have done everything possible to keep breastfeeding). Parents often blame themselves, even when external factors have made breastfeeding difficult. These kinds of emotions can overshadow the postpartum period and get in the way of a mother being able to enjoy her baby.

Shame: Breastfeeding in front of other people is a very public display of who you are as a mother – you're saying something about yourself and the choices you've made when you sit in a café or attend a support group and breastfeed. You can feel an authentic sense of 'this is who I am.' But if breastfeeding difficulties rule out feeding your baby in public in the way you wanted it's not uncommon to feel shame – shame that you are not feeding your baby in what you believe to be the *proper* or *correct* way. You may feel that people will judge you for that. The feeling of shame can be compounded by being in the company of other breastfeeding mothers and as a result some women will intentionally isolate themselves when breastfeeding is difficult.

Anger: Anger is a very normal response when breastfeeding is hard. You may feel angry that no one told you breastfeeding could be this hard and anger at how difficult it has been for you to get the evidence-based support from healthcare professionals. And you may also feel angry and frustrated at receiving conflicting advice from healthcare professionals – one person telling you one thing, another telling you something completely difficult. There may be times when it feels like no one understands what you're going through.

Sadness: The loss of a longed-for breastfeeding relationship can leave you feeling profoundly sad. It can be difficult to understand yourself and why you feel so strongly. We don't really talk about the deep embodied desire that many mothers feel to breastfeed – it's not even so much that they consciously want to breastfeed, but that they feel a longing in their bodies. It could be primal or instinctive, or perhaps it's conditioning. But it can be a powerful feeling, and the unmet expectations of that desire can leave you feeling a deep well of sadness.

Trauma: Trauma is an on-going distressing response to a very stressful event or situation, like shockwaves that continue to reverberate for weeks, months or even years after the event. It can be experienced in different ways – emotionally, psychologically, physically, spiritually or subconsciously. It's not an exaggeration to say that severe breastfeeding difficulties or a breastfeeding journey ending before you wanted it to can be traumatic for a mother. The situation can be compounded by insensitive or unhelpful encounters with healthcare professionals and by a lack of support from family members. Trauma can also be compounded by social isolation and a feeling that you are on your own. It is a subjective experience, so what constitutes trauma for you, may not be traumatic for someone else. Symptoms of trauma include

- Feeling overwhelmed
- Feeling anxious and on edge
- Feeling alone and like no one understands what you've been through

- Difficulty sleeping
- Mood swings
- Constantly replaying events or interactions in your mind
- Feeling very sad and full of self-blame
- Feeling like you've lost control and had something taken away from you
- Avoiding friends or certain situations for fear of being triggered

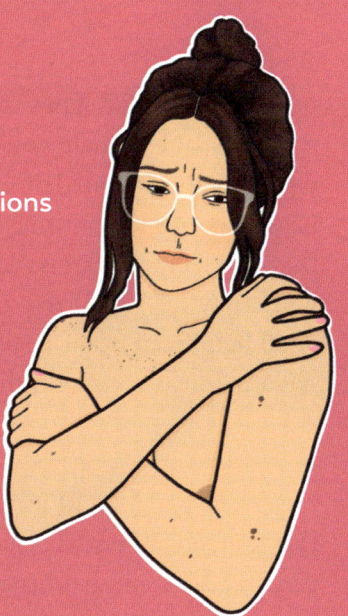

If you experience any of the above emotions, you are not overreacting. You are not being selfish or unreasonable. These emotions are normal responses for anyone experiencing breastfeeding difficulties. Give yourself permission to feel and accept all that comes up for you when breastfeeding is hard. You *will* find a way to work through these emotions. You are not on your own. Many mothers feel this way when faced with breastfeeding challenges and the loss of an expected vision of breastfeeding. It's OK to really, really want to breastfeed. And it's OK to have complicated feelings when it doesn't turn out as you had hoped. The important thing is that you acknowledge your experience for what it is, talk to someone and access the help and support you need.

Getting Help and Support

If you are finding breastfeeding difficult, if you had to end your breastfeeding journey before you wanted to or if you're struggling with some of the emotions discussed in the above section, it's important that you find help as soon as you can.

Professional Breastfeeding Support: Can you get help and support from an IBCLC? They may not be able to fix everything, but they should be able to help you find a way to feed your baby and support you emotionally. If your IBCLC suggests a care plan to help you continue breastfeeding or continue to provide milk for your baby, it is important that you feel the plan is manageable and that it doesn't get in the way of you enjoying your baby. In addition to IBCLC support, you may also need help from other healthcare professionals, for example if your baby has a medical condition that is affecting feeding.

Voluntary and Peer Support: Sometimes mothers who have significant breastfeeding difficulties avoid breastfeeding support groups because they perceive them as places where all the mothers present are enjoying *perfect* breastfeeding journeys. This is not the case. Breastfeeding support groups are as much about social support as they are about support to breastfeed, and they are friendly and welcoming spaces for everyone. No one is going to judge you, if anything a breastfeeding support group is where you will receive the greatest amount of empathy and support,

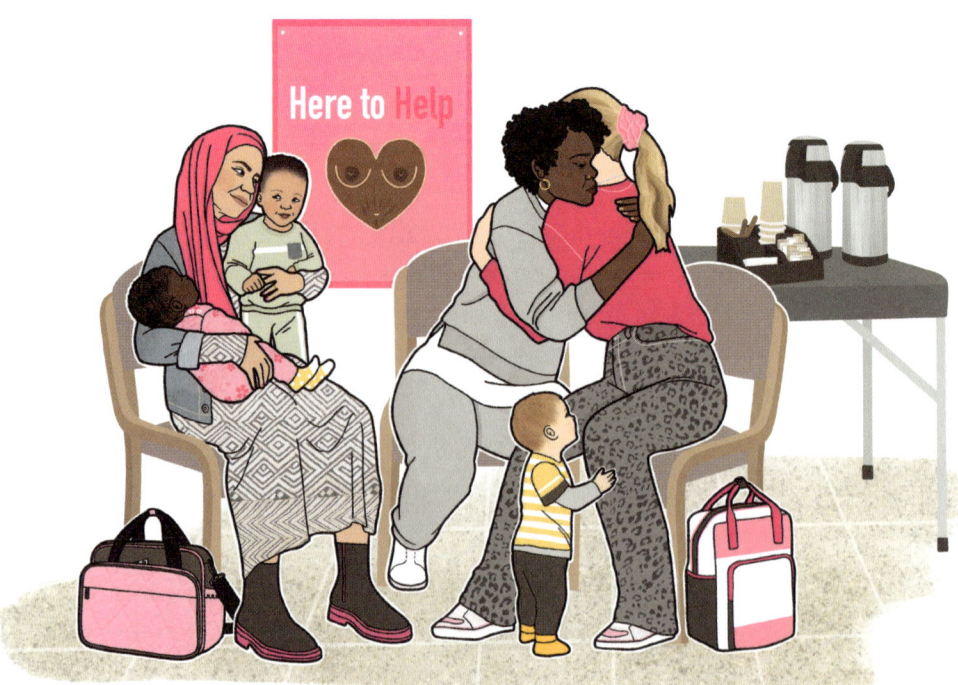

irrespective of how you are feeding your baby. Additionally, attending a breastfeeding support group could give you the opportunity to speak one-to-one to a trained supporter – someone who will listen, empathise, offer evidence-based information and just hold space for you. Being able to talk to someone like this can help you to process your feelings and give you greater clarity on your situation. And sometimes talking things through can help you figure out what you want to do or how you can help yourself.

Talk to People who have experienced similar problems: Talking to someone who has experienced similar problems to you and who *gets it* can be very validating and reassuring. Whether it's reflux, low supply, a non-latching baby, pumping for a preterm baby, there are other mothers who have been there and who will understand what you're going through. You could ask at a local or online breastfeeding support group if they know anyone who has had a similar problem or see if you could find a specialist support group on social media.

> *Some of the emotional burden of breastfeeding difficulties is relieved by having contact with and sharing experiences* **with other women having similar problems**
>
> Spannhakke et al, 2021

Mental Health Supports: Breastfeeding difficulties can affect you emotionally and can impact your mental health. You may need to talk to a psychotherapist or counsellor, see a psychiatrist, and/or take medication. The important thing is that you reach out for help and don't diminish what you are experiencing. Talk to your GP, your health visitor or your public health nurse so that they can refer you to appropriate perinatal mental health supports in your area. You matter and your mental health matters.

Healing and Acceptance

A difficult breastfeeding experience is usually a journey that culminates in finding some degree of healing and acceptance. And often with that sense of having overcome something difficult is a sense of pride and inner strength. I've seen this many times with mothers I've worked with. Even though they may always feel a little sad that breastfeeding wasn't how they wanted it to be, they get to a place where they are able to acknowledge all their efforts and feel proud of what they've managed to overcome.

Part of your healing journey may mean reframing how you nurture and connect with your baby. There are so many ways to bond, communicate with and nurture your baby. Nurturing is not just about milk. You can nurture and enjoy your baby in the following ways

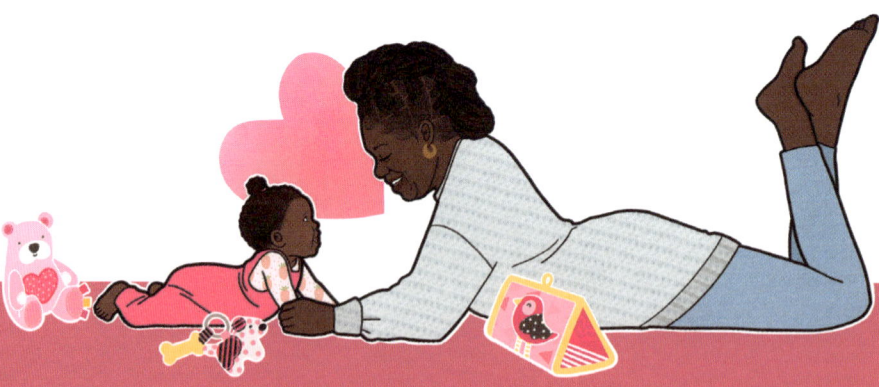

- ♥ caring touch or massage
- ♥ holding, cuddling or rocking them
- ♥ playing with them
- ♥ talking or singing to them
- ♥ bottlefeeding in a loving way
- ♥ co-bathing and enjoying skin-to-skin contact
- ♥ wearing them in a sling
- ♥ going for walks with them in their pram

When you do any of the above, you are also building your baby's brain! Even just doing skin-to-skin contact releases biochemicals which help with brain development.

No matter how you feed your baby, you are the best mother or parent they could have. You know them better than anyone else and they want you above anyone else.

Another thing that may help you through a time when breastfeeding is difficult, is trying to understand things from your baby's perspective – this may be particularly useful if your baby cries a lot, refuses to latch or has a feeding aversion. There is a concept in Dialectical Behavioural Therapy called *mentalisation* – in simple terms this is the ability to understand your own thinking and what your baby is thinking. It's about trying to see things from your baby's perspective and letting them know that you understand them. What is your baby experiencing? What are they feeling? What appears to be upsetting them? What are they trying to communicate with you? Can you try to see what they are seeing? When you do this, it can help you to find some meaning in how they are behaving and it may also reassure your baby that you hear them, that you understand and that you are there for them.

For example, let's say you're trying to get your baby to latch. They refuse. They get upset. You get upset. Take a few moments and breathe. Meet your baby where they are at, look into their eyes and say something like

> *'I can see you're upset, it's ok.*
> *I can see that something is difficult for you.*
> *You don't want to latch right now, do you?*
> *That's ok. I'm here for you. No matter what.*
> *Here, let me give you a big hug!'*

Just articulating these words can help to keep you in the moment and bring you into your baby's experience and feelings. They see that you are calm and they get the message that you are trying to understand them. This can help your baby feel safe and accepted. It may also help you to accept the kind of feeding journey you and your baby are having, even if it's not the one you wanted.

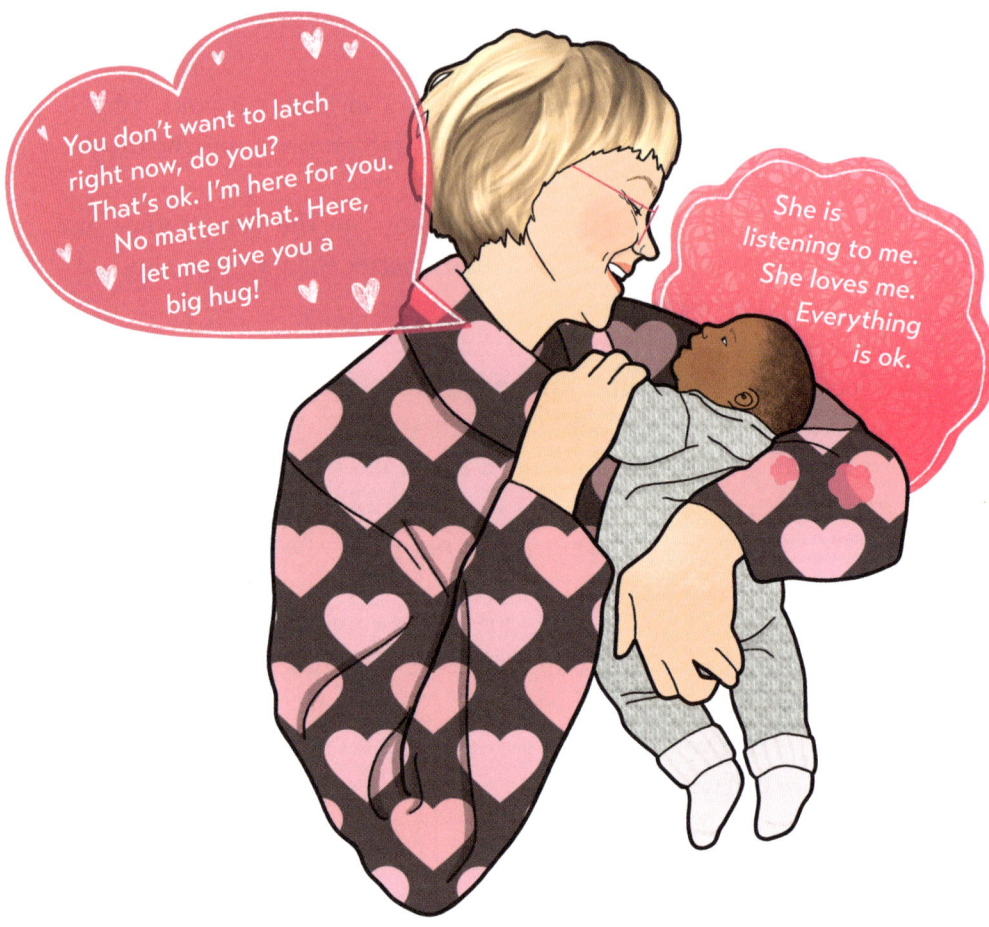

Mentalising can help you to understand your baby and remain close and connected to them, no matter what feeding difficulties you face together.

Finding acceptance of your difficult breastfeeding journey takes time. Most parents will have to work through complicated feelings of anger, disappointment and grief, before being able to let go and fully embrace the path that breastfeed has taken them on. Try to be gentle and patient with yourself. Things that may not make sense now, may become clearer in time. A feeding experience that may feel like failure now, may in time end up as an achievement that you're proud of. Your perspective of what *success* looks like will change and evolve over time, and you will get to a place of accepting what *is* rather than what *should be*.

Some parents I have worked with report that they found the concept of radical acceptance helped them embrace and accept their breastfeeding journey. Radical acceptance is the practice of trying to fully accept things as they are. Instead of wishing a situation was different and viewing it through a lens of personal inadequacy, we allow ourselves to be willing to fully experience ourselves and all that life is throwing at us. The philosophy behind radical acceptance is that it can give you a sense of control and prevent you from getting stuck in self-judgement and negative emotions like anger and sadness. The writer Tara Brach says

> *As we lean into the experience of the moment – releasing our stories and gently holding our pain or desire – Radical Acceptance begins to unfold. The two parts of genuine acceptance –seeing clearly and holding our experience with compassion– are as interdependent as the two wings of a great bird. Together, they enable us to fly and be free.*

Mindfulness is another technique that can help you move through and accept challenging experiences. You don't have to follow any complicated techniques, just take a few moments when you can and

- Sit and close your eyes.
- Feel your body become still.
- Allow your breath to settle.
- Relax your shoulders.
- Notice all the different physical sensations in your body – your body in contact with the chair, your lips touching, your feet on the floor, air in contact with your skin.

- Again notice your breath. Observe three long slow in breaths and out breaths.

- Come back to being aware of your body. Notice any sensations.

- Be aware of sounds around you.

- Gently open your eyes.

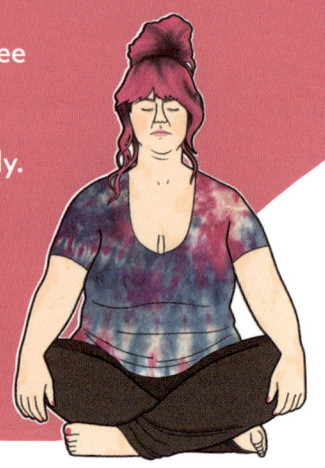

How do you feel? Has two minutes of mindfulness made any difference? Could you make a habit of doing this? It doesn't have to be at set times, you can do it anytime, anywhere. You can also practice mindfulness as you go about your day – it is simply a practice of paying attention which takes you out of your own tangled thoughts and feelings, even for a few short moments.

Finally, another step in finding healing and acceptance for some parents who have had a difficult breastfeeding experience and been let down by suboptimal support is giving feedback, making a complaint or having a debriefing session with staff at their maternity hospital. Whatever you decide to do, it can give you an opportunity to get grievances off your chest, to be heard and to feel like you are helping to improve services for other parents. For some parents, giving feedback can help them achieve closure on the upset (and even trauma) that poor breastfeeding support has caused them.

CHAPTER 14
Low Milk Supply

Milk supply is one of the most common concerns among new breastfeeding mothers and not having enough milk is the number one reason they give for stopping breastfeeding early than intended. This is despite the fact that most mothers *can* make enough milk for their babies. So why all the fuss? Is there really such a thing as low milk supply? Why do mothers worry about it? This chapter will answer these questions and provide information on how various types of low milk supply can present and how they can be addressed.

The reality is that some women will struggle to make enough milk to exclusively breastfeed. That does not mean they can't breastfeed. With help and support they can have very happy breastfeeding journeys. Breastfeeding doesn't have to be all or nothing.

Producing enough milk to feed your baby is important. The stakes are high – not having enough milk means your baby may not get sufficient calories to grow optimally. This is why there is a big emphasis on ensuring you do what you need to in the early weeks postpartum to establish good milk production (ie, lots of frequent breastfeeding or milk removal). Once milk production is established, it's a demand and supply situation – your baby feeds or you pump (this creates the *demand*), and your body gets the message to make more milk (*supply*). A slow-down in the frequency of milk removal or a reduction in the volume being removed at feeds or pumps, can result in a reduction in milk production.

Low Milk Supply can be categorised as *Perceived*, *Secondary*, or *Primary*. It can also be due to *Delayed Lactogenesis II* (a delay in your milk *coming in* or increasing in volume) – see Chapter 4. If you have a concern about your milk supply it is important to get skilled support and determine which of these aforementioned types it might be.

Perceived Low Milk Supply

As the name suggests, *perceived* low milk supply is an unfounded belief that you're not making enough milk for your baby. It is very common among breastfeeding parents. If you are worried that you're not making enough milk, it is important to rule out perceived low milk supply before considering other causes. Reasons for believing you are not producing enough milk are

- *cluster feeding -* it can be so intense sometimes, especially if your baby is going through a growth spurt, that it can cause you to question whether you have enough milk

- *lack of confidence* – it can make you doubt your ability to make enough milk for your baby

- *an expectation that your baby should be feeding according to a schedule* – breastfed babies don't like schedules! There might be three hours between some feeds and at other times there could be just one or two hours between feeds

- *a lot of nighttime waking and feeding* – it's normal and probably isn't because you don't have enough milk

- *your baby wanting to be held a lot* – this is also very normal

- *your baby wanting to go back to the breast after having had what seemed like a good breastfeed –* sometimes babies want to go back for a little bit of comfort or dessert

- *your baby guzzling milk from a bottle -* also not a sign that you don't have enough milk

These are all normal baby behaviours! Really what perceived low milk supply comes down to is a gulf between expectations of what breastfeeding is going to look like (that your baby will feed every three hours) and the more chaotic and unpredictable reality. If you are worried about not making enough milk, answering yes to the following questions, it is unlikely that you have low milk supply:

- Does your baby have sufficient nappy output (two-three dirty nappies plus six-seven wet nappies per 24 hrs)?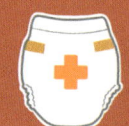

- Is your baby gaining weight appropriately? (ie, back to birth weight between weeks 2 and 3 and there after gaining somewhere in the region of 170-240g per week).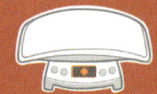

If you have answered no to one or both of these questions, it's *possible* that your milk supply is low. But bear in mind there are many other reasons why your baby might not be gaining appropriately or having sufficient nappy output – for example, they might not be breastfeeding enough times per 24 hours or they might not be transferring milk well. This is why it is important to get skilled support to help you figure out what is going on and how to address it.

The best way I can recommend you develop confidence in your ability to make enough milk for your baby is to attend a breastfeeding support group or spend time with other breastfeeding mothers. When you see other nursing dyads, you learn about normal newborn behaviour and get a better feel for what early days breastfeeding looks like.

Primary Low Milk Supply

Primary low milk supply is caused by some underlying or *intrinsic* factor related to your anatomy and/or physiology. Causes of primary low milk supply include breast reduction surgery and hormonal conditions such as PCOS and insulin resistance. By far the number one cause of primary low milk supply that I see among my clients is insufficient glandular tissue (IGT).

> **How many mothers have primary low milk supply?**
>
> That's a good question. Unfortunately, there's very little epidemiological research on primary low milk supply so it's hard to say just how many mothers are affected, but probably four to six percent.

IGT, also called mammary hypoplasia is a lack of glandular or milk-making tissue in one or both breasts. Little is known about the cause of IGT, but women who have it will often report that their periods were irregular or painful during puberty and/or that they were overweight as a teenager. Many women who have IGT also have PCOS. There is some evidence that IGT can be caused by genetic factors. If you have IGT, your breasts will probably have some of the characteristics associated with the condition:

- Wide spacing
- Tubular shape
- Bulbous areolas
- Asymmetry
- Stretch marks

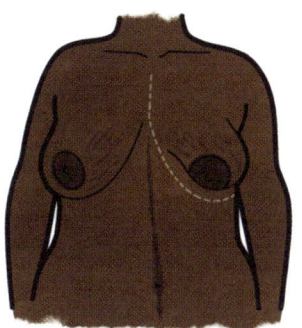

These characteristics can be identified during pregnancy. They suggest that milk supply might be an issue, but there is no way to tell with certainty how much milk you will make once your baby is born. Another factor which suggests that milk supply might be an issue is lack of breast changes during pregnancy.

There isn't always an obvious cause of primary low milk supply, despite thoroughly investigating all possibilities. But whatever the cause, most women who have primary low milk supply can partially breastfeed while also supplementing their baby with extra milk (expressed breastmilk, infant formula and/or donor milk).

Factors that can contribute to Primary Low Milk Supply

Condition	Lactation
Insufficient Glandular Tissue	A lack of milk-making tissue in one or both breasts. Probably the most common cause of PLMS.
Polycystic Ovarian Syndrome (PCOS)	Many women with PCOS can make enough milk to exclusively breastfeed. But some will struggle to make a full supply, especially if they also have other conditions such as insulin resistance, IGT, or obesity.
Sheehan's Syndrome	This condition is rare in developed countries. It can result from a severe postpartum haemorrhage. The blood loss causes damage to the pituitary gland and renders it unable to produce prolactin, the main hormone involved in milk production.
Breast Surgery/ Injury	Lots of women can make enough milk after breast surgery, but if the 4th intercostal nerves or ducts have been cut, or if glandular tissue has been removed (due to breast reduction), lactation capacity may be affected.
Thyroid Dysfunction	Most women who have hypothyroidism or hyperthyroidism can make enough milk to exclusively breastfeed if their conditions are well managed. However, there are some studies done on rats which suggests that thyroid dysfunction can affect milk production and breast development. Hypothyroidism can affect oxytocin levels and as a result, milk may be a little slower to letdown.

Obesity, Diabetes and Insulin resistance	These conditions can influence the hormones involved in breast growth/development and milk production. This does not mean that you won't make enough milk for your baby if you are obese, have diabetes or insulin-resistance, but that you have a higher risk for low milk production.
Radiation Treatment for Breast Cancer	Post-operative radiation treatment in women who have had breast cancer results in the treated breast being unable to make much milk postpartum. Mothers can, however, feed from the untreated breast.
Chemotherapy Treatment for Breast Cancer	Previous chemotherapy treatment for breast cancer can significantly impact the ability of the breasts to produce sufficient milk.

Please note: This is not an exhaustive list of factors that can contribute to PLMS. Research on how lactation works is ongoing and we are still learning! Hopefully in years to come we will have a better understanding of all the factors that affect lactation and how to address PLMS. If you are affected by any of the above conditions, arrange an antenatal consultation with an IBCLC and get help early in the postpartum period if you run into problems.

How do you know you have Primary Low Milk Supply?

You will probably have some of the risk factors for primary low milk supply, such as minimal breast changes during pregnancy, breasts that have the appearance of IGT and/or one or more of the underlying factors that are listed in the table. Usually, PLMS becomes apparent in the first few weeks postpartum when your baby struggles to regain their birth weight, gains weight very slowly and has scant nappy output. Some mothers notice that their milk appears to be slow to come in or that their breasts never feel very full.

If you are concerned that you have primary low milk supply, it is really important that you get skilled and individualised breastfeeding support from an IBCLC as soon as you can. An IBCLC will do a thorough assessment and help you to figure out how to supplement your baby, optimise your milk supply and continue breastfeeding in a way that works for you.

Breastfeeding with Primary Low Milk Supply

You *can* breastfeed if you have PLMS. Breastfeeding does not have to be exclusive to be rewarding, enjoyable and to have significant health benefits for you and your baby. It can be difficult to accept that you have PLMS but one way of thinking about it that some mothers find helpful is to bear in mind that you are giving your baby *everything* you have. You cannot give more than that.

Below I have listed the things which I feel are important for anyone who is breastfeeding with PLMS:

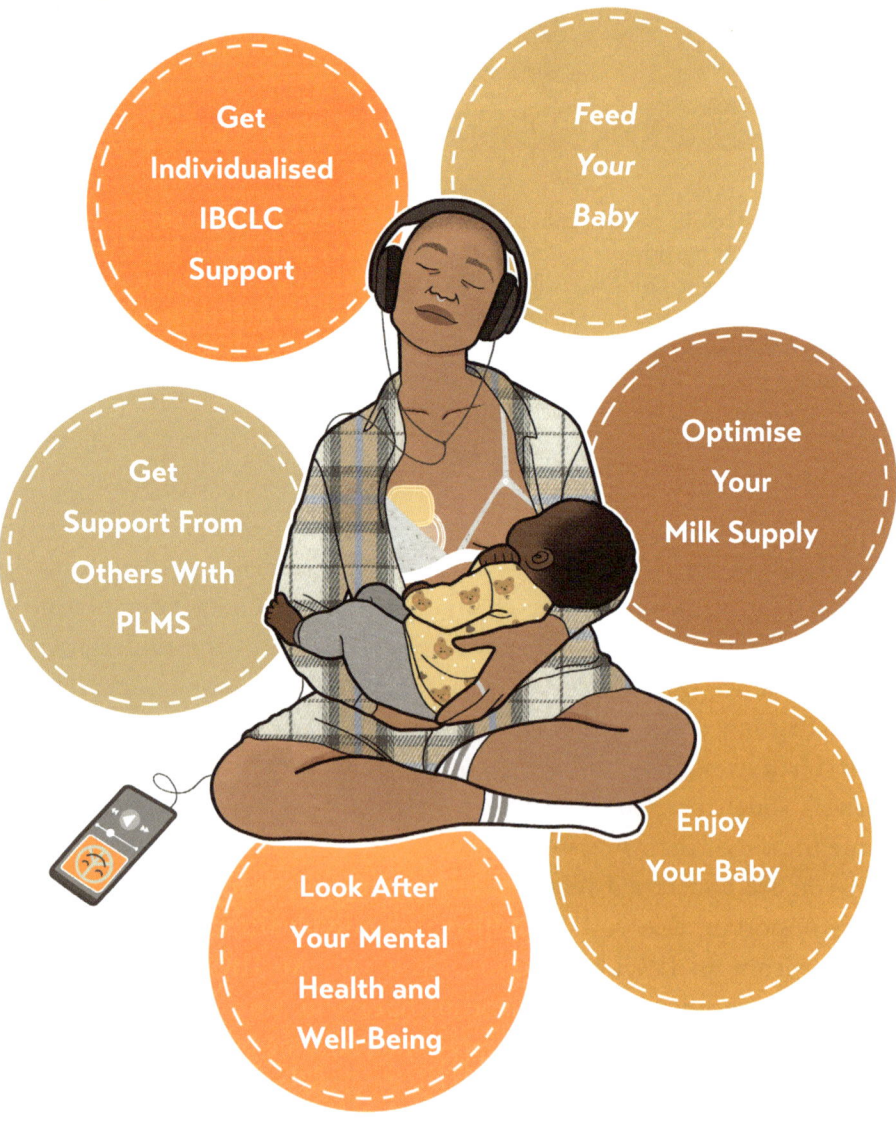

Individualised Support from an IBCLC

Individualised breastfeeding and lactation support is important for parents who have PLMS. This means working withing with someone who listens to you and who is prepared to help you find a way forward with your feeding journey that

- Aligns with what matters most to you and your feeding goals
- Works for your family
- You feel is manageable
- Will be sustainable
- Supports your mental health and wellbeing

The plan might be to breastfeed at every feed and supplement by bottle with infant formula a few times a day. Or it might be to breastfeed using an at-the-breast supplementer and pump a few times a day after feeds. Or the plan might have a focus on double-pumping. There is no one right way to approach breastfeeding with PLMS. Some mothers I work with express a strong desire to avoid pumping at all costs, while others are determined to maintain some pumping while they continue to breastfeed. Whatever plan you come up with should be sustainable and manageable.

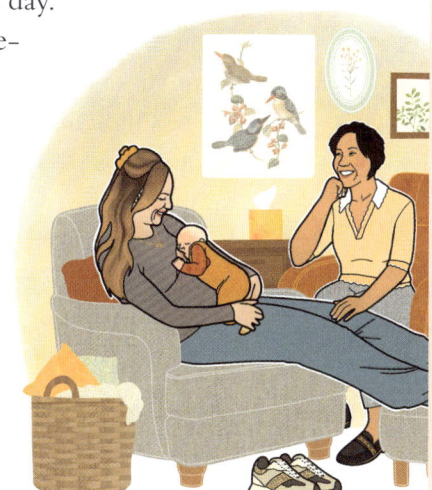

Feed Your Baby

Yes, I'm stating the obvious, of course you are going to feed your baby. The most important thing is to ensure your baby gets enough milk. Sometimes it can take time and some degree of trial and error to determine just how much extra milk your baby needs, and how you will combine breastfeeding with supplementation. Consideration needs to be given to what kind of milk you give your baby and *how* you give it to them. Do you give pumped milk, informally shared donor milk or infant formula (or a combination?) And how do you give it, by bottle or using an at-the-breast supplementer (or both)? Usually when I work with a mother who has low milk supply and advise supplementation, I will suggest giving a particular volume of milk every day for a week and then evaluating how that has worked. If the baby has gained a lot of weight, we might calibrate the volume down, but if the baby's weight has been below what we had hoped for, we'll calibrate the volume up. In this way, we determine an approximate volume of extra milk that the baby needs per 24 hours. This volume is not set in stone. As your baby grows and goes through growth spurts and developmental leaps, you might need to increase the volume for a time. Or there may be days when your baby doesn't need quite a much. It can be difficult at times figuring out how much extra milk to give, and for some mothers, anxiety inducing as they fear that giving more supplemental milk will lead to a decrease in their milk supply. I've heard many mothers describe breastfeeding and supplementing as being like "a balancing act" of trying to keep supplements to a minimum while trying to maximise breastfeeding. Try to take each day as it comes and reach out for support and reassurance when you need it.

> *If your baby needs extra calories, infant formula is a safe and an appropriate option. It does not take away from the benefit your baby gets from live cells in breastmilk. Sometimes supplementing with infant formula enables you to continue breastfeeding for longer.*

When to give your baby supplemental milk? Mothers are often advised to give a set amount of supplemental milk after every breastfeed, for example 40ml of formula, eight times a day. Your baby might not need this volume after every breastfeed as there are times of the day when you will be producing more milk, such as night-time and/or the morning. You baby might only need supplements from mid-morning or lunchtime – try to gauge this by looking at your baby. Do they seem to be asking for more after a feed or do they seem satisfied? It isn't always easy to tell, but be open to the possibility that your baby might not need supplementation after every feed (or might not need the same volume). For example, they might need 20ml after morning feeds and double that after afternoon and evening feeds. What matters is the total volume of milk your baby drinks per 24 hours. Being able to just breastfeed for some feeds means less work for you in terms of preparing supplemental feeds and cleaning and sterilising equipment.

Community-based Milk Sharing:

Some parents choose to supplement their babies with expressed breastmilk from other mothers. If you choose to do this, you will find useful information on the Eats on Feets website (www.eatsonfeets.com). The Human Milk 4 Human Babies Facebook pages and groups enable parents who wish to donate and receive milk to connect with each other.

Optimise Your Milk Supply

The main way you can optimise your milk supply is to encourage your baby to do lots of breastfeeding, assuming they are able to remove milk effectively. Try to get your baby to feed from both breasts at each feed or do switch nursing (switch frequently from one breast to the other during a feed – this helps to increase the volume of milk your baby drinks). Breast compressions can also help your baby to get more milk.

Another way to increase or optimise milk production is triple feeding – a regime of breastfeeding, pumping and supplementing. The extra milk removal from pumping, in addition to breastfeeding, can help to optimise milk production: more milk out = more milk made. However, pumping is not always necessary and some mothers with primary low milk supply choose not to pump and instead just focus on breastfeeding. Whether or not you pump is best decided in consultation with an IBCLC.

There are times when triple feeding can be necessary for a short time to increase milk production, but in the longer term, it isn't sustainable for most parents as it can negatively affect their mental health and get in the way of their enjoyment of the postpartum period. If you have been advised to triple feed, ask your IBCLC or healthcare professional how long they recommend you should do it. Triple feeding should always have a timeframe. Also, bear in mind that triple feeding doesn't have to be all or nothing. You could do one or two pumps a day rather than after every feed. Whatever you decide on should be manageable and not lead to overwhelm. In my practice, I see a lot of parents who have been advised to pump after every feed, for an unspecified length of time, and they generally end up exhausted and feeling as if they are on a hamster wheel. Please note: if your baby is unable to feed directly at the breast or is not transferring milk efficiently, regular pumping will be necessary to protect your milk supply.

Galactagogues are another option which can be considered to help optimise milk production. These are herbs, foods or medications that are said to increase milk production. Taking galactagogues will not result in significant increases in milk production but alongside adequate breastfeeding and/or pumping they might help to bump production up just a little bit. Read more about galactagogues in Chapter 15.

Enjoy Your Baby

When you have primary low milk supply, efforts to protect breastfeeding and increase milk production can become all-consuming and leave very little time to play with your baby or do fun things like go to a baby massage class. This is something to think about when you work

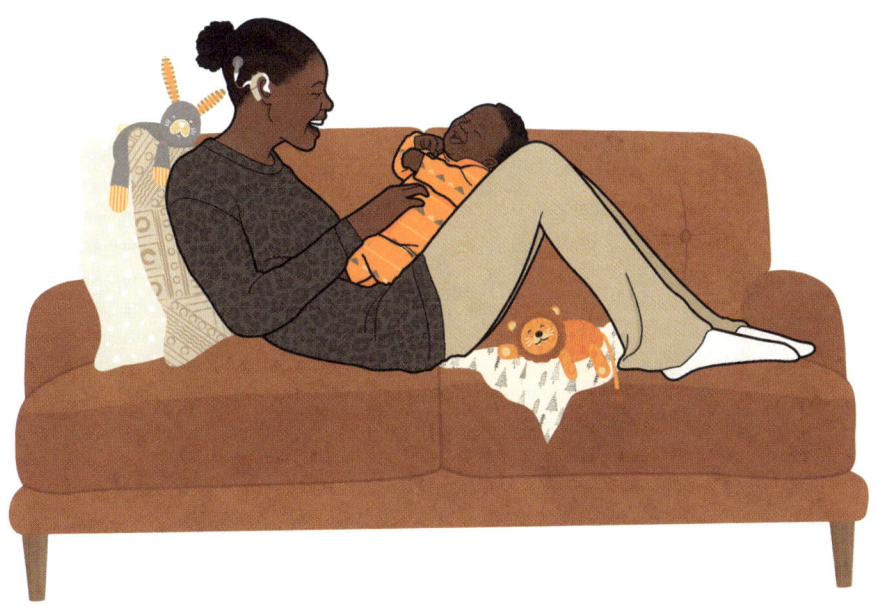

with an IBCLC on a care plan – does the plan allow for downtime? Or will it completely dominate your fourth trimester? It is important to have time in the day that is not taken up with feeding or pumping, so you can simply enjoy being with and getting to know your baby. Just chatting to your baby, cuddling them and playing with them are important forms of nurture too – it's not all about the milk.

Look after Your Mental Health and Well-Being

There is ample research which shows that breastfeeding difficulties such as primary low milk supply can negatively impact a mother's mental health and put her at greater risk of postnatal depression or anxiety. So, it's important that you have supports in place – support from a partner, from friends and family, peer breastfeeding supports – and that you know when to ask for help. If you are worried about your mental health, don't hesitate to chat to a healthcare provider about it. The sooner you get help the better. It's also important to be attuned to how breastfeeding and the efforts you may be putting into optimising your milk supply are affecting you. Acknowledge when you're feeling overwhelmed or exhausted, and when you need a break. If it's all too much, make changes. Talk to your IBCLC and tweak the plan to allow for more sleep, or less pumping or whatever it is you feel you need. Try to be gentle with yourself. In my experience, I find that mothers who have primary low milk supply tend to put huge pressure on themselves to do everything they can to protect breastfeeding and maximise their milk supply. But it is often to the detriment of their mental health and well-being.

Get Support from others with PLMS

When mothers first discover that they may have primary low milk supply, they are often shocked. They may have assumed they would be able to exclusively breastfeed and absorbed the narrative that low milk supply is very rare. This can make them feel alone and marginalised and they may feel reluctant to attend local breastfeeding support groups for fear of being judged. They may also feel disinclined to be around other mothers who they perceive to be having a perfect breastfeeding journey. However, I have found from working with many mothers with primary low milk supply that they derive huge benefit from peer support from other mothers who also have PLMS. The mothers report that they feel less alone, validated, listened to and seen. They also really value hearing other mothers' stories and picking up practical tips. Social media can be a great way to connect with other women who have PLMS. There are some dedicated low milk supply pages and groups. Or you could ask your IBCLC or a breastfeeding counsellor if they could point you in the right direction.

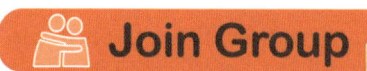

> *Some of the emotional burden of breastfeeding difficulties is relieved by having contact with and sharing experiences with other women having similar problems*
>
> Spannhake, 2021

At-the-Breast Supplementation (ABS)

At-the-breast supplementation is an alternative to bottle-feeding which involves giving your baby extra milk from a tube *while* they are latched and feeding at your breast. Some parents love it, some not so much, but it's worth considering if you are breastfeeding with PLMS.

Please note: ABS will only work well for babies who can latch well.

Benefits of ABS	Disadvantages of ABS
◊ It can help to protect the breastfeeding relationship as all the feeding is done at the breast ◊ It can help to optimise and increase milk supply (extra stimulation of nipple) ◊ Can foster bonding and attachment ◊ Babies are less likely to overfeed (compared to bottle) ◊ Some parents find ABS easier and less time-consuming than bottle-feeding ◊ It avoids the use of bottles and teats	◊ It can be tricky at the start. May require some getting used to. ◊ Some parents may be self-conscious using ABS. ◊ Spillage of milk can be an issue ◊ Not all babies will be happy to feed at the breast with ABS ◊ Sometimes older babies will pull at the tube

There are a number of different ABS products on the market, but before you purchase one I suggest you try using a 05Fr paediatric feeding tube with a feeding bottle (a homemade nursing supplementer). An IBCLC should be able to provide you with one of these tubes and help you get set up and get a feel for whether ABS will be an option for you and your baby.

How to use:

1. Put the supplemental milk in a bottle. Make a small incision in the teat (or push the teat to one side) and thread the tube through the opening.

2. Watch your baby while they breastfeed. When the flow of milk appears to slow down, gently insert around 2cm of the tube into the corner of your baby's mouth while they continue to suck.

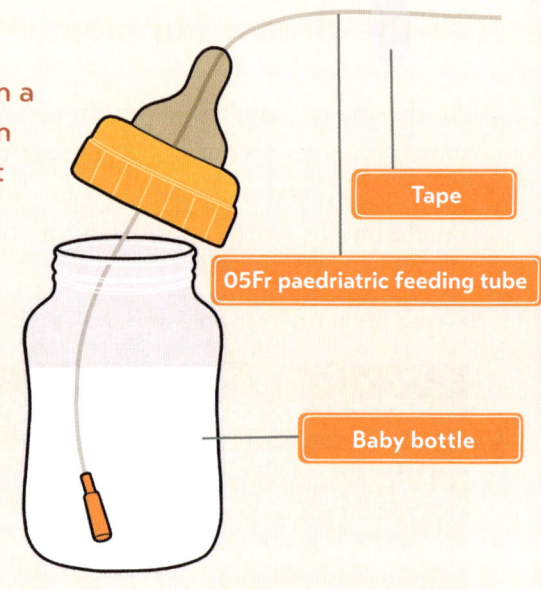

3. The higher you hold the bottle the easier it will be for your baby to get the milk flowing, so there will be some trial and error to start to find the optimal positioning of the bottle. Your baby should be able to get milk while sucking, but not be overwhelmed with milk or feed too fast.

4. Once your baby has settled into a nice sucking rhythm, you can use a little piece of medi-tape to hold the tube in place.

How to clean (you'll need a syringe):

1. After feeding, use a syringe to flush the tube with cooled boiled water.

2. Flush with hot soapy water.

3. Flush with warm water.

4. Dry the tube by pushing air through with the syringe a couple of times.

5. Place in a ziplock bag and store in the fridge.

PVC tubes can be used for approximately one week. Over time the PVC degrades and hardens.

Some mothers love supplementing with 05FR tubes and choose to continue using them for the duration of their breastfeeding journey. Others opt for one of the supplementers you can buy online such as the Medela SNS, the Haakaa Feeding Tube or the Lact-Aid System (it has to be imported from the US). Chat to your IBCLC and/or other mothers who have PLMS to help you decide if ABS is for you and if so, how you will do it.

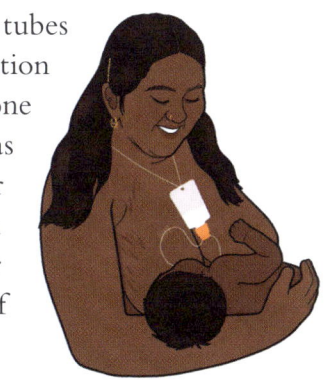

Secondary Low Milk Supply

Secondary Low Milk Supply is caused by *extrinsic* factors, meaning the causes are not related to your anatomy or physiology. When you have secondary low milk supply, something else is interfering with your potential to make enough milk for your baby. For example, one common cause of secondary low milk supply is if a baby does not breastfeed frequently enough to establish or maintain a full milk supply – in other words, insufficient milk removal. Things like scheduling feeds or supplementing with infant formula can result in less breastfeeding and lower milk production. The table below outlines possible causes of secondary low milk supply:

Not Enough Breastfeeding	Suboptimal Milk Removal	Medications/ Hormones
Scheduled/timed feeds	Submucosal cleft palate	Pseudoephedrine (Sudafed)
Just feeding on one side per feed	Tongue tie	Bupropion (Wellbutrin)
Not enough breastfeeds per 24 hrs	Recessed Chin	Certain antipsychotics
Supplementation with infant formula	Sleepy/late-preterm baby	Birth control
Giving baby a soother to stretch out the time between feeds	Sick baby, genetic condition	Smoking
		Postpartum Haemorrhage (PPH)
		Return of periods

Birth Control – Birth control pills that contain oestrogen and progestin can negatively impact milk production. However, most women find that the progestin-only mini pill does not result in a drop in milk production. Intrauterine devices (IUDs) are thought not to affect milk production, but a small number of mothers report that they do.

So how do you know if you have secondary low milk supply? You will probably experience many of the behaviours in the previous section on perceived low milk supply, but you will also probably notice

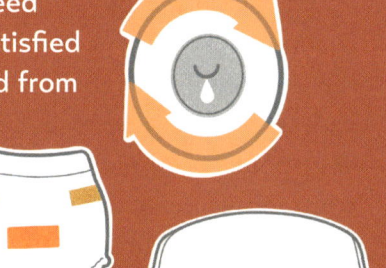

- that your baby appears to want to feed very frequently and doesn't seem satisfied after feeds, even when they have fed from both breasts

- a decrease in nappy output

- a drop in your baby's rate of weight gain

If you think you have secondary low milk supply, it is important to seek skilled support to help you determine what the issue is and how to increase milk production. Mothers who experience secondary low milk supply can usually regain full milk production.

Things you can to do increase your milk supply include

More breastfeeding! – Sometimes all it takes is a couple of extra feeds per 24 hours to turn things around. Try and get in a couple of extra feeds here and there, even for just a few minutes.

Switch Nursing – This is a term that is used to describe switching breasts more frequently during a feed. Rather than leaving your baby on one breast for a feed, switch them to the other breast as soon as they start to slow down or become sleepy. You might switch two or three times per feed. Doing this can help your baby to take more milk in one breastfeed.

Breast Compressions – This is another way to help your baby get more milk when they breastfeed. Look at your baby feeding. When they seem to slow down, gently squeeze and hold your breast for a few moments, then release. Doing this squeezes a little bit of milk out and encourages your baby to do more sucking. Watch how your baby responds to the compressions.

Skin-to-Skin – Try to do some skin-to-skin with your baby. This gives your baby an opportunity to hang out and breastfeed and can encourage the flow of oxytocin and this can positively impact milk production.

Take a Breastfeeding Holiday – The idea with a breastfeeding holiday is that you take a couple of days to focus on doing lots of close contact, cuddles and breastfeeding with your baby.

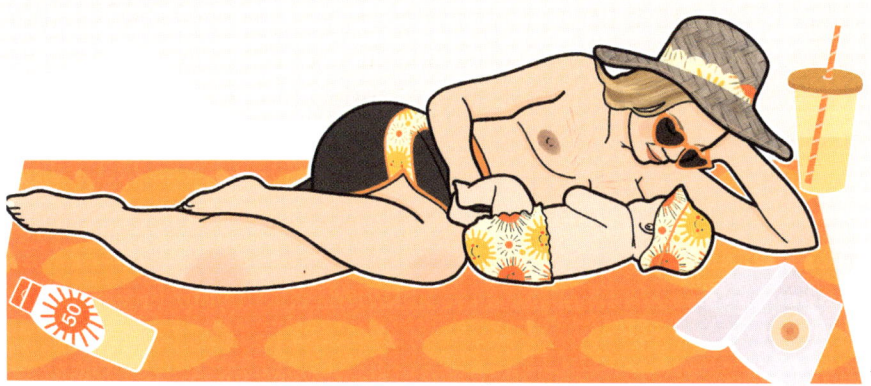

Other measures that some women try to increase their milk supply are pumping and taking some kind of galactagogue, ie, a herb or medication that is said to increase milk production. Simply taking galactagogues without increasing milk removal will not be effective in increasing milk supply. But taken in conjunction with the above measures, they might help. There is some evidence that taking 10mg three times daily of Domperidone per day (brand name Motilium) for a couple of weeks can help to bring your milk supply up, especially if you had a full milk supply and something happened to cause it to drop. Talk to an IBCLC about whether herbal galactagogues and/or Domperidone would be helpful for you.

If your baby is unable to remove milk effectively when they are breastfeeding, doing some pumping for a time might be necessary. Get some support with this to help you find a way to introduce pumping that is manageable for you. Any extra milk you get from pumping, you can feed to your baby.

If you can manage to increase your milk supply with all or a combination of the above measures, you may not need to supplement your baby. If supplementation is necessary, it might only be for a short time. An IBCLC will be able to help you determine if supplementation is needed, and if it is how much milk to give and for how long.

Using Infant Formula

Women who have low milk supply often struggle with the idea of supplementing their babies with formula as they may perceive it as bad, harmful and a threat to breastfeeding. It may take time to reconcile your use of infant formula if your intention had been to exclusively breastfeed. You might have to find a way to reframe it, from being the enemy of breastfeeding to being a safe product that provides your baby with the extra calories they need and allows you to continue breastfeeding. If you are supplementing with infant formula, your baby continues to benefit from the incredible live cells in your breastmilk.

Which formula to use? The range of different formulas sitting on the supermarket shelves can be mind-boggling – there are different brands, different stages, ready-made formula, powdered formula, goat's milk formula and specialised formulas for reflux and allergies. If your baby is less than six months, you should use a stage one formula. The brand you choose is up to you, but bear in mind that there is no brand that is superior to other brands as they all must comply with the same regulations on manufacture and composition. Mothers who are supplementing with small volumes often find the ready-made formula quite handy, but if you are giving larger volumes, using powdered formula would be more cost-effective.

How to prepare formula? It is important that you follow the instructions on the packaging of the powdered formula you're using. Sterilise the equipment you use. Make up a feed using boiled water that has been allowed to cool for 30 minutes. Formula preparation machines are not recommended due to concerns about their safety. Many of them don't heat the water up sufficiently to kill the bacteria in powdered formula.

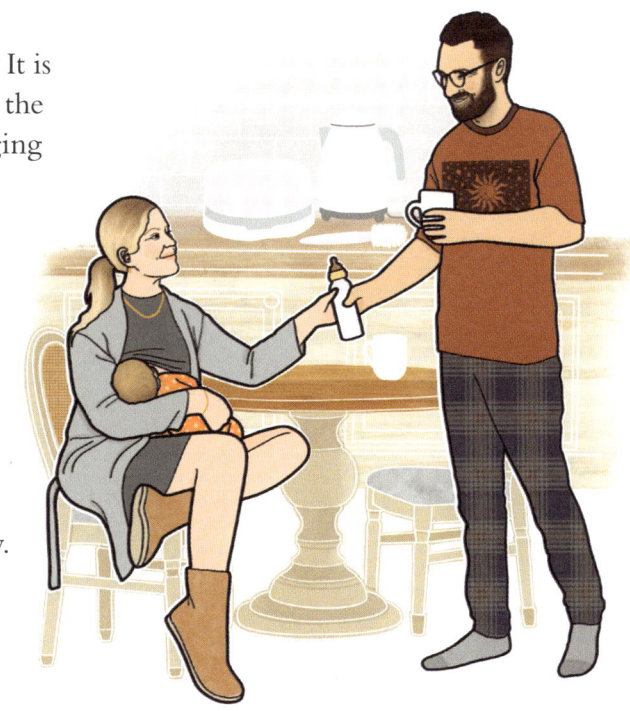

How much formula to give? This is something that an IBCLC or skilled breastfeeding supporter can help you determine. It will depend on how much milk you are producing and how much milk your baby needs for optimal growth. It can sometimes take a little bit of trial and error to arrive at an approximate volume per 24 hours. Bear in mind that this volume can change – for example, if your supply increases you might be able to reduce the volume of formula, but if your baby goes through a growth spurt you might need to increase it. You might not need to supplement at all feeds. Your own milk supply is probably bigger in the morning, so you may find that there are a couple of feeds where you don't need to supplement. Some mothers find that they can get through the night with just breastfeed and then give their baby supplements during the day. Everyone is different.

For how long will you have to keep using formula? It depends! Many mothers find that sometime between six months and twelve months they can stop supplementing. Again, a lot depends on what your milk supply is like and also how quickly your baby takes to solids. Some babies don't really get to grips with solids until they are closer to nine months.

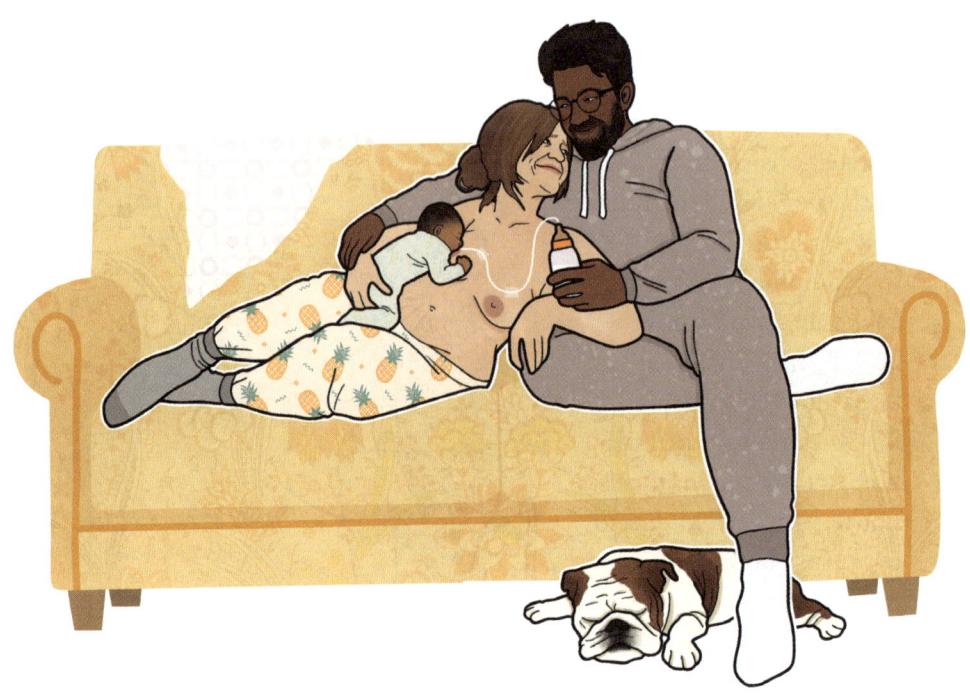

Can you mix formula and breastmilk? Yes, you can. Just be careful not to mix small volumes of breastmilk with large formula feeds because if your baby doesn't finish the feed you will have wasted some of your precious milk!

The First Steps Nutrition website is an excellent source of evidence-based information on all aspects of infant formula use: www.firststepsnutrition.org

The Emotional Impact of Primary Low Milk Supply

Being unable to exclusively breastfeed in the way that you had expected and having to supplement with infant formula can be a huge shock, and can result in a whole gamut of difficult emotions such as anger, grief, shame, guilt and sadness. The experience of having PLMS can also put you at an increased risk of postnatal mental health challenges such as anxiety and depression. Some mothers may find themselves becoming completely pulled into an obsessive focus on the numbers and on pumping, particularly those who may be autistic, neurodiverse or very left-brained. There isn't a quick way to process the emotional impact of having PLMS. Most mothers find it is a journey of working through the shock and the emotions to get to a place of healing and acceptance. It takes time. And requires sensitive and empathetic support from others – IBCLCs, healthcare professionals, partners, family, friends, volunteer supporters and/or other mothers with PLMS.

I've talked about the emotions around having a difficult breastfeeding experience in Chapter 13. Here I outline the journey towards healing and acceptance, because hard as it is, there is light at the end of the tunnel!

The First Three Months - The Emotional Whirlwind: This is probably the hardest time. You have to process the fact that you can't exclusively breastfeed, you may struggle to access the information and support you need, it's likely you will get conflicting advice from various sources and you will be confronted with a lot of unexpected emotions. Many mothers get caught up in an exhausting regime of triple feeding, where almost every waking hour is taken up with something to do with feeding or increasing supply. You throw everything at making breastfeeding work and feel an ever-present anxiety that you'll lose your milk supply or sabotage your breastfeeding relationship. It's hard. I don't think there's an easy way to avoid the emotions and feelings that come up when you're in this space, but the experience is definitely made easier by having skilled and peer support.

Three to Six Months – Making it Work: Usually breastfeeding with PLMS is easier during this period. The emotions you experienced during the first three months don't completely leave you, but you will probably be better able to deal with them. By now you will probably have a better understanding of PLMS and how you can balance breastfeeding and supplementation. You might still be doing some pumping but you will hopefully have found a way to work it into your day without feeling overwhelmed by it.

Six to Nine Months - Starting Solids: It's a huge achievement to get to six months and be still breastfeeding! While it is probably a lot easier than it was in the first few months, there are still some challenges during this time. Often mothers are given blanket assurances that they will be able to stop supplementing with infant formula altogether when their baby starts solids, or that they will be able to drop supplements during the night. This is not always the case. It can take time to get your baby established on solids, to gradually reduce supplementation and to figure out what your baby needs. This might be a good time to check back in with your IBCLC or talk to other mothers with PLMS who have some experiences they can share with you. Many mothers find that by nine or 10 months they can stop supplementing as their baby can get enough calories through direct breastfeeding and solid food. But some mothers will need to continue supplementing with extra milk.

Nine to Twelve Months – Finding Acceptance: I have found from working with mothers who have PLMS and from research I've conducted, that mothers really only start to find some degree of acceptance of having PLMS during this time. They start to realise how much they have done for their baby, the effort they have put in to providing milk for them, and how far they have come from the emotional upset and shock of the first few months. As they reflect, they are better able to acknowledge what they have achieved and start to feel proud of their efforts. Around this time, some mothers start to think about the possibility of having another baby and what breastfeeding with PLMS might look like second time around, and what they might do differently. It's normal to feel a mix of fear and hope when you think about breastfeeding a second baby. Whatever kind of experience you have it will be different, and you will be better equipped to deal with whatever it throws at you.

CHAPTER 15

Drugs, Food and Alcohol

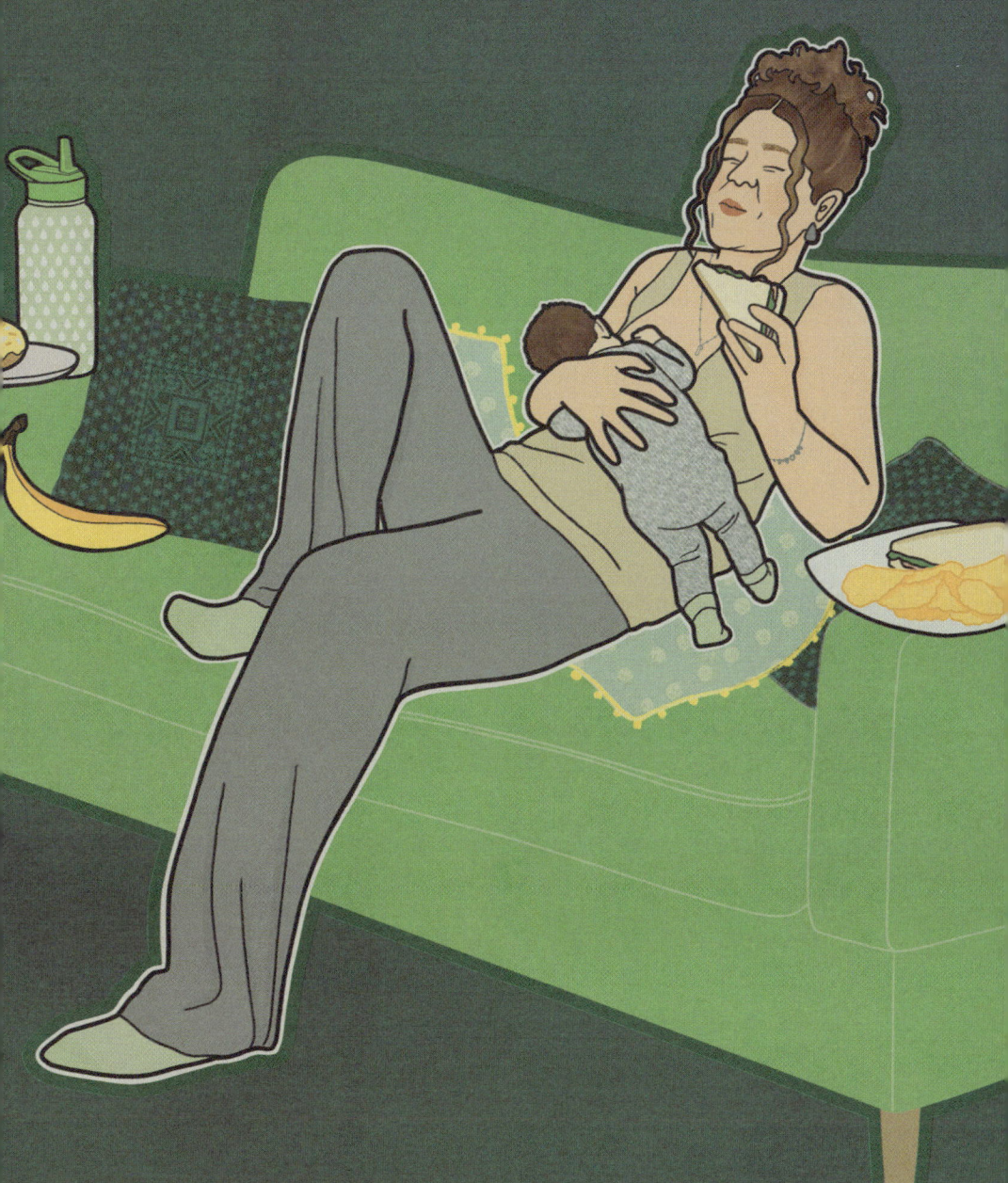

This chapter will tell you most of what you should know about lactation and over-the-counter and prescription medications, MRIs and ultrasounds, food, alcohol, cannabis and galactagogues. It will also point you in the direction of some trusted sources of online information to help you make evidence-based decisions.

Medications

Most medications are safe to take while you are breastfeeding and do not affect your milk supply. While drugs can pass into your breastmilk in small amounts, usually less than one percent a drug is passed to your baby. Only in very rare circumstances does a mother need to interrupt or discontinue breastfeeding due to taking a particular medication.

The information in this chapter is intended only as a guide and cannot replace medical advice from a healthcare professional (HCP) regarding your use of medications while breastfeeding. Always consult with an HCP if you are unsure about taking a particular medication and/or seek further information from The Breastfeeding Network website or helpline in the UK or St James's Hospital National Medicine Information Centre in Ireland. Some HCPs might be a little over-cautious in advising against continuing to breastfeed while you take certain medications, so don't hesitate to seek a second opinion if you've been advised to pump and dump or discontinue breastfeeding.

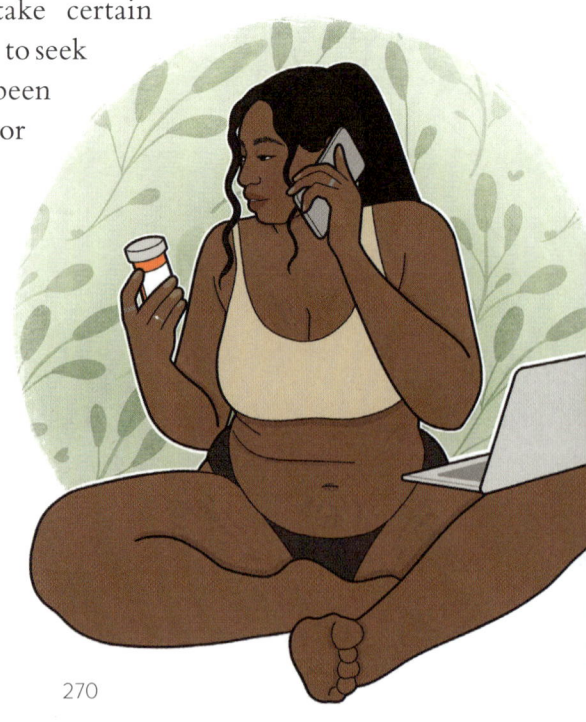

How much of a Drug you take is transferred into your Breastmilk?

This depends on a number of different factors – it's complicated, but here's a simplistic overview of some of those factors:

- **The size of the drug molecule (molecular weight)** – Drugs that have small molecules pass more easily from your bloodstream into your breastmilk, while drugs with large molecules are less likely to pass into your breastmilk.

- **The Milk-plasma ratio** – Plasma is the fluid in your blood which transports constituents such as red and white blood cells and platelets around your body. The milk-plasma ratio represents the amount of a drug in plasma relative to the amount that transfers into breastmilk. All drugs have different milk-plasma ratios.

- **Degree of Protein binding** – There are proteins suspended in plasma. Some drug molecules stick to these proteins, making it difficult for them to pass into breastmilk. Other drug molecules do not stick to proteins and are therefore pass more easily into breastmilk.

- **The Half-life of the Drug** – This is the time that it takes for the serum concentration of a drug to decrease by 50%. Drugs with a short half-life clear quickly through your system and if you are breastfeeding, are preferable to drugs with a long half-life. Paracetamol and Ibuprofen have short half-lives.

- **Bioavailability** – This is the percentage of a drug that passes into your circulation after your take it. The oral bioavailability of the baby is also a consideration – their stomach acid can degrade some drugs and limit how much passes into their bloodstream.

- **Fat Solubility** – Drugs which dissolve more easily in fat pass in higher concentrations into breastmilk.

- **Lactogenesis II** – Drug molecules pass more easily into breastmilk (colostrum) *before* milk starts to come in.

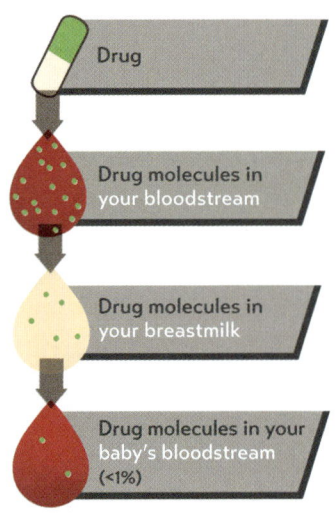

There are many other factors to consider when making a decision about taking a particular medication when you are breastfeeding – things like the age and weight of your baby, the timing of feeds, the volume of milk your baby consumes, and potential side effects for your baby. Talk things through with your HCP and look to trusted sources on medications and breastfeeding for information.

Is Botox® Safe when you're breastfeeding?

While there are no studies on onabotulinumtoxinA (Botox®) and breastfeeding, is thought to be safe when breastfeeding because it does not enter the bloodstream and would therefore be unlikely to pass into breastmilk. Caution may be advised if your baby is preterm or a neonate.

Commonly used Medications and Breastfeeding

Antibiotics	**Most antibiotics are safe to take while breastfeeding.** Your baby might have more liquid poos while you take an antibiotic, but this is not a reason not to take the drug.
Antidepressants	**Most antidepressants, such as selective Serotonin Re-uptake Inhibitors (SSRIs), are safe to take while breastfeeding.**
Antihypertensives (Blood Pressure Medications)	**These drugs are generally safe to take when breastfeeding,** but you might be advised to monitor your baby for drowsiness or poor feeding while taking them.

Antihistamines	**Non-sedating second-generation antihistamines are the preferred choice for breastfeeding mothers.** They can be taken safely for short periods of time. Taken long-term they can cause a baby to be drowsy. **First-generation sedating antihistamines should be used with caution.** Bed-sharing is not recommended, and babies should be monitored for drowsiness and irritability. **Prolonged use of antihistamines can cause a drop in milk supply.** Doxylamine (Cariban®) is commonly prescribed for hyperemesis. If you are nursing an older infant and taking Doxylamine, monitor them for signs of drowsiness or irritability. Doxylamine is not recommended for mothers who are nursing preterm babies or those less than one month of age.
Pain Killers/ Analgesics	**Paracetamol and Ibuprofen are safe to take when breastfeeding.** Aspirin is not recommended. Opioid painkillers are sometimes prescribed to mothers who have had a c-section. They are safe to take for short periods, but you may be asked to monitor your baby for feeding difficulties, sedation and breathing difficulties.
Anaesthetics	**Local anaesthetics are considered safe for breastfeeding mothers.** **In the case of General Aesthetic, a mother can resume breastfeeding once she is awake and alert.** There is no need to pump and dump.
Mood-Stabilising Medications	Decisions on the use of mood-stabilising or antipsychotic medications should be taken in consultation with your healthcare providers. **Some of these drugs are not considered compatible with breastfeeding.**
Antiseizure Medications (ASM) for Epilepsy	**Most ASMs are considered safe for breastfeeding mothers with epilepsy.**

Asthma Inhalers	Asthma inhalers are safe to use when breastfeeding.
Topical Acne Treatments	These treatments are poorly absorbed by the skin so very little of the active ingredients pass into breastmilk. Don't apply on your breasts and wash your hands well after use.
Domperidone	**Domperidone is safe to take when breastfeeding.** Read more about Domperidone on page 283.
Steroids	Steroids are safe to take when breastfeeding. However, high doses can cause a transient dip in milk production. Prednisolone is a corticosteroid used in the treatment of asthma, irritable bowel syndrome and Rheumatoid Arthritis. **It is considered safe for breastfeeding mothers in doses up 40mg daily.**
Decongestants	Decongestants do not pose a risk to babies, but **they can have an impact on milk supply so should be avoided by breastfeeding mothers.**
IVF Medications	**Letrozole is NOT compatible with breastfeeding as it poses risks to the baby.** There is limited information on other drugs and hormones used in IVF treatments. Discuss options with your healthcare providers. The closed Facebook group 'Breastfeeding Mums undergoing Fertility Treatment/IVF' www.facebook.com/groups/bfduringivf/ is a good place for information and support from other mothers.
Cancer Chemotherapy	**Many drugs used to treat cancer are toxic and therefore not compatible with breastfeeding.** There may be situations where a mother could pump and dump while undergoing treatment and resume breastfeeding a few days afterwards. These decisions can be made in consultation with your care team and by seeking guidance on specific medications from LactMed or the reference book 'Medications and Mother's Milk' by Dr Thomas Hale.

Radiology

In my experience, lactating parents are commonly given incorrect information about Magnetic Resonance Imaging (MRI) scans, mammograms and ultrasounds, X-rays and computed tomography (CT) scans done. These procedures *can* be done while you are breastfeeding and there is no need to pump and dump.

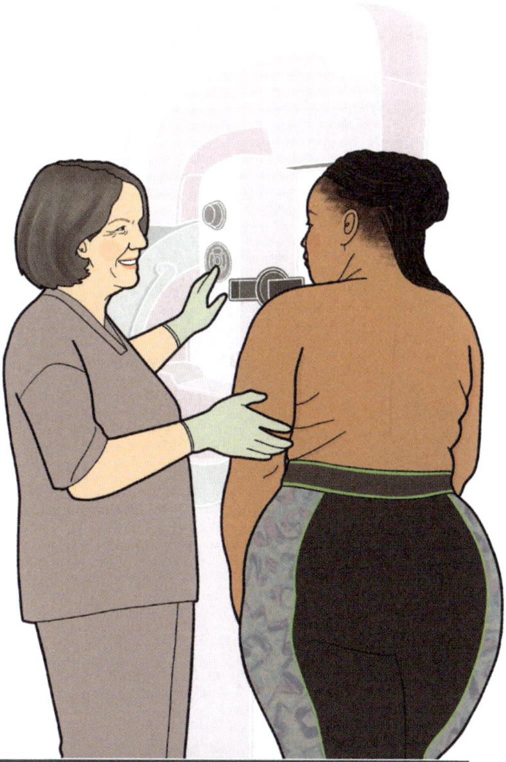

Is it safe to continue breastfeeding?

Procedure	Safe to Breastfeed?	Note
Mammogram	✓	Empty your breasts beforehand to improve the sensitivity of the test.
Ultrasound	✓	Empty your breasts beforehand to improve the sensitivity of the test.
X-ray	✓	Common X-rays are completely safe.
CT scan	✓	It is safe to continue breastfeeding after a CT scan with an iodinated contrast.
MRI	✓	Also considered safe. Only tiny amounts of the gadolinium contrast are absorbed by the baby.
Angiogram	✓	Completely safe.

Nuclear Medicine Scan	X	If possible, nuclear medicine scans should be delayed until the parent has stopped breastfeeding.
		Radioactive particles from the nuclear agent can pass into breastmilk so breastfeeding must interrupted for a time to avoid exposing your baby to a dose of radiation. The length of time that you have to stop breastfeeding for can vary, depending on the type of agent used. You can discuss this with the nuclear medicine specialist performing the test. www.trashthepumpanddump.com has detailed information on nuclear medicine scans and breastfeeding.
		Milk that you pump while breastfeeding is interrupted can be stored in your freezer. Over time it will lose its' radioactivity so you will eventually be able to give it to your baby.

Food

You don't need to eat a special diet to make nutritious milk that is perfect for your baby. Your breastmilk is synthesized from constituents in your bloodstream so, what you eat does not significantly affect its composition or your baby's health. And there are no foods that you should avoid. You will probably be a bit hungrier than usual (most breastfeeding women will need 300-500 extra calories a day) so it's a good idea to have plenty of snacks on hand. You may also find yourself thirstier than usual. A lot of breastfeeding mothers like to have a water bottle to drink from when they're breastfeeding, especially in the early days.

You might have heard old wives tales about having to avoid certain foods when you're breastfeeding, for example, that you should avoid cabbage, broccoli or spicy foods as they can make your baby gassy. This is not true. Or you might have been told that you have to drink plenty of cow's milk in order to make milk – also untrue! Have you heard that you should avoid carbonated drinks as they could carbonate your milk? You guessed it, this is also untrue. All you need to do is eat a normal, balanced diet. Eating a variety of foods and flavours can flavour your milk and increase the likelihood of your baby accepting similarly flavoured food when they start on solids.

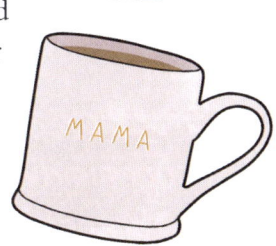

What about coffee? You can drink coffee when you are breastfeeding, however, it is recommended that you limit your intake to around 300mg per day (two to three cups). Some mothers find their babies are not sensitive to caffeine, while others find it can make their babies irritable – try and get a feel for what works for you and your baby.

Mothers often have concerns about Cow's Milk Protein Allergy (CMPA). This condition affects very few babies and omitting dairy products from your diet is rarely necessary. If there is a history of allergies in your family, or if you are concerned about allergic symptoms in your baby, talk to an IBCLC and/or your GP and seek a referral to a paediatric dietitian.

There is some evidence that eating peanuts during breastfeeding along with the early introduction of peanuts when your baby starts eating solid foods might play a role in preventing peanut allergies. Avoiding allergenic foods (such as cow's milk and eggs) during pregnancy and breastfeeding does not prevent food allergies in infants.

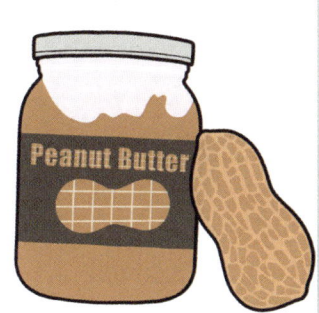

If you eat a vegetarian or vegan diet, you will need to ensure that you are getting enough iodine, Vitamin B12, Vitamin D and iron so that these nutrients are present in adequate levels in your milk. The milk of vegan and vegetarian mothers who meet these nutritional requirements is nutritionally equivalent to the milk of non-vegetarian mothers.

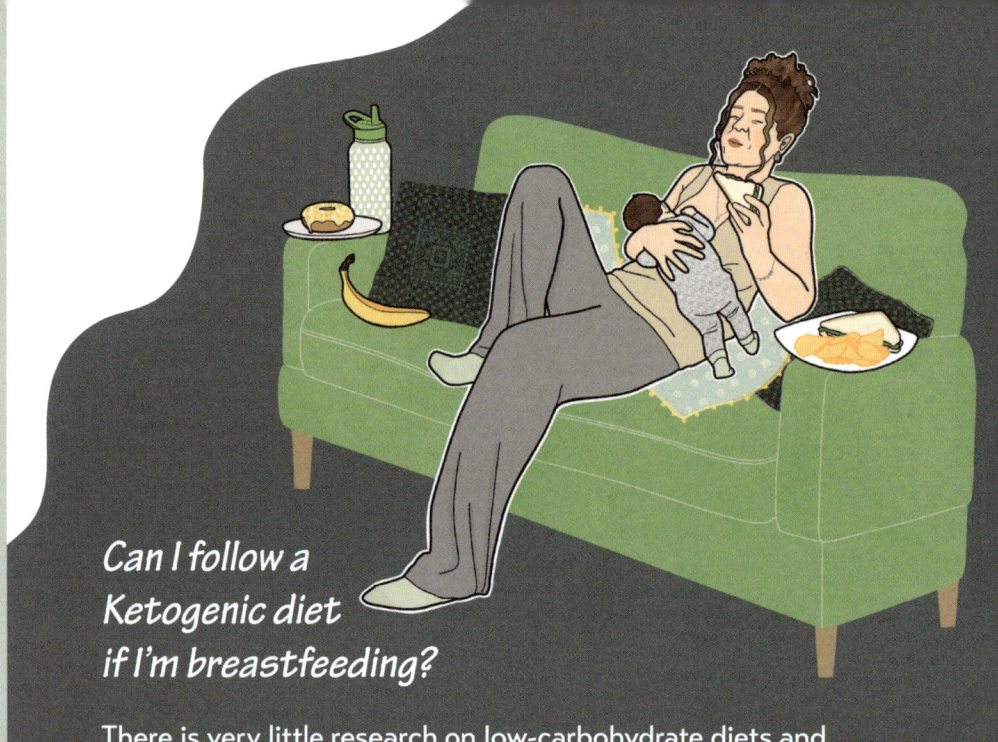

Can I follow a Ketogenic diet if I'm breastfeeding?

There is very little research on low-carbohydrate diets and breastfeeding, but there have been case studies of breastfeeding mothers who became very ill after following strict Ketogenic diets. It is thought that the increased energy demands of lactation coupled with restricted intake of carbohydrates led to ketoacidosis, a life-threatening condition whereby the body produces dangerously high levels of ketones and the blood's pH level becomes too low (acidotic). So, for now, the recommendation is that it is best not to follow a strict Ketogenic or low-carb diet when breastfeeding.

Alcohol

Alcohol passes easily into your breastmilk, but this doesn't mean you can't have a drink when you're breastfeeding. One unit of alcohol (a glass of wine or beer) clears from your bloodstream within an average of two hours from when you first start drinking. Two units of alcohol would take about four hours to clear, and so on. Once the alcohol has cleared from your bloodstream, it will have cleared from your breastmilk also. There are other factors that can influence the level of alcohol in your bloodstream and milk:

The amount of alcohol in your drink

Whether or not you eat something

How much you weigh

How long it takes you to finish your drink

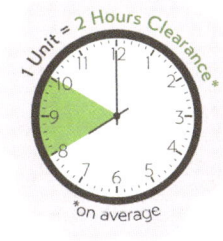

This means that you can have an occasional drink and not worry about harming your baby. If you have one drink, you can safely breastfeed your baby approximately two hours after you have finished your drink. Alcohol levels in your bloodstream peak 30 – 90 minutes after you have started drinking. To limit the amount of alcohol that you expose your baby to through breastfeeding, try to time feeds so that you feed your baby immediately *before* having a drink, and then feed them approximately two and a half to three hours later when the alcohol has cleared from your system (assuming you have had only one drink). Also consider the age of your baby. It is probably best to avoid alcohol in the first couple of months when your baby is very small. Older babies can metabolise alcohol more quickly than a younger, smaller baby.

What if your baby needs to feed before alcohol has cleared from your system? You could feed your baby milk that you expressed prior to having a drink. Even if you don't have expressed milk and your baby needs to feed, the risk to them is still quite low.

> This website has a handy Breastmilk Alcohol Content Calculator: www.milk-facts.co.uk

Do you need to *Pump and Dump*?

This term describes the practice of expressing breastmilk and pouring it down the drain instead of feeding it your baby. It is a common assumption that mothers should do this if they have consumed alcohol. But this is not the case. Pumping and dumping does not reduce the amount of alcohol in your bloodstream – only time will do that.

Other considerations if you drink alcohol:

- **If you drink alcohol, it is not safe to co-sleep with your baby** because doing so puts them at an increased risk of SIDS.

- If you've had quite a bit to drink – so many units that it would be unsafe for you to feed your baby – you may need to express milk for comfort and to protect your milk supply.

- If you get drunk (which of course is never a good idea), your baby should be cared for by another adult who is sober.

- If you are concerned about your drinking habits or if drinking alcohol is negatively affecting you, consider seeking help. There are many organisations that provide support for people who think they have a problem with alcohol. You don't have to hit "rock bottom" to need help for problem drinking.

Cannabis

There is limited research on cannabis use in breastfeeding mothers. The main psychoactive component in cannabis, tetrahydrocannabinol (THC), is very fat-soluble. This means that it stays in your system for longer and take weeks to clear from breastmilk. Studies on the effects of maternal cannabis use on breastmilk composition and on infants are inconclusive, but health guidelines recommend that cannabis use should be avoided by breastfeeding mothers and that cannabis should not be smoked by anyone in the vicinity of the baby.

Galactagogues

Galactagogues are herbs, food or drugs that are thought to have properties that help to increase milk production. Most mothers make plenty of milk for their babies and don't need to take anything to boost milk production. However, if you are struggling with milk supply, taking a galactagogue *might* help as part of an overall plan (which optimises milk regular removal with breastfeeding and/or pumping) to increase your supply.

Foods and Herbs

There is little evidence that certain foods or herbal galactagogues are effective in increasing milk production, but that's not to say they don't have any effect. Many mothers report that taking certain herbs and foods result in them making more milk. If you are interested in taking an herbal galactagogue, it would be best to work with an IBCLC to determine what herb might be most appropriate for you. You could also consider working with a Chinese medicine practitioner or an herbalist. These are some of the most commonly used herbs and foods for increasing milk production:

Fenugreek: There is some evidence that taking fenugreek leads to a small increase in milk production in mothers who already have a good milk supply, but unfortunately there are no studies on fenugreek use by mothers with low milk production. Fenugreek is not recommended for mothers who have type 1 diabetes or hypothyroidism as it can affect hormone levels in the body. Will fenugreek work for you? Maybe, maybe not. One thing to be mindful of when taking this herb is its pungent smell!

Moringa: Moringa oleifera leaf (in powder or capsule form, aka Malunggay) is thought to increase milk production by raising prolactin levels, but as with other galactagogues, there is little evidence to support this. It is considered safe to take and even if it doesn't increase your milk supply, Moringa is regarded as a nutritionally dense super food and anti-oxidant, so it might benefit you in other ways.

- ***Goat's Rue:*** Goat's Rue is an herb (nothing to do with goats) that is believed to improve milk production by stimulating the growth of glandular milk-making tissue in the breasts. It is usually recommended for mothers who have insufficient glandular tissue (IGT), polycystic ovarian syndrome or insulin resistance, and for people who wish to induce lactation.

- ***Shatavari:*** Shatavari is a type of wild asparagus plant used in Ayurvedic medicine. It is thought to help with milk production by increasing prolactin levels but there is little evidence for this.

- ***Torbangun:*** Torbangun has traditionally been given to postpartum women by Bataknese people in Indonesia as it is believed to enhance milk production. There are a few studies which have found Torbangun to be an effective galactagogue, but they are low quality. Some breastfeeding professionals recommend Torbangun for mothers with IGT.

- ***Lactation Cookies:*** These are biscuits/cookies containing certain ingredients that are said to increase milk production, for example oats and brewer's yeast. However, there is no evidence that consuming lactation cookies leads to an increase in milk production. They can make good, healthy snacks though so by all means enjoy lactation cookies - just don't expect that they will result in increased milk production.

- ***Oats:*** There is little evidence that eating oats increases milk production, but in any case, porridge is a great, nutritious start to the day.

There are many other herbs and foods which have reputed lactogenic properties. These include barley, brewer's yeast, garlic, quinoa, fennel, flaxseed, linseed, coriander, cumin, dill seed, blessed thistle, ashwagandha, aniseed, caraway seed, milk thistle and red raspberry. If you'd like to learn more about herbs and foods for lactation, I suggest you read the book 'Mother Food' by Hilary Jacobsen.

Please Note:

Some herbal galactagogues can interact with prescription drugs. If you are taking a prescription drug, talk to your GP or IBCLC to see if the herbal galactagogue you plan to take is suitable for you.

When you take an herbal galactagogue, it can take up to a week before you notice any impact on your milk supply.

When taking a herbal supplement, pay attention to any possible undesirable side-effects.

Pharmaceutical Galactagogues

There are no over-the-counter or prescription drugs that are licensed for increasing milk production. However, some drugs are known to affect milk production as a side-effect. The drug that is most commonly prescribed (off-licence) to people in the UK and Ireland for lactation is Domperidone (trade name Motilium).

Domperidone is an over-the-counter medication that is commonly used to treat nausea and stomach upset. One of the possible side-effects of Domperidone is raised prolactin levels, which in turn can lead to a small increase in milk production. Studies have found Domperidone to be effective in increasing milk production in mothers of both preterm and full-term babies, but no studies have considered its' efficacy in increasing milk production in mothers with primary low milk supply. Taking Domperidone can help in situations where a mother previously had a full supply and something happened that caused it to drop, but it is unlikely to increase milk production for mothers with IGT.

Before you consider taking Domperidone, talk to your GP and work with an IBCLC on other measures to increase your milk supply.

The recommended the dose of Domperidone for increasing milk production is 10mg three times daily for two weeks. Taking larger doses for longer periods does not result in a bigger increase in milk production, and is not recommended. Very small amounts of Domperidone pass into breastmilk.

Potential side effects of Domperidone are:

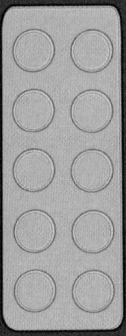

Dry mouth

Headache

Constipation

Upset stomach

Low/depressed Mood

Palpitations

Domperidone should not be taken with certain medications (such as Fluconazole, Erythromycin and SSRI anti-depressants) as doing so can cause a *prolonged QT interval*, or irregular heart rhythm. And it should not be taken if you have a family history of cardiac arrythmia or sudden death syndrome.

Gradual weaning off Domperidone is recommended. The Infant Risk Centre at Texas Tech University recommends that if you are taking 30mg of Domperidone a day you should reduce your dose over a two-week period by taking 20mg a day for one week, then 10mg a day the following week.

References

Domperidone for increasing breast milk volume in mothers expressing breast milk for their preterm infants: a systematic review and meta-analysis BJOG, LE Grzeskowiak, LG Smithers, LH Amir, RM Grivell: *International Journal of Obstetrics and Gynaecology*, 2018; 125(11):1371-1378

What Evidence Do We Have for Pharmaceutical Galactagogues in the Treatment of Lactation Insufficiency? – A Narrative Review, LE Grzeskowiak, et al, *Nutrients* (2019)

CHAPTER 16
Outside the Box Lactation

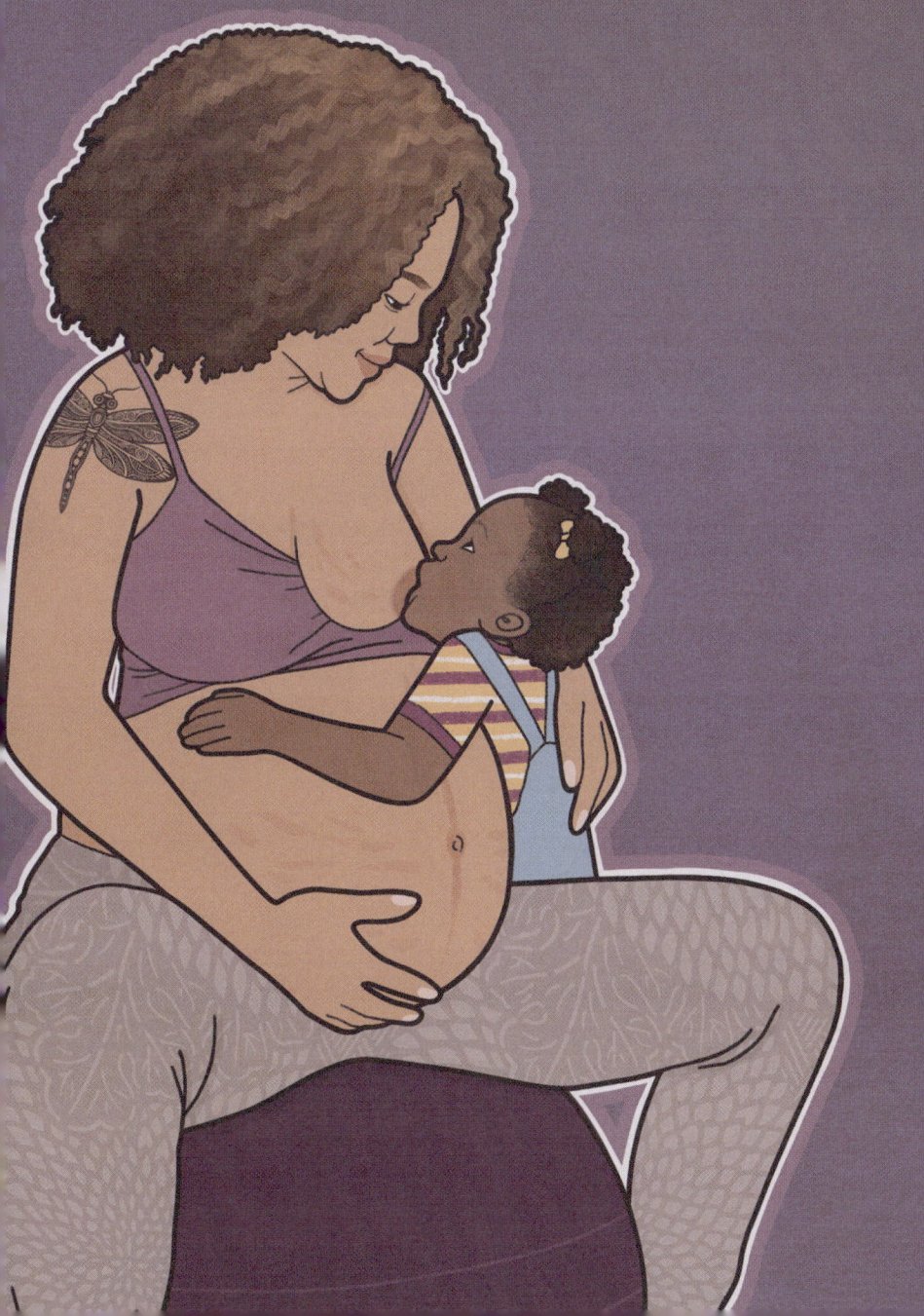

This chapter describes some less common breastfeeding or lactation scenarios. Parents often struggle to access evidence-based support when their lactation journey does not fit with the stereotype that most people imagine when they think *breastfeeding*. But breastfeeding and lactation can mean and be different things to different people.

Breastfeeding while Pregnant

Can you breastfeed when you're pregnant? Yes, you can! There is no clear evidence that breastfeeding while pregnant is related to birth outcome or miscarriage risk. However, if you have had miscarriages in the past or are having a high-risk pregnancy, seek guidance from your healthcare team about continuing to breastfeed.

If you breastfeed during pregnancy

- Your breasts and nipples may feel quite tender during the first trimester. This might make breastfeeding uncomfortable.

- Pregnancy hormones can cause a dip in milk production. This can be a factor in some infants self-weaning.

- The taste of your milk changes during pregnancy. This is can also be a factor in infants self-weaning.

- The milk that you produce during your pregnancy continues to be nutritious and beneficial for your infant.

- Your body can support your growing foetus, provide milk for your infant and stay healthy so long as you eat well and look after yourself.

- There is no correlation between breastfeeding during pregnancy and lower birth weights.

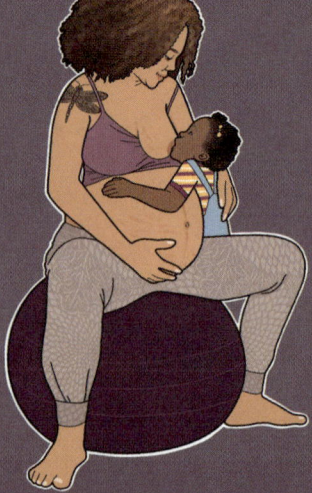

Some mothers love the experience of breastfeeding during pregnancy and feel that it helps them maintain a nurturing bond with their infant during a time of change. For other mothers, it may not be such a pleasant experience. Some find that breast sensitivity can make breastfeeding painful or that pregnancy hormones can cause some degree of breastfeeding aversion. Go with what *feels* right for you.

Tandem Breastfeeding

Tandem breastfeeding is when you feed a newborn baby while also continuing to feed an older sibling. There are benefits – it can help your toddler adapt to the changes that come with having a new sibling, it can help you maintain a strong connection with your toddler and it helps to ensure you have a good milk supply. Also, toddlers can be very helpful if you become engorged!

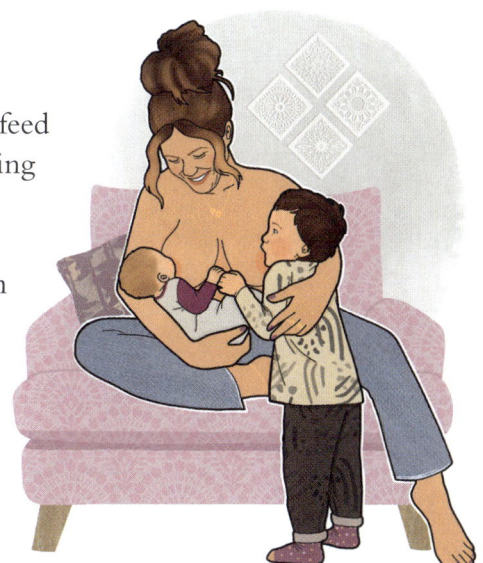

Here are a few tips to help you manage tandem feeding:

◊◊ *Prioritise the new baby.* Ensure they are getting enough milk by feeding them first, or at the same time as your toddler.

◊◊ It's okay to have some *boundaries for your toddler* to help them understand that the new baby needs to breastfeed first, or that there may be times when you say no to breastfeeding.

◊◊ *Be flexible* and give yourself some time to figure out how tandem feeding is going to work for you. You might love it or you might find it overwhelming.

Relactation

Relactation is when a mother restarts milk production after a break of weeks, months or even years. There are a number of reasons why a mother might decide to relactate:

- Regret or unresolved feelings about stopping breastfeeding
- Breastfeeding had to be interrupted due to illness and medical treatment
- A desire to provide breastmilk for a sick baby or family member
- Wanting to breastfeed an adopted baby
- In a lesbian relationship, a woman (who has previously breastfed) may wish to co-nurse a baby that her partner has given birth to

While relactation is possible, it isn't always easy. It takes time, patience, commitment, and support from a partner and/or family. It is important to have realistic expectations when you are trying to relactate. There are no absolute guarantees that you will get the results you want. Some mothers will manage to reestablish lactation but may struggle to get their baby to resume direct breastfeeding, while in some cases a mother will be unable to achieve a full milk supply but will succeed in getting her baby back to the breast. Also, some mothers who attempt to relactate decide at some point in the journey that it's not for them. I find from my work with these mothers that even if they decide not to continue with relactation, they gain a sense of having gotten something out of their system through giving it a go, and rarely regret having tried. Sometimes it's about the journey, rather than reaching the goal.

Relactation is generally easier if you previously had a full milk supply and if the time that has passed since you stopped lactating is relatively short. If you decide you would like to relactate, it is advisable to have the support of a an IBCLC and/or an experienced voluntary breastfeeding supporter.

How to Start the Relactation Process

Before you start the process of relactation, give some consideration to what your goals are. Is it to get your baby feeding at the breast or is it more about the milk? How will you feel if relactation doesn't give you the results you want? Have you talked through your wish to relactate with your partner or family? Do they understand why relactation is important to you? Have you debriefed what caused you to stop breastfeeding?

These are some factors that could help you to relactate and re-establish direct breastfeeding:

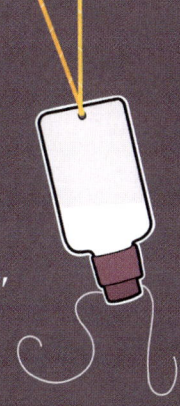

- *Breastfeeding using an at-breast supplementer* – if your baby is willing to latch, you could start giving them supplemental milk at the breast. The stimulation of your nipples will help to encourage your body to start making milk again.

- *Pumping* – If your baby is not latching, initiating double pumping (ideally 8 – 10 times per 24 hours, but as often as you feel you can manage) will help to restart lactation. Combine the pumping sessions with massage and hand expression. Warm your breasts and the flanges before pumping. It can take time before you start producing milk.

- **Skin-to-skin** *with your baby* will help to encourage the flow of oxytocin and may entice your baby to latch and suckle if they aren't already doing so.

- **Co-bathing –** This can be a lovely calming way to do skin-to-skin with your baby. For some mother and baby dyads, it can be a healing, rebirthing sort, back to basics sort of experience that can result in a non-latching baby showing willingness to breastfeed.

- **Tell your Baby about your wish to Relactate –** Your baby won't understand, but they may intuit some of the sentiment you convey.

- **Sleepy Feeds –** If your baby is continuing to have milk in a bottle, giving them time snuggled in close your breasts after feeds could help to establish a positive association with being at the breast and encourage them to latch (non-latching babies may be more willing latch when they are half-asleep).

- **Domperidone –** Some mothers choose to take Domperidone to help increase milk production. There is more information about Domperidone in Chapter 14.

- **Online Support –** There are relactation-specific support groups on Facebook (search 'relactation' under Groups). US-based IBCLC Alyssa Schnell runs a free online support group for parents relactating and inducing lactation www.alyssaschnellibclc.com/signup.

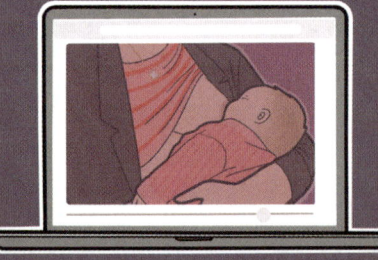

- **Patience –** Be patient with yourself and with your baby. It can take weeks and even months to get to a place you are happy with. It might not unfold in the way that you had hoped, so try to be accepting of the outcomes and of feelings that arise during the process. Some mothers find it helpful to keep a journal.

Please note: These are general guidelines. Working with an IBCLC with help you create a tailored plan.

Getting an older baby back to the breast can be challenging. A couple of ways that mothers I have supported found helped were

- showing the baby breastfeeding videos on YouTube
- co-sleeping for a few hours in the early morning
- attending a breastfeeding support group where the baby can see other babies breastfeeding

Any amount of milk you produce or any skin-to-skin or nursing your baby does is a win. Relactation does not have to be all or nothing.

Induced Lactation

Induced lactation is a term that describes the process whereby a non-birthing parent who hasn't previously breastfed or lactated, follows a protocol to encourage their body to start producing breastmilk. Induced lactation is most commonly practiced by parents who wish to breastfeed an adopted baby, or a baby born to a surrogate mother. Non-birthing parents in a same-sex relationship or transgender women may also sometimes choose to induce lactation so that they can have a breastfeeding relationship with their baby.

How do you induce lactation?

There are different protocols for inducing lactation, but they all involve three main steps:

1. **Prepare the Body to start making milk:** This happens two to six months before you baby arrives or is born. It may involve breast massage and pumping or taking a combination of lactogenic herbs and/or medications. The herb mostly commonly recommended to help breasts prepare for lactation is Goat's Rue. The Newman-Goldfarb protocol stipulates taking birth control pills (to trigger

the kind of breast growth that happens during pregnancy) and Domperidone.

2. **Start to Make Milk Before Baby Arrives:** This stage starts one to two months before your baby arrives and involves breast massage, pumping, and hand expression. Some protocols recommend continued use of herbs and Domperidone. Milk that you produce during this stage can be frozen and given to your baby when they arrive.

3. **Breastfeed and Continue to Make Milk:** When the baby arrives, you breastfeed them using an at-the-breast supplementer. You might also continue to pump and take herbs and/or Domperidone.

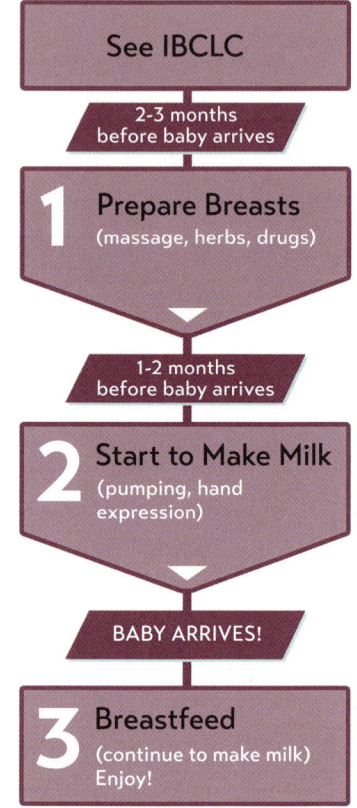

Please note: I've simplified the steps involved in inducing lactation here. If you want to induce lactation, work with an IBCLC and your GP to determine the most appropriate protocol for you. I also recommend you read the book *Breastfeeding without Birthing* by Alyssa Snell and Google 'Newman-Goldfarb Protocol.'

Induced lactation may not result in you having a full milk supply, but this doesn't mean you can't have a long-term breastfeeding relationship with your baby. Many parents breastfeed and supplement at the breast or by bottle. Breastfeeding is not just about food. Even if you make very little milk, both you and your baby can benefit from the emotional nurturing that happens when your baby is at the breast.

If you induce lactation, the first milk you make will be mature breastmilk. You will not produce colostrum. If you would like your baby to have colostrum, you could ask the surrogate mother to express colostrum antenatally or during the first couple of days postpartum.

Inducing lactation is a big undertaking. It requires commitment, time, patience and support from your partner and/or family members. Some people find it emotionally and physically exhausting, but it can also be very rewarding as it can result in you having a breastfeeding relationship with your baby that you might not otherwise have had.

Co-nursing in Same-Sex Relationships

A non-birthing parent in a same-sex lesbian relationship can relactate (if they have previously breastfed) or induce lactation so that they can be involved in breastfeeding or providing milk for their baby (or babies). Being able to breastfeed may help them with bonding and positively influence how they feel about themselves as a parent and how they feel about their body (particularly if they were unable to become pregnant).

When the baby is born, it is important for the birthing parent to do most of the breastfeeding in the first few weeks in order to establish a good milk supply. Once their milk supply is established, the non-birthing parent can get more involved with breastfeeding. It's going to be up to each couple to figure out what co-nursing is going to look like for them. It might end up being half and half, or it might be a case that the non-birthing parent just does a few feeds per day. Or one parent might pump milk and store it for future use. It's okay to not be sure how it's going to work out – feel your way along and give yourself latitude as a couple to learn as you go.

A great resource for people wishing to induce lactation is the Breastfeeding Outside the Box podcast. I would also recommend finding support within the LGBTQI+ community and working with professionals who understand your needs as a family.

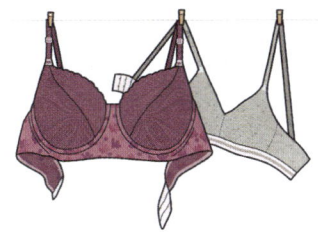

Trans and Nonbinary Lactation

We've all become much more aware over the last number of years that not everyone identifies with the gender they have been assigned at birth, and with the concept that both gender identity and orientation can be fluid. What this means for those of us who work in the lactation field is that we've had to shift how we conceive of breastfeeding, from a heteronormative practice that only cis women who have given birth can experience, to something that potentially any parent or primary caregiver can do. Some parents prefer not to use the word breastfeeding to describe how they feed their babies and instead opt for terms such as *chestfeeding, bodyfeeding, nursing, human milk feeding or just feeding*. In 2016 a gay transgender man, Trevor McDonald, wrote a memoir about his experience of male pregnancy, gender dysphoria and chestfeeding with donor human milk (using an at the breast supplementer). This book created much more awareness of what it is like to be a chestfeeding transgender parent.

Transgender women can also nurse their babies. Although they cannot become pregnant, they can induce lactation – some even manage to achieve a full milk supply. The milk that transgender women produce is nutritionally equivalent to the milk that cis women produce and is 100% safe for their babies.

There are many different factors that influence how much milk a person can produce, be they transgender, cisgender or non-binary. They include

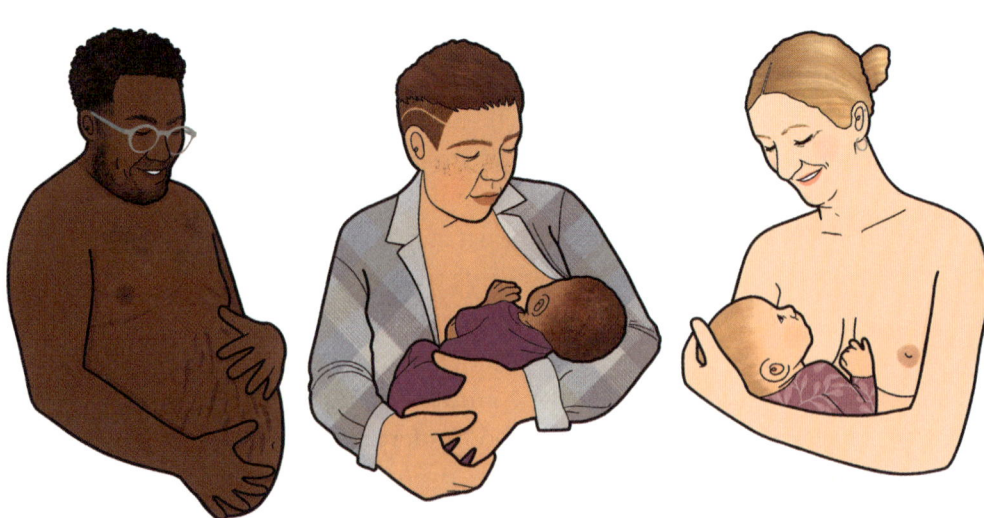

- Whether they are the gestational parent
- The amount of glandular tissue they have (even trans men who have had top surgery can have some amount of glandular tissue)
- Specific techniques that were used for breast/top surgery
- Hormone therapy and medications the person is taking
- Whether they have had genital affirming surgery
- Levels of endogenous hormones
- What happened during puberty – was it experienced as a male or a female?

It's complicated and not always easy, but there are numerous possibilities for lactation. Whatever the outcome, chest, breast or body feeding is not just about milk. It's about nurturing and connection too. If you are a non-binary or trans parent and wish to make milk for your baby and/or chest/breastfeed them, seek out skilled support from an IBCLC and healthcare professionals who provide gender-inclusive care to people in the LGBTQIA+ community. Support and information from other trans and nonbinary parents is available from a closed Facebook group called 'Birthing and Breast or Chestfeeding Trans People and Allies.'

Breastfeeding Twins

Can you breastfeed twins? Yes, you can! Women can even breastfeed triplets! Human bodies can do amazing things. Most women who have multiple births can make enough milk to exclusively feed their babies, so long as they have adequate support. It is more difficult in the early days than establishing breastfeeding for a singleton baby, but it does become easier over time.

Some tips for before you have your babies:

 Attend a breastfeeding class* and/or a one-to-one antenatal session with an IBCLC.

 Check out breastfeeding support groups and join the 'Breastfeeding Twins and Triplets Support' Facebook group.

 Inform your care providers that you intend to breastfeed.

 Twins are more likely to be preterm, late preterm or early term, and born by c-section. Talk through these scenarios with your care providers.

 Consider expressing colostrum antenatally. Ask about the policies in your maternity hospital for mothers expecting twins or triplets.

 Talk to your partner about your wish to breastfeed. Let your family and friends know that you're planning to breastfeed, and that it matters to you.

 Line up support for the postpartum period. You are going to be busy caring for your babies. Can you enlist help from other family members or hire a postpartum doula?

 Try to maintain realistic expectations of yourself in the postpartum period. Your time will be taken up with caring for your babies and feeding them. It's okay if that's all you do for a few months!

 Buy the excellent 'Breastfeeding Twins' book by Kathryn Stagg.

After Your Babies have Been Born

If your babies are born prematurely, they will have to spend some time in the NICU. They might be tube-fed initially. If this is the case, it is important that you establish your milk supply so that you can provide colostrum and milk for the babies while they are in the NICU and so that you will have an adequate milk supply further down the line. How to do this? In the first 48 hours, hand express every two hours, and then switch to double pumping every three hours. The staff in the NICU will support you with this. They will also help you to transition to direct breastfeeding when your babies are ready to do so.

If your Babies are born a little early but don't have to go to the NICU (for example if they are 35-38-ish weeks) they might be able to do skin-to-skin and have their first feed at the breast. However, even though your babies might initially look and behave like full term babies, they will probably need some help with feeding in the first weeks. This is because they are not developmentally ready for full breastfeeding (a lot of important brain growth happens in the last couple of weeks in utero) – they may be sleepy, a little bit jaundiced and not be able to feed well enough to get the milk they need or to establish your milk supply. If this is the case you will have to express extra milk to supplement your babies with, while you continue to breastfeed. This is a short-term measure, to ensure that your babies get enough milk and that you protect your milk supply, until such time that they are ready to exclusively breastfeed.

If your Babies are Born Full Term, or close to Full Term (38/39-ish + weeks) they may be able to do skin-to-skin with you and have their first feed at the breast. If they are both able to feed well (a midwife or IBCLC will help you assess how they are feeding), it's possible that you can just continue with direct breastfeeding. You might be able to feed both of them together from the get go, but very often mothers will feed their babies one at a time to start, as they build their own confidence in breastfeeding and get to know how each baby is breastfeeding. Feeding the babies on demand in the early weeks will help to build your milk supply.

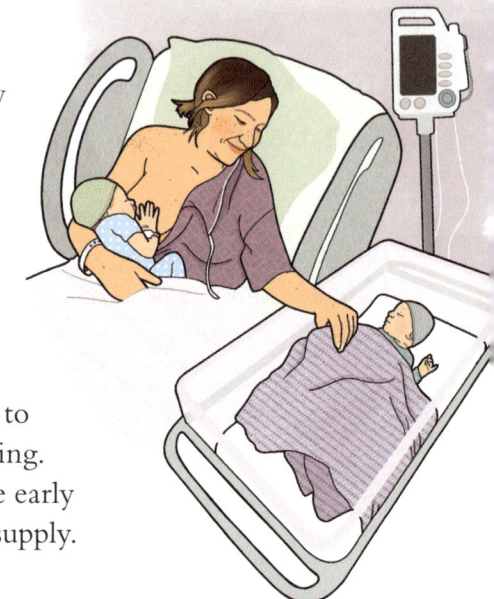

Success doesn't look the same for everyone. As a mother of twins you might

- Exclusively breastfeed both babies
- Exclusively pump milk for your babies
- Breastfeed one baby and bottle-feed the other baby
- Breastfeed and supplement your babies with formula
- Breastfeed for a short time and then switch to formula feeding

Whatever way you feed your babies, any amount of breastmilk or breastfeeding is a win!

Tandem Feeding

Tandem feeding is feeding both babies at the same time. If you are able to master it, it saves time. It might not always be possible in the first few weeks, but it is

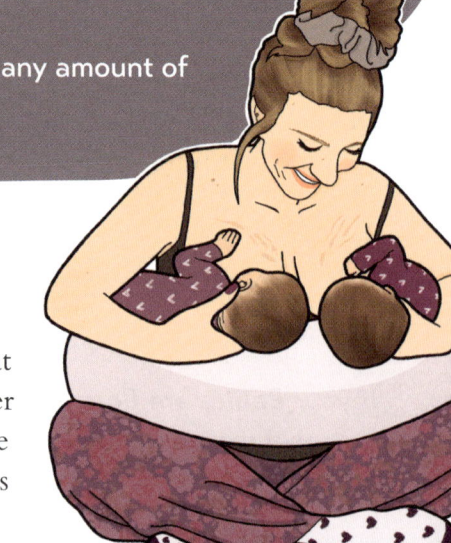

definitely worth trying it. There will be times when one baby wants to feed and the other doesn't, but even doing some tandem feeds can make life a little easier. Alternate the babies on your breasts (ie, don't assign one breast to each baby). Some mothers find that using a good twin nursing cushion can help with tandem feeding.

Triple Feeding

Many mothers who have twins start off their feeding journey by *triple feeding* – doing a mix of breastfeeding, pumping and bottle-feeding. This may be necessary for a time until both babies are developmentally ready and have the stamina to just breastfeed. While you are triple feeding, it's important to get help with a manageable plan that you're able to follow.

If you are tandem feeding your routine might look something like this (every three hours):

1. Breastfeed the babies
2. Give the babies a supplement by bottle (one at a time, or at the same time if you have someone to help)
3. Double pump for 15-ish minutes

If you are feeding your babies one at a time, your routine could look like this:

1. Breastfeed baby 1
2. Breastfeed baby 2 while a helper else gives baby 1 a bottle supplement
3. Double pump while your helper gives baby 2 a bottle supplement

The whole breastfeed/bottlefeed/pump cycle should take under an hour. See Chapter 10 for more tips on triple feeding.

Triple feeding is a temporary measure to ensure your babies get enough milk and that you protect your milk supply. It should have some kind of timeframe. This is something you can discuss with your IBCLC, or whoever is supporting you with breastfeeding.

Lactation After Loss

Whether it's through miscarriage (0-20 weeks), perinatal death (20 weeks-birth), neonatal death (birth-28 days) or the loss of an older infant, the loss of a baby or infant is devastating and immensely difficult for parents to make sense of. Amid the grief, shock, and emotional distress mothers may have to deal with the reality that their bodies will continue to lactate (if lactation has already been established and they have been providing milk for their baby) or that their milk will come in a few days after the birth of their baby (in the case of a perinatal or neonatal death). A decision about how to manage lactation while grieving is an intensely personal one that can be facilitated by sensitive support from a bereavement midwife and/or IBCLC. Some parents will choose to suppress lactation while others will opt to express their milk and donate it to a human milk bank. There is no right or wrong. It's about trusting what your heart and your body tell you is the right thing for you.

Suppressing Lactation after Loss

It can sometimes come as a shock to mothers that their bodies will start making milk after the loss of their baby. There is no way to stop this happening but there are measures you can take that will make the process as gentle as possible. Your healthcare team will support you with this.

If you have experienced a miscarriage, a perinatal death or your baby dies before your milk comes in the following measures will help to suppress the onset of full milk production and keep you comfortable:

- Wear a snug-fitting bra day and night.
- Try to touch your breasts as little as possible.
- Use breasts pads to soak up milk.
- Place cabbage leaves (straight from the freezer) in your bra to help relieve engorgement.

- Apply ice packs or cold compresses to your breasts if they feel very warm. This can reduce pain and engorgement.

- Ibuprofen or paracetamol will also help to reduce pain.

- If your breasts feel very full, hand express a little bit of milk – just enough that you feel more comfortable.

- Stay hydrated.

- Herbs like peppermint, sage and parsley can help to downregulate milk production.

If you have been breastfeeding or pumping for your baby when they die, you will need to reduce your supply over a period of time by gradually reducing the amount of milk you express from your breasts. An IBCLC will provide you with an individualised plan that will enable you to do this safely, so that you don't get mastitis and that your hormone levels can return to normal gently – reducing your supply too quickly can result in a sharp drop in mood. At each pumping session, remove as much milk as you need to feel comfortable. Over time the volume of milk you need to pump to feel comfortable will reduce. You can also try to drop a pumping session every few days. The time that it takes to completely stop lactation will vary for individuals, but many women find it takes approximately two weeks.

In some situations medications (Bromocriptine or Cabergoline) can be taken by a mother to prevent or suppress lactation. This can be discussed with your care team.

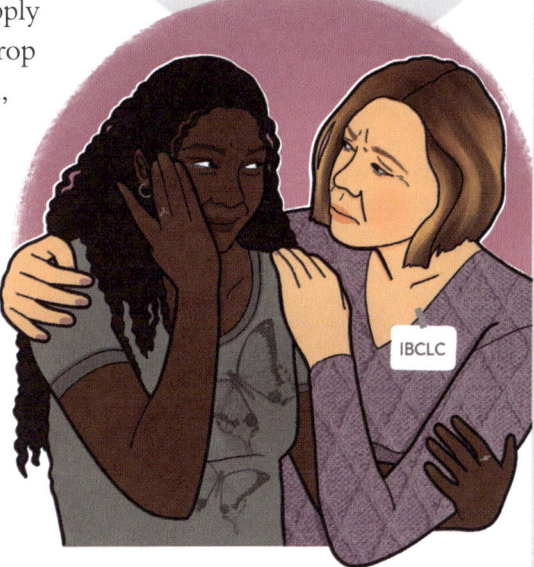

Expressing and Donating Milk after Loss

Some parents choose to donate their milk to a milk bank after the loss of their baby. They may find comfort in knowing that their baby's milk can help sick or premature babies who need life-saving donor milk. Some mothers may find expressing and donating milk helps them to get through the grief and shock of the first few weeks after their baby's death. One mother whose baby girl died when she was a few weeks old describes her experience of expressing and donating milk:

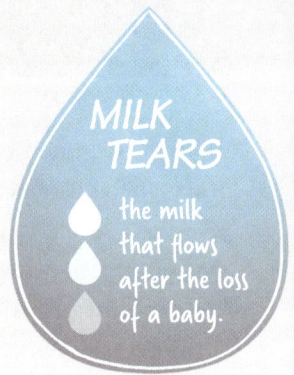

It validated who I was, a postnatal mother... It allowed me to come to terms with her death while protecting me from the potential hormonal crash that can come with early weaning. I grieved but I wasn't depressed, and I attribute that in part to my expressing.

(Deering, 2018)
https://womenshealthtoday.blog/2018/01/14/milk-tears

MILK TEARS – the milk that flows after the loss of a baby.

Breastmilk Keepsakes

Some mothers like to commemorate having provided milk for their baby or having donated to a milk bank by commissioning a piece of jewellery made using some of their breastmilk. Another option to create a lasting memory is to have milk infused into a blown glass bowl or paperweight. Northern Ireland artist Helen Hancock creates beautiful glass objects using breastmilk. Her website is www.breastbowl.com.

> *Without support, parenting an infant can be hell. Shared, it has moments of heaven.*
>
> (Julie Philips, 2022)

CHAPTER 17

Maternal Conditions/ Illnesses and Breastfeeding

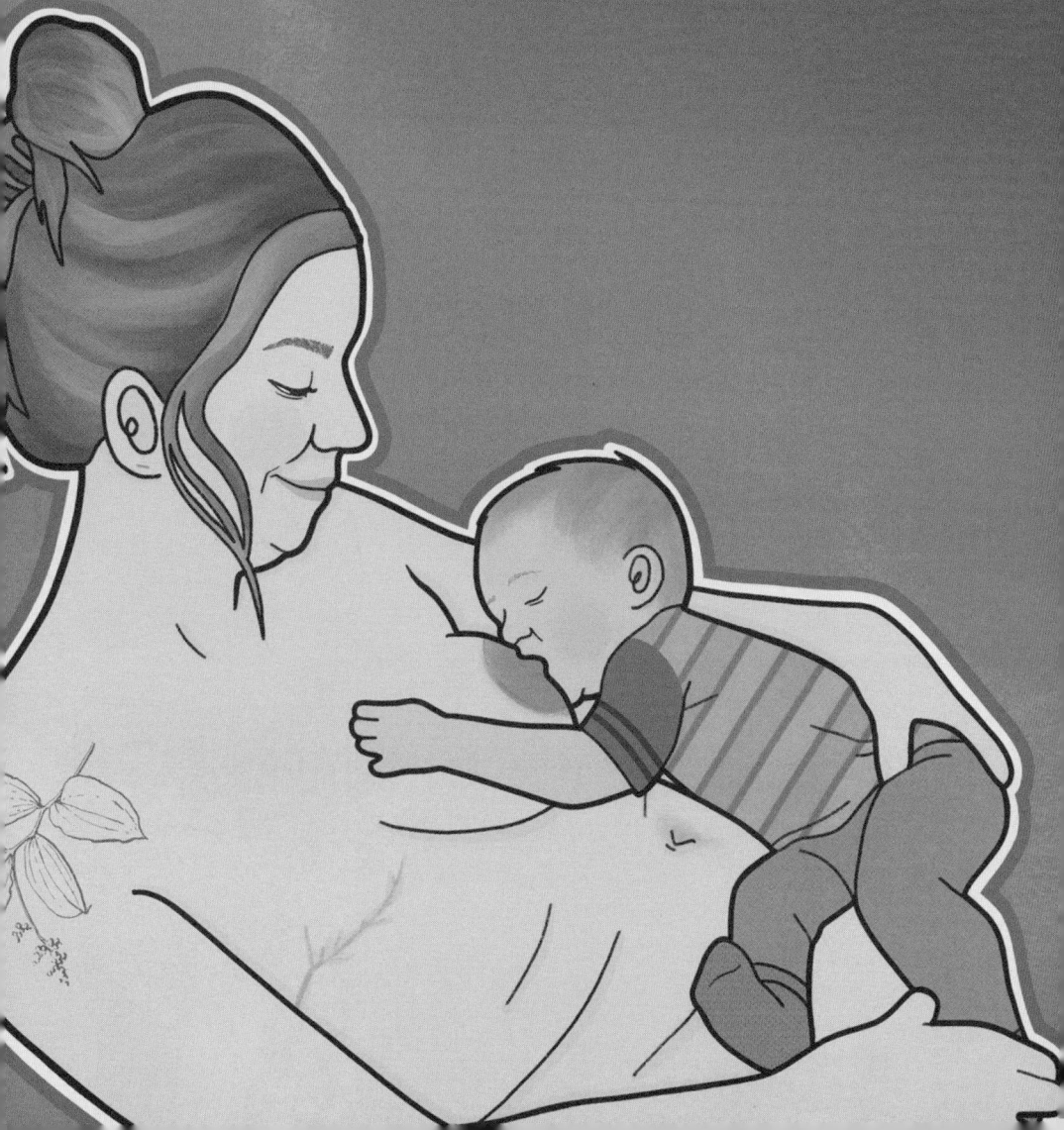

There are very few maternal illnesses or conditions that prevent you from being able to breastfeed. But there are some that may require a little bit of management and support. Even if you don't experience problems with breastfeeding, attending a face-to-face breastfeeding support group will provide you with emotional, social and practical support, all of which are important when you're managing a life-long illness or chronic condition and adapting to the challenges of new parenthood. Breastfeeding might not look like exactly how you imagined it would. It might mean partially breastfeeding or breastfeeding for a shorter time than you had intended. It might even mean deciding early on that you don't want to breastfeed. You have to do what's right for you.

In this chapter I've outlined some of the most common maternal conditions that I see among my clients, along with some suggestions for how to manage breastfeeding and lactation.

Type 1 Diabetes

You can breastfeed if you have type 1 diabetes. Breastfeeding can have a positive long-term effect on your glucose metabolism. And while any amount of breastfeeding will be good for your baby, exclusive breastfeeding for six months will reduce their risk of developing obesity or type 1 diabetes in later life. If you have type 1 diabetes

Consider antenatal expression of colostrum. Babies born to mothers with type 1 are at a greater risk of having low blood sugar levels in the first few days postpartum. Antenatally expressing colostrum means you're less likely to have to supplement with infant formula.

Be aware that your milk might be a little slower to come in than usual. It could be day five rather than day three. Lots of skin-to-skin, frequent feeding and hand expression can help to bring your milk in sooner.

You will need less insulin when you are breastfeeding – it might take some time to determine how much less but your healthcare team can help you. Hypos are more likely in the first few weeks as your body adjusts and you work out new insulin to carbohydrate ratios or basal levels, so have plenty of snacks to hand.

Epilepsy

Women with epilepsy can safely breastfeed while continuing to take anti-seizure medications, but there are some additional challenges:

- **Small amounts of the anti-seizure medications prescribed for epilepsy** get into your breastmilk, but most are considered safe when breastfeeding. This is something you can discuss with your healthcare team. They may ask that you observe your baby for signs of sleepiness, irritability, jaundice or poor weight gain.

- **Some medications such as Phenobarbital can make babies sleepy.** If this is the case with your baby, you might be advised to partially breastfeed and supplement with some formula.

- **Sleep deprivation is often a concern among mothers with Epilepsy as it can be a trigger for seizures.** Talk to your partner and an IBCLC or skilled breastfeeding supporter about figuring out a plan for optimising your sleep while you are breastfeeding. It might mean your partner giving the baby an infant formula or expressed breastmilk supplement during the night, so you get an extended stretch of sleep. Whatever you decide, there is always a way to provide milk for your baby while minimising the risk of having a seizure.

Autoimmune Disorders

Autoimmune disorders are conditions in which the immune system attacks and damages body tissues because it can't tell the difference between healthy and harmful cells. They affect more women than men and include rheumatoid arthritis, lupus, inflammatory bowel disease, multiple sclerosis, Raynaud's disease, coeliac disease, fibromyalgia and hypothyroidism. These conditions will all present in different ways for different people, but common symptoms are fatigue, pain and inflammation. You *can* breastfeed if you have an autoimmune condition. Your body will be able to make nutritious milk for your baby and you won't pass on your condition to your baby through your milk. Any amount of breastfeeding you do will help to build your baby's immune system and reduce their risk of developing autoimmune conditions when they are older. These are some factors to consider if you have an autoimmune condition and intend to breastfeed:

- **If you are taking medications to manage your symptoms, they are probably compatible with breastfeeding.** Discuss this with your medical team.

- **Think about lining up some extra support for when your baby is born.** Even if you are not breastfeeding, being postpartum and dealing with broken sleep on top of managing a serious health condition is difficult, so don't be shy about asking for help.

- **Some women experience remission from their symptoms when they breastfeed.** This is thought to be related to lactational amenorrhea (not having periods).

- **Some women may experience a flare up of their symptoms after they have their baby.** Hopefully this won't be the case for you, but it is advisable to be attuned to how you're feeling and to contact your healthcare providers if you feel something's not right.

- **It's OK to feel unsure about breastfeeding.** You could give it a go and just feel your way along. Some mothers will breastfeed for a short time, some for a longer time. Some will exclusively breastfeed, some will partially breastfeed. Only you can know how to balance providing milk for your baby with managing your condition.

- **Investigate breastfeeding support before your baby arrives.** You could meet with an IBCLC and attend a local support group. These people will be your support network once your baby arrives.

Breast Cancer

If you've had breast cancer previously, you can breastfeed from the unaffected breast. It is unlikely that the affected breast will go through normal breast changes during your pregnancy, and unlikely that it will produce milk once you have your baby. This may be due to either a mastectomy or a lumpectomy followed by radiation therapy. Breastfeeding on the affected side using a supplemental nursing system is not recommended. According to the US breast surgeon Katrina Mitchell "A nipple preserved in a nipple-sparing mastectomy still has ductal tissue through which the infant mouth or latch trauma could cause problems with underlying reconstruction (such as a breast implant). Reconstructed nipples are purely cosmetic, and extended suckling could cause tissue damage and infection."

Some women find that they can produce enough milk from the unaffected breast to exclusively breastfeed, while others find that they need to supplement. Get help early to optimise your milk supply and see what happens! A little bit of hand expression and/or pumping in addition to breastfeeding could help to increase your milk supply.

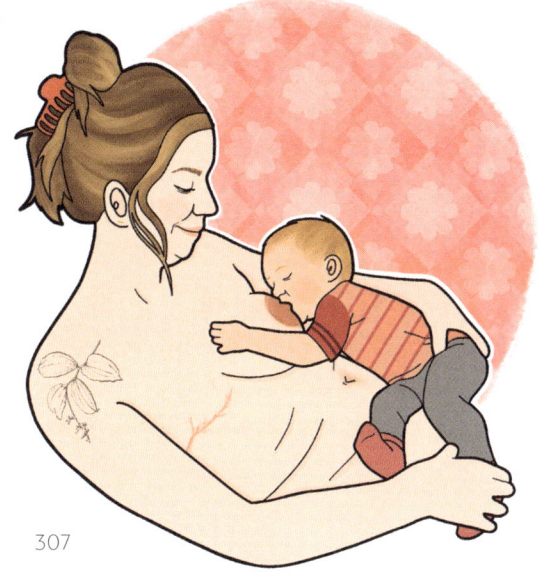

Breastfeeding does not increase the risk of you getting breast cancer again in the future. It is actually linked to a lower risk of developing both breast and ovarian cancer.

Yes, you will look a little lopsided while you are breastfeeding from just one breast! But this is temporary. After a few months of breastfeeding, the breast you are feeding from won't be quite as large, and when you stop breastfeeding it will revert to its pre-breastfeeding size.

What if you've had chemotherapy? Chemotherapy can result in lower milk production in both breasts, so you might have to supplement.

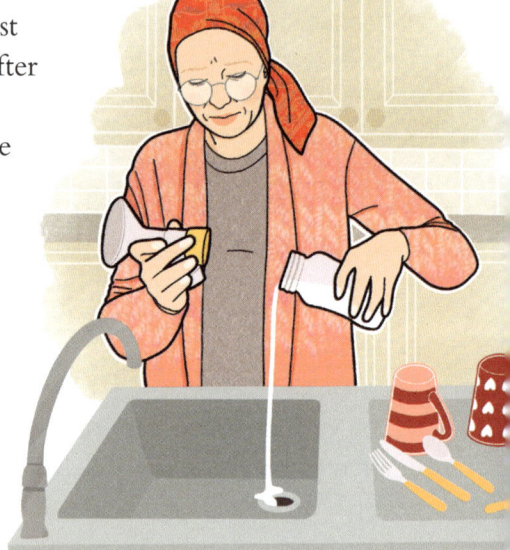

Chemotherapy: If you are diagnosed with breast cancer while breastfeeding and you need to receive chemotherapy or anti-oestrogen drugs, you will have to stop breastfeeding your baby. These drugs can pass into your milk and harm your baby. It may be possible to pump and dump your milk while you undergo treatment, and then resume direct breastfeeding when your care team advise that it is safe to do so.

Anti-oestrogen therapy: Some women will be advised to take anti-oestrogen therapy after chemotherapy treatment. Breastfeeding is not safe while taking this kind of hormone therapy but it might be possible to delay the treatment to allow you to breastfeed for a specified duration.

Breast Screening: MRI's, mammograms and ultrasounds can be done while you are breastfeeding. It is recommended that you breastfeed or pump immediately before the procedure to reduce the density of your breasts and improve the sensitivity of the scan.

Phenylketonuria (PKU)

Mothers who have PKU can breastfeed and make nutritionally perfect milk for their babies. PKU cannot be transmitted to a baby through breastfeeding. Women who have PKU are able to consume more protein when pregnant and breastfeeding. From around week 16 of the pregnancy when the baby's liver starts functioning, it processes phenylalanine on behalf of the mother. And during breastfeeding, the mother's increased need for calories and shifting hormone profile, mean she can consume more protein – over time she will have to gradually come back down to the amount she was able to eat before she became pregnant.

Hospital Admission

If you are admitted to hospital while you are breastfeeding, it might not be possible to have your baby with you. A little bit of planning needs to go into how you manage the situation, maintain your milk supply and keep your baby fed.

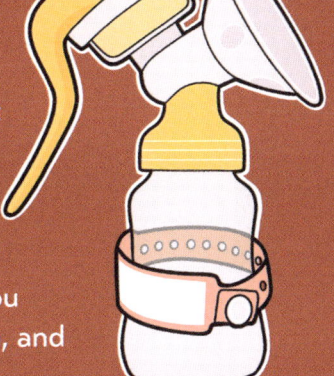

- If you know in advance that you will be apart from your baby, you can start pumping and freezing milk that they can have while you're in hospital.

- Ask in the hospital about access to a pump and facilities for storing milk. Explain that you are a breastfeeding mother and that you will need to be supported to continue pumping while apart from your baby. It might also be worth asking to see the hospital's breastfeeding policy (if they have one).

- If the hospital is unable to provide you with somewhere to safely store your milk, you will need a cooler bag to put pumped milk in, and someone to bring it home for you.

- If possible, have someone bring your baby to you for breastfeeds after you have been admitted.

- If you receive any instruction to pump and dump your milk (due to medications you are receiving), seek out a second opinion or refer to the Breastfeeding Network website.

- Pumping and dumping after a general anaesthetic is not necessary. You can safely feed your baby once you are awake.

- Being apart from your baby and having to pump can be stressful. Try not to worry. Sometimes mothers find that their supply dips a little while in hospital, but if you have previously had plenty of milk, your supply is likely to increase once you resume breastfeeding.

CHAPTER 18
Infant Conditions/Illnesses

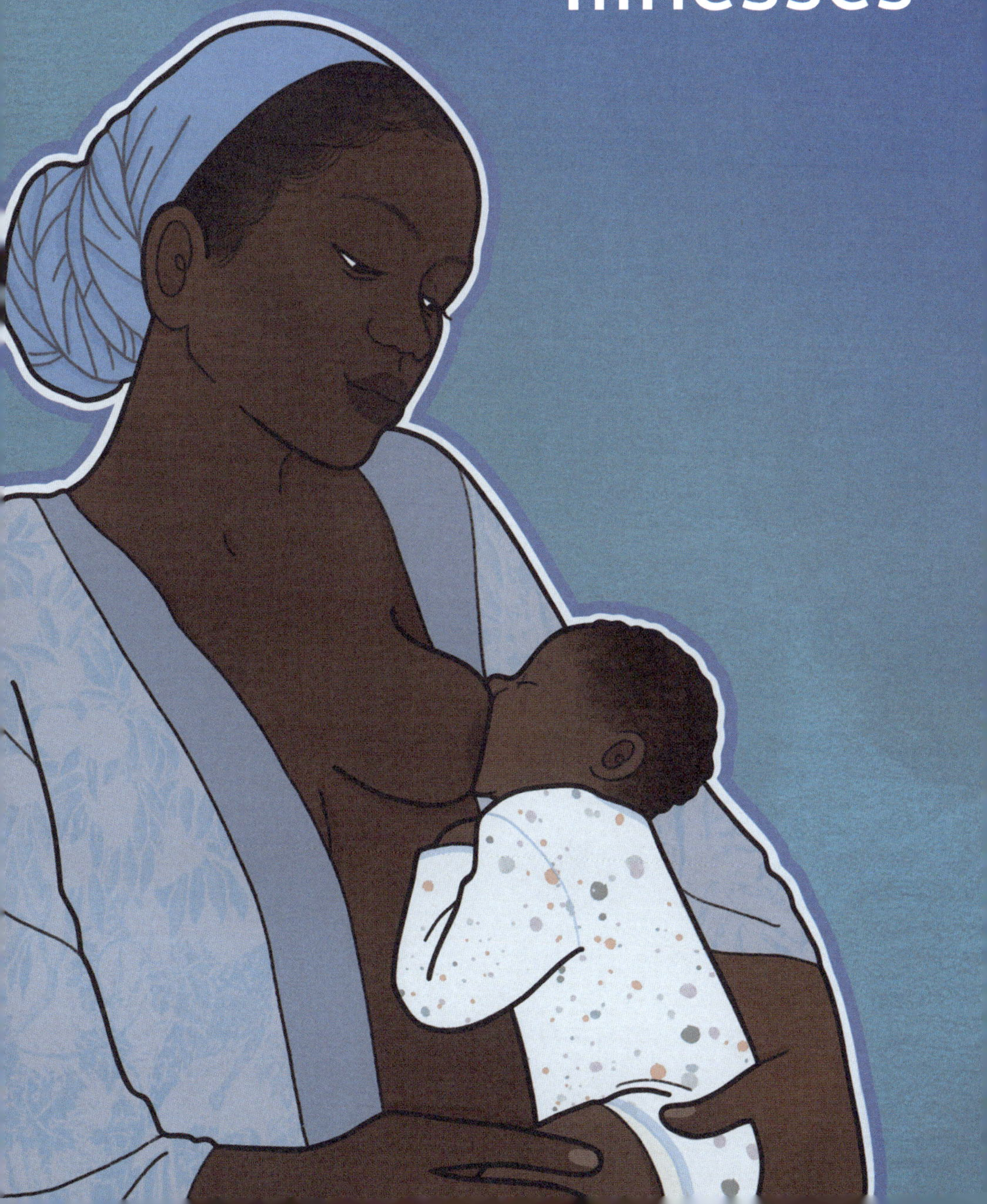

Please note: The information contained in this chapter is not intended as medical advice. If your infant has been diagnosed with an illness or condition, they will receive the best care possible from paediatric medical staff. You will need individualised lactation support to help you continue providing milk for your infant. The goal of this chapter is to provide you with some helpful tips as you navigate a difficult time and offer some words of support and encouragement.

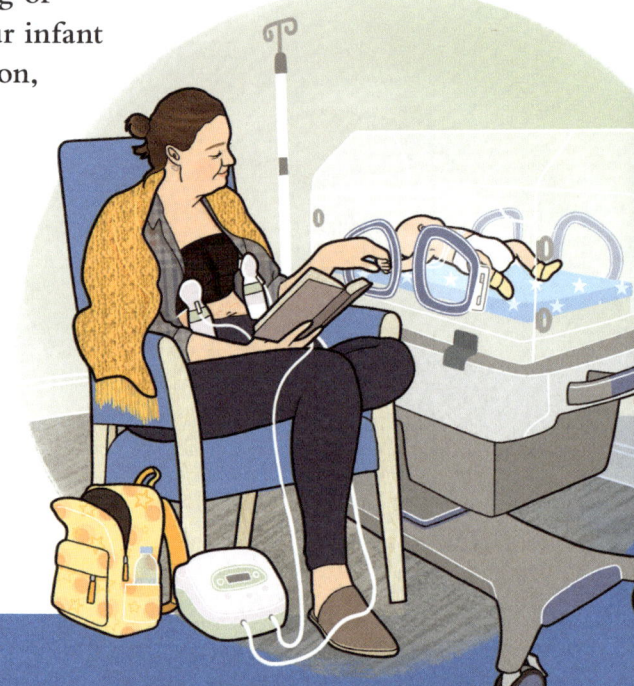

If you are breastfeeding or providing milk for your infant with a medical condition, hopefully your care team will encourage you and support you in whatever way you need. Breastfeeding or the provision of breastmilk should be regarded as an important aspect of your infant's care. These are some of the reasons why:

- Breastmilk is easily digested
- Breastmilk can help to support your baby's immune system and prevent infections
- Breastmilk has a lower allergenic load than other milks/foods
- Breastfeeding can provide pain relief for babies
- Breastfeeding can provide comfort and connection for you and your baby
- Providing milk for your baby can help you to feel involved in their care
- There may be specific benefits for your infant depending on their condition

Baby Backwash Theory: *Your milk is custom-designed for your baby. When they breastfeed, a small amount of their saliva gets drawn into your breast. If they have been exposed to an infection, your body will detect it in their saliva and then produce milk with cells to directly target that infection. Magic!*

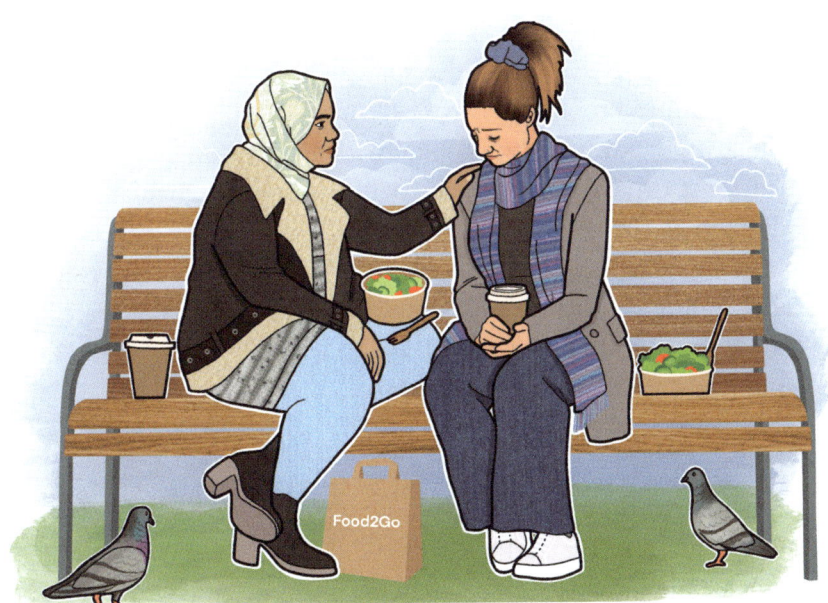

Look after Yourself

Coming to terms with a serious diagnosis and caring for your baby as they undergo treatment can be overwhelming and stressful. It can be upsetting if you are unable to feed your baby directly at the breast, and exhausting trying to exclusively pump and maintain your milk supply. An added challenge is being apart from older children for long periods if your infant is in hospital. So don't forget to look after yourself. Eat as well as you can and try to get a little bit of outside time every day. Call a voluntary breastfeeding supporter – they will be able to provide you with empathy, support and encouragement, as well as some practical tips around breastfeeding and pumping. If you search *Breastfeeding the Brave* on Facebook you will find a support group for parents breastfeeding their infant through a serious illness.

RSV/Bronchiolitis

RSV (respiratory syncytial virus) is the biggest cause of lower lung infections among infants worldwide. Breastfed infants are less likely to get RSV, but if they do get it their infection will be less severe and their hospital stay shorter than if they had not received any breastmilk. They are also less likely to need respiratory support or supplemental oxygen if admitted to an intensive care unit.

If your baby is admitted to hospital with RSV, they may need to be tube fed for a time while they are being treated, particularly if they have developed Bronchiolitis (a lower respiratory tract infection that results in a dry cough and wheezing). It is important that you start double pumping to protect your supply and continue to provide milk for your baby. Ask in the hospital about access to a multiuser pump, a space where you can pump and a place to store your milk. Exclusively pumping can be difficult at first if you have only ever breastfed your baby, but with practice and support it will get easier. Try to focus on measures that will help oxytocin to flow – massage, being close to your baby, relaxing music, closing your eyes and doing mindful breathing. Also remind yourself that the situation is temporary and that your baby will be able to resume direct breastfeeding when they are well enough. Even if your milk supply does dip, you should be able to get it back to where it was before your baby became ill.

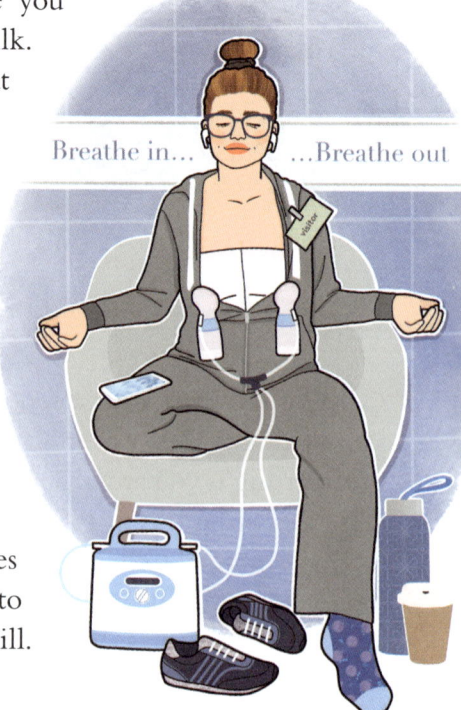

Breathe in... ...Breathe out

Laryngomalacia and Tracheomalacia

Laryngomalacia is an upper airway condition that is characterised by a sharp, high-pitched noise (stridor) when your baby breathes in. The noise is caused by a soft or underdeveloped epiglottis (the little flap of tissue that prevents food from entering your airway) collapsing over the larynx on the in-breath. This noise often doesn't become apparent until a few weeks postpartum. Most babies with laryngomalacia can breastfeed without significant difficulties, but some will struggle to coordinate sucking, swallowing and breathing. Adjustments to positioning can help babies cope with the flow of milk. Mothers often find that being in a reclined position when feeding with their baby facing them and with their head extended to open their airway can work well. If the flow of milk is very fast, you might need to pace the feed by taking your baby off for a little breather after every four or five sucks. Occasionally a baby with laryngomalacia will need to be bottled fed for a time. The symptoms of laryngomalacia gradually disappear sometime between six months and two years of age.

Tracheomalacia is a developmental defect in the trachea whereby the rings of cartilage around the tracheal wall are softer than normal. This results in the airway collapsing on the out breath, resulting in an expiratory stridor. Babies with tracheomalacia often develop wheezing and reflux. The same adjustments to positioning that can be helpful for laryngomalacia can also be helpful for babies with tracheomalacia. Because of the extra effort that babies with tracheomalacia exert when breathing, their weight gain is sometimes slow. If this is the case, you may need to express milk and supplement. Tracheomalacia is far less common than laryngomalacia.

Gastro-oesophageal Reflux Disease (GORD)

Many babies have reflux (gastro-oesophageal reflux GOR) ie, they regurgitate or spit up some milk after feeding. This is normal baby behaviour and in the majority of babies, is not something to be concerned about. Very occasionally, reflux can cause significant issues for a baby, such as poor weight gain, apnoea (stopping breathing), ear infections, excessive crying and intense distress. In these cases, the term gastro-oesophageal reflux disease (GORD) is used to describe the condition. If you suspect that your baby may have GORD, it is important to seek medical help. I would also suggest seeking support from a lactation consultant who can help you to continue breastfeeding. Measures that can help are giving your baby small frequent feeds, keeping them upright after feeding, wearing your baby in a sling, gentle touch and massage, and talking to your baby. Also, be mindful to look after yourself. Dealing with GORD can be very stressful. You will be better able to care for and regulate your baby if you are having your own needs met. Also, bear in mind that your baby's digestive system is immature – over time as it develops and matures, their symptoms of GORD will lessen.

Type 1 Diabetes

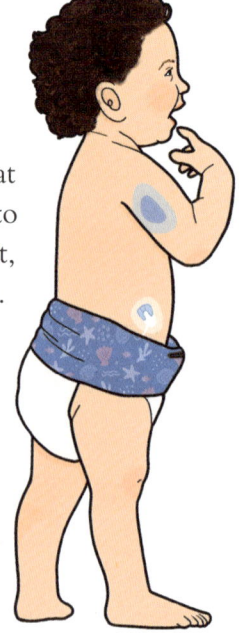

Type 1 diabetes is an autoimmune condition that can develop at any age. When a person has type 1 diabetes, their pancreas stops producing insulin. This means that their body cannot convert carbohydrates in food into energy that cells in the body can use. And as a result, glucose levels in the blood stream become very high. These high blood glucose levels will lead to symptoms associated with type 1 diabetes – a high thirst, needing to pee a lot, weight loss, feeling tired and irritable and a ketone smell off the breath (a bit like nail polish remover). Type 1 diabetes is managed using insulin therapy, most commonly delivered subcutaneously by an insulin pump. Insulin converts glucose into energy that the body can use to function normally.

You can continue to breastfeed your infant if they are diagnosed with type 1 diabetes. Your milk will continue to nourish them and provide them with immune protection. Your medical team will help you to figure out appropriate insulin to carbohydrate ratios, and approximately how many carbs will be in an average breastfeed (on the basis that breastmilk contains seven grammes of carbs per 100ml). If your baby is still exclusively breastfed, the volume of milk they take at the breast will be higher than if they are well established on solids. Your care team might suggest weighing your baby before and after a full breastfeed to determine an approximate feed volume. There may be a little bit of trial and error to start with – don't worry, this is normal, even in infants who are not being breastfed.

Down Syndrome

Babies who have Down Syndrome can and do breastfeed. Support to establish breastfeeding is very important. Some babies will latch and feed without difficulty from day one, but most will need help with feeding. Common breastfeeding challenges in the early weeks with Down Syndrome babies are sleepiness, low tone (which can make latching and sucking difficult), weak suck and tongue protrusion. You might need to exclusively pump for a time, while bottle-feeding your baby expressed milk. With time and growth, and possibly some oral motor exercises, your baby's feeding skills will

The Dancer Hand position can be helpful to use with babies with Down Syndrome as it helps to stabilise their jaw and increase the intraoral vacuum which in turn improves milk transfer. You place your thumb and index finger either side of your baby's jaw and use your other three fingers to support your breast.

improve and they may be able to transition to breastfeeding. Be patient with them. And seek both professional and volunteer breastfeeding support to help you with latching and positioning. It is best to avoid breastfeeding positions in which your baby's head is extended back as this can cause their tongue to stick out even further and make latching more difficult.

Breastfeeding helps to strengthen your baby's facial muscles, tongue and lips. This supports speech development and helps to improve coordination.

Cystic Fibrosis

Cystic fibrosis (CF) is a genetic condition that primarily affects the lungs and digestive system. Exclusive breastfeeding is recommended for babies who have CF, for all of the reasons that it is recommended for other babies, but especially because it helps to support lung function, lowers the risk of respiratory infections and increases the diversity of the gut microbiome. If you are breastfeeding your baby with CF, you will be required to give them pancreatic enzymes before each feed. Usually mothers will mix the enzymes (which come as granules) with a little bit of expressed milk and give this to their baby on a spoon. Your baby might also need salt and vitamin supplements.

Some breastfed babies with CF might need additional calories if their weight gain is slow. If this is the case, you may be able to pump some milk and use it to supplement. Or you might choose to supplement with infant formula. Whatever you decide, you should be supported to continue breastfeeding. Working with an IBCLC will help you to optimise your milk supply and ensure your baby is transferring milk well when they're breastfeeding.

Phenylketonuria (PKU)

PKU is a genetically inherited condition that is characterised by elevated levels of the essential amino acid phenylalanine (PHE). People with PKU must eat a special low-protein diet. If your baby is diagnosed with PKU (through newborn screening), you can partially breastfeed them, while supplementing with a specialised PHE-free formula. In the days after your baby is first diagnosed, their PHE-level will have to be stabilised by reducing or stopping breastfeeding and giving them large volumes of PHE-free formula. You will need to pump to protect your milk supply. Once your baby's PHE-level normalises, you can resume breastfeeding in combination with PHE-free formula supplementation.

Your care team will help you to determine what ratio of breastfeeding to formula will be appropriate for your baby. There are different approaches to combining breastfeeding with PHE-free formula: some parents will give their baby a prescribed volume of formula before or during every breastfeed (using a bottle or at-the-breast supplementation) while others will alternate breastfeeds with formula feeds.

Your baby's PHE levels will have to be monitored carefully. It may feel stressful at times – hospital appointments, the on-going monitoring, trying to determine breastmilk intake and balancing breastfeeding and PHE-free formula feeds – so don't lose sight of the immense benefit that breastfeeding confers to your baby and yourself. Try to connect with other mothers who have breastfed babies with PKU.

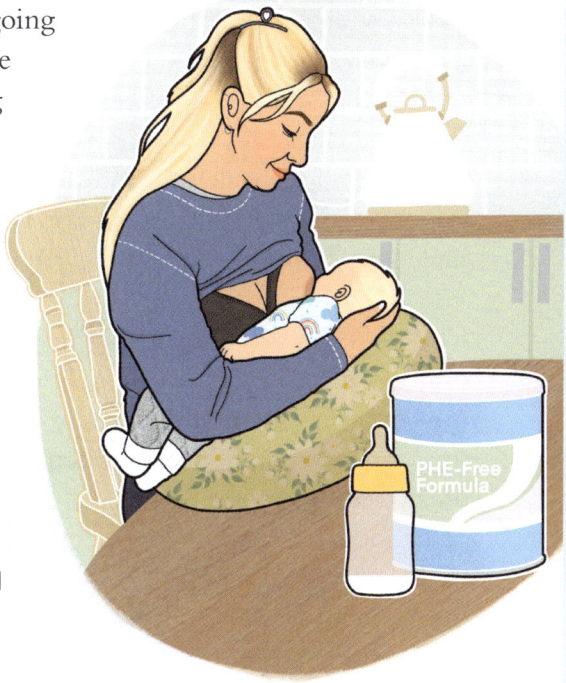

Please note: Babies who have PKU are more susceptible to thrush, be aware of the signs in your baby and yourself (see page 151).

Cancer

Breastfeeding helps to protect infants against infections and lowers their risk of developing non-communicable diseases and some childhood cancers, but unfortunately it does not completely eliminate the possibility of them getting cancer. It is a shocking and frightening diagnosis for any parent to receive. It is upsetting to see your infant undergo invasive procedures and treatments. There can be so much going on that you don't have any control over, but one thing that you (and only you) can do is make milk for your baby. There will be times when they may not be able to feed at the breast or when their appetite is poor. They might even have to have an NG feeding tube inserted. No matter how they are being fed, remind yourself that your milk provides them with infection-fighting cells and is the most easily digested food they could have. Your breastmilk even contains HAMLET (human alpha-lactalbumin made lethal to tumour) cells which kill tumour cells.

Cleft Lip and Palate

Babies with a cleft palate or lip (or both) often struggle to breastfeed. They may not be able to create enough suction to transfer sufficient milk at the breast, they often have difficulty latching and breastmilk can leak through their nostrils. But breastmilk is important for babies who have a cleft lip and/or palate – for all the reasons that it is important for other babies, but also because it reduces their risk of ear infections (which they are more prone to than other babies).

Cleft Palate: A cleft (opening) in a babies' palate makes it difficult for them to create suction, so this makes effective milk transfer when breastfeeding difficult. If the cleft is very small or narrow or if it is submucosal, breastfeeding (or partial breastfeeding) might be possible if they baby can manage to get a good latch with a big mouthful of breast tissue. Babies with a larger cleft will have to be bottle-fed, so this will mean exclusive pumping for mothers who want to provide breastmilk. A type of feeding bottle called a *SpecialNeeds*

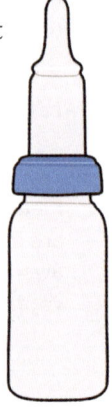

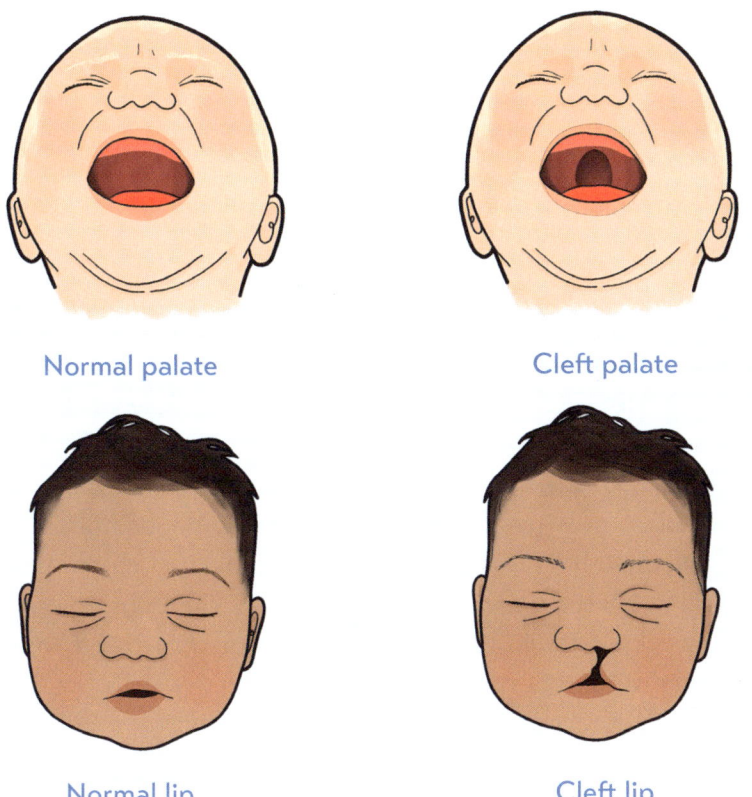

Normal palate Cleft palate

Normal lip Cleft lip

Feeder or *Haberman Feeder* is often used to feed babies with a cleft palate. It allows them to get milk out by compressing their jaw and gums, rather than requiring them to create a vacuum. Cleft palates are usually repaired between 6 and 12 months, so sometimes these babies can successfully transition to direct breastfeeding. If your baby is unable to transfer milk at the breast, you may still be able to put them to the breast for comfort or *non-nutritive sucking*. Upright positions are recommended.

Cleft Lip: Some babies with a cleft lip may be able to breastfeed (or partially breastfeed) if the mother's breast can be moulded into their mouth to create a seal. A lot depends on the size of the cleft, the shape of the mother's breasts and nipples, and the breastfeeding position used. An upright breastfeeding position usually works best and Dancer Hand position can help to provide stability for the baby's mouth.

Cow's Milk Protein Allergy (CMPA)

If your baby has symptoms which suggest an allergy – vomiting, blood in their stool, diarrhoea, rashes, irritability – you should be referred to a paediatrician and/or dietitian who can investigate and support you to continue breastfeeding while implementing measures to ease your baby's symptoms. CMPA is not common in exclusively breastfed babies, but occasionally it can present, particularly if there is a history of allergies in the family.

If CPMA is suspected, you might be advised to follow an *elimination diet* whereby you remove cow's milk products from your diet, but only if there is strong evidence that allergens in your milk are the problem. There are specific protocols that should be followed in situations where a baby has an allergy. Generally, it is recommended that suspected allergens are eliminated one at a time, for a period of two-four weeks. Switching to a hydrolysed or soya-based formula (which contain none of the live immune-protective cells that are in breastmilk) is not recommended.

Please note: there are other foods (such as soybeans, eggs, nuts, fish, shellfish and wheat) which can cause allergies. Working closely with a dietitian will help you identify the allergens that may be causing symptoms in your baby.

CHAPTER 19

Breastfeeding Beyond the Fourth Trimester

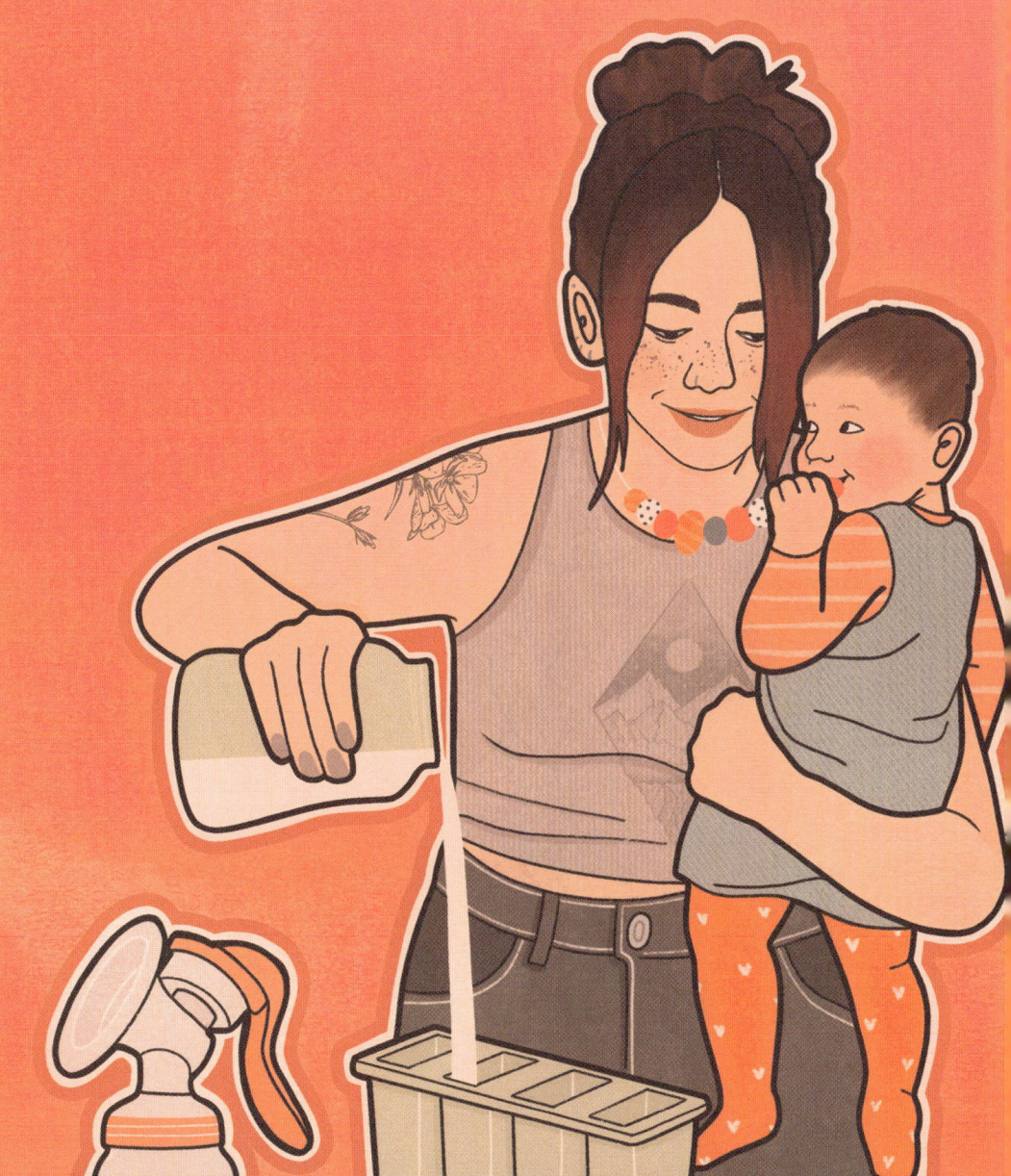

When it comes to breastfeeding education, the emphasis is usually on getting started and the first few weeks. This is undoubtedly the most difficult time for most new lactating parents. And while things generally do get easier after a few weeks, there may still be some challenges to navigate on your breastfeeding journey. There will be times when you're completely rocking it and times when you feel like you don't know what you're doing. Support is key, at every stage, whether you find it online, face-to-face at a group, among friends or in a book. In this chapter I address some of the common challenges that parents face with breastfeeding beyond the first few months.

Sleep Struggles

Probably the burning question for most parents as their babies hit twelve weeks is "when will they sleep through the night?". It certainly was for me with my first baby. I had read a baby care

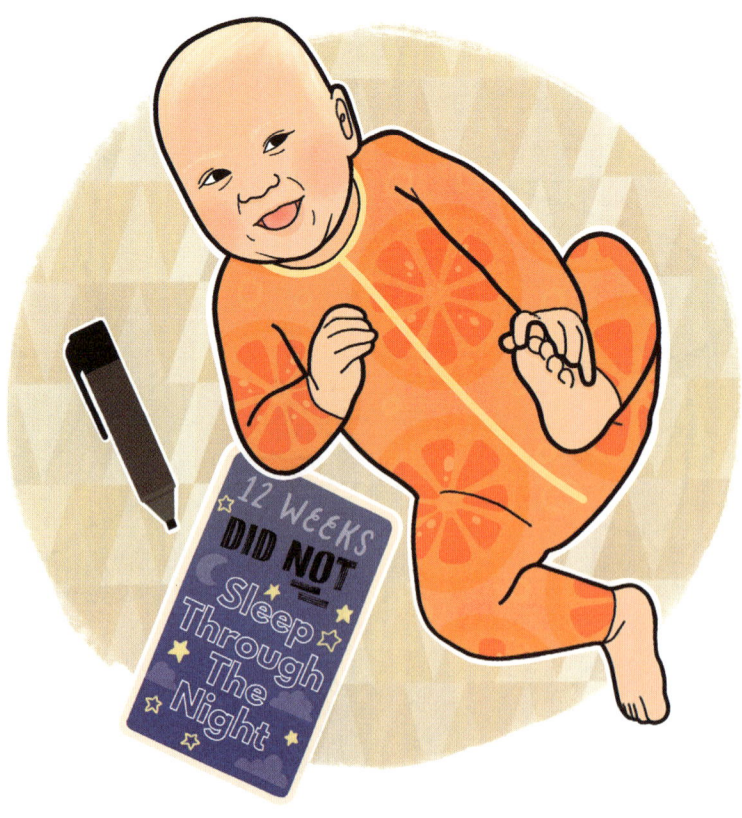

book which stated that babies should start sleeping through the night from twelve weeks. I fully expected that my baby, who had been waking and breastfeeding a few times a night since birth, would magically start sleeping through the night once he turned twelve weeks. But he didn't. He continued doing what he had been doing and there was no dramatic change in his nighttime routine. I was disappointed and felt like I had failed in getting him to reach that *sleeping though the night* milestone. It's the question that everyone asks isn't it, "is he sleeping through the night?" – like it is absolutely the most important goal you have as a parent of a new baby. But, actually the reality is that most babies still wake a few times a night right up to one year of age. The science tells us that this kind of night-time waking is normal. So, if you're wondering if your baby should be sleeping through the night by now or if there's something you should be doing to encourage this, the answer is no on both fronts. If your baby is waking and feeding during the night, congratulate yourself that they are doing what is developmentally normal for breastfed babies.

It is hard, there's no denying that. It can help to attend a breastfeeding group where you can listen to other parents talk about their babies' nighttime habits. It can also help to get a nap in during the day when you can and to get out for a walk and some fresh air. Expect that you'll still get people asking if your baby is sleeping through the night. Have an answer ready for them "yes, thank you he is" or "oh no of course he isn't! He's only five months old, so he still needs to have a few breastfeeds during the night" – whatever you feel is the easiest way to shut down a conversation you may not want to have.

Remember that all babies are different. Some will sleep for five to six hour stretches from two months (these babies are few and far between), while others won't sleep for longer stretches or through the night until they're toddlers. Trust that your baby will sleep for longer stretches or through the night when they are ready.

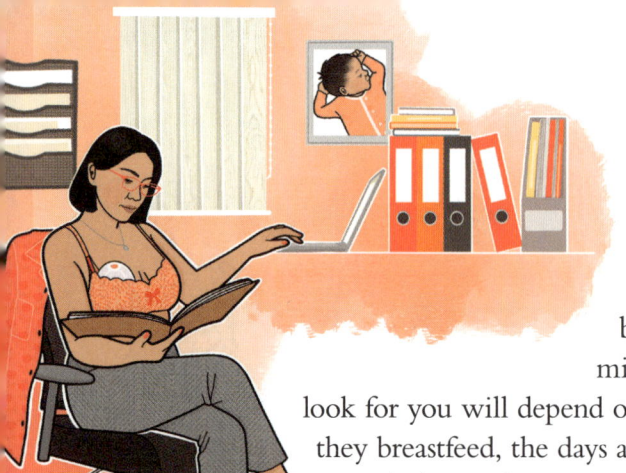

Back to Work

Lots of mothers return to work either full time or part time and find a way to keep breastfeeding or providing milk for their baby. How it will look for you will depend on your baby's age, how much they breastfeed, the days and hours you work, and your workplace. These are a few things to consider before you go back to work:

- Will you need to provide milk for whoever is caring for you baby while you're at work?

- Will you need to pump to maintain your milk supply during work hours?

- Is there a space in your workplace where you can pump? Is there a fridge where you can store milk?

- Have you spoken to your employer and ascertained your rights and their legal obligations?

- You might not need to pump – a lot depends on your hours and the age of your baby.

Mothers often feel apprehensive about how they will manage their return to work – not just breastfeeding, but how they will feel about being apart from their infant, worries about how their infant will cope with the new routine and concerns about how things will work out with their childcare provider. There are a lot of unknowns. While you can put some plans in place there will be a certain element of figuring it out as you go along, and that's okay. One thing you don't want to do is spend the last few months of your maternity leave stressing about *what-ifs*.

It can take parents around a month or two to settle into the new routine and get a better handle on how to manage breastfeeding and work. It can often look different to how you had planned so having a little bit of flexibility is a good idea. With the change in routine and longer than usual separation from you during the day, it is likely that your baby will feed more during the night – for a while at least. Expect that the change might be difficult at the start. You will probably be tired. It's a lot – parenting a small infant *and* working outside the home, so be gentle with yourself and rest assured that it will get easier.

The Law and Returning to Work and Breastfeeding

IN THE UK:

You should inform your employer in writing if you are breastfeeding. Your employer must:

 provide a suitable space where you can rest, breastfeed or pump

 provide somewhere for you to safely store milk

 conduct a risk assessment to ensure that your working conditions are suitable

IN IRELAND:

You should inform your employer in writing if you are breastfeeding. Your employer must

 Give you one hour off each day to pump or breastfeed (until your infant turns two). This time can be taken as a one-hour break, two 30-minute breaks or three 20-minute breaks

 Either provide you with a suitable space where you can breastfeed or pump or reduce your working hours with pay if a suitable space is not available

Exercise

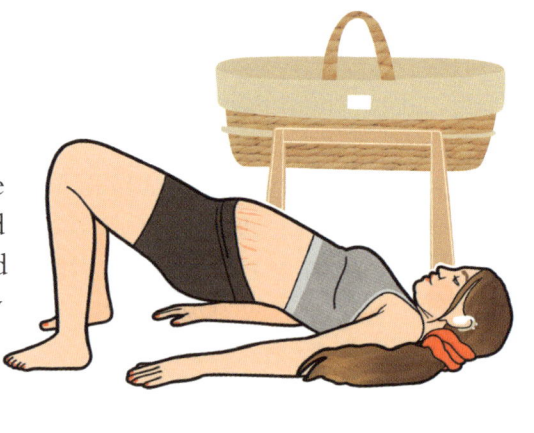

Resuming some kind of gentle exercise in the postpartum period is beneficial for physical and mental health. You will know when the time is right for you to start getting more physically active. It might be at six weeks postpartum, it might be at four months postpartum. There are many variables which will determine when is the right time, including the time that YOUR body needs to recover from giving birth and your level of fitness before you had your baby. Start slowly. Be gentle with yourself. Walking is a great way to get active again. And consider doing some kind of postnatal class such as yoga or pilates to help strengthen your pelvic floor.

Does exercise affect milk production? If you are consuming enough calories and staying sufficiently hydrated, and also continuing to breastfeed or pump to meet your baby's needs, exercising will not affect milk production. It won't affect the nutrient composition of your milk either. You can exercise regularly and make plenty of nutritionally perfect milk.

What about lactic acid? Lactic acid is a chemical created in your body when you exercise (formed when carbohydrates are broken down). It fuels cells when you're exercising and plays a role in fighting infections. Moderate exercise does not increase the level of lactic acid in breastmilk, but high-intensity exercise can result in higher lactic acid levels in your milk for up to an hour afterwards. It can make your milk taste a little more salty than usual. If your baby doesn't like the taste, wait for around an hour after you exercise to feed them.

Staying comfortable and avoiding blocked ducts. Ideally, breastfeed or pump before you exercise and wear a supportive sports bra. Start off gently. Listen to your body.

Return of Periods

Most breastfeeding mothers get their period back somewhere between nine and eighteen months, but everyone is different. Some mothers who are exclusively breastfeeding will get their period back after a few months, while for others it could be years. The more breastfeeding you do (including during the night), the less likely your period is to return.

If your baby starts to breastfeed less frequently or starts solids, starts to sleep for longer stretches at night or if you reduce the amount of pumping you're doing, the hormones that tell your body to menstruate will increase, and your period is more likely to resume. Other factors that can influence when your period returns are your individual hormonal and physiological profile and your Body Mass Index (BMI). Women who are overweight or obese are more likely to get their period back sooner

Can you get pregnant before your period returns? Yes. You could ovulate before you get your first period after having your baby. However, if you are adhering to the criteria for the Lactational Amenorrhea Method (page 132) in the first six months postpartum, there is a low risk of this happening.

Can having your period affect milk production? Yes. Hormonal changes can result in a *temporary* dip in milk production when you have your period.

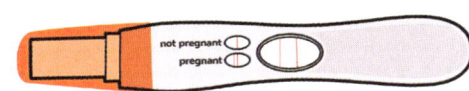

Starting Solids

Introducing solid foods to your baby can seem like a monumental milestone for parents, and it is! It is the end of one chapter – exclusive milk feeding – and the beginning of another. Babies do not go from exclusively breastfeeding to having three square meals overnight. Starting solids is a process during which babies

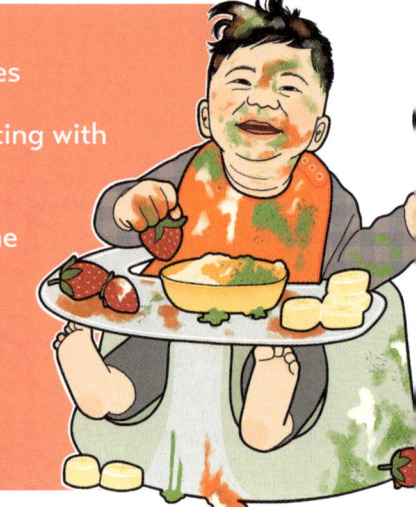

- learn about food tastes and textures
- learn about the social aspect of eating with family
- discover the joy in being given some autonomy to feed themselves
- develop fine motor skills and hand eye coordination when handling food and eating

Is your baby ready to start solids? The recommendation from the World Health Organisation is that babies start solid foods when they are six months old. This is a guideline. Some babies will be ready a little bit earlier, some a little bit later. Your baby is probably ready to start eating solid food if they can

- Sit upright and hold their head steady
- Pick up pieces of food and put them in their mouth
- Chew and swallow food and not push it back out of their mouth with their tongue

Starting your baby on solids before they are ready can put them at an increased risk of developing allergies, increase their risk of becoming obese in later life and put them at a risk of choking if they can't yet swallow effectively.

What food should you give your baby? Some people advocate starting with purees, others recommend doing baby led-weaning and starting which chunks of food that babies can suck or chew on. The important thing is that there is some iron in the foods that your baby starts eating. From around six months your baby's natural iron stores start to dwindle, and they need iron from other sources. Foods that are rich in iron include meat, beans, lentil and dark leafy greens and tofu.

Should you start with purees or do baby-led weaning? What do you want to do? What do you think would be best for your baby? Do some research on both and see what feels right. Some parents do a mix of both. Breastfeeding parents often opt for baby-led weaning as they like the idea of giving their baby autonomy over how they eat – a little bit like responsive breastfeeding where you follow your baby's cues.

How much food does your baby need? Very little to start with. Breastmilk (and/or formula) will continue to be their main source of nutrition, and the most nutrient dense food they will eat. Babies might start by eating once a day and just having a few mouthfuls of something. Try not to put pressure on yourself to get your baby eating big meals. Give them time to adjust to eating solid food and try to follow their lead. Between six months and twelve months your baby will gradually increase their intake of solid food and reduce their intake of milk, such that solids take over from milk as the main source of nutrition.

How do you balance breastfeeding and solid foods? Breastfeeding doesn't suddenly become less important on the day that your baby starts eating solids. It is still your baby's main source of nutrition and continues to provide immune protection. Breastfeed your baby before you offer them solid food. Try to follow their lead. If you are going at a nice, relaxed pace with solids, your supply will gradually decrease to meet your baby's needs. Continue to breastfeed your baby whenever they want to be fed.

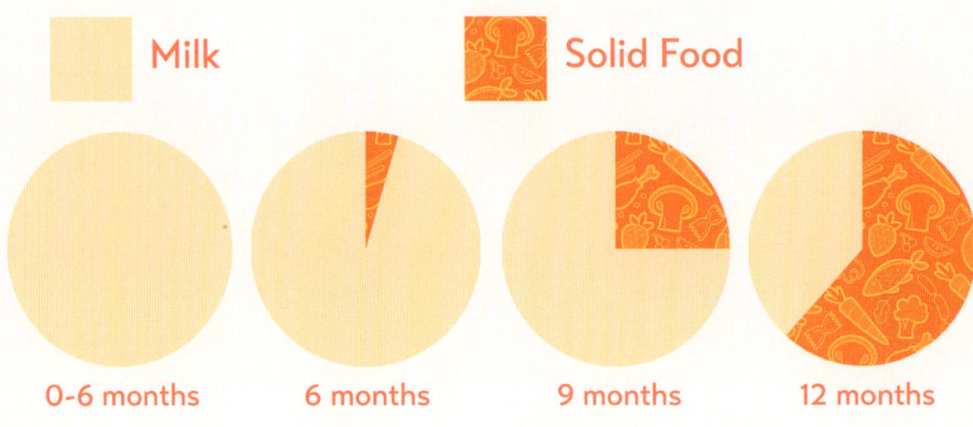

* this graph is for illustrative purposes only: each child is different and their ratio of breastmilk to solid food may differ

Should you give your baby other liquids? You can offer your baby water in a sippy cup. Or cow's milk (the latest recommendation from the WHO says cow's milk can be given to infants from six months of age, if they are getting enough iron from other sources). How much water or cow's milk you offer your baby may depend on your breastfeeding goal.

Starting your baby on solids is not an exact science. How you do it should depend on WHO and national guidelines, your baby's readiness, and what you feel is going to work best for your family.

Teething

Most babies start teething sometime between four and six months and cut a first tooth at around six months, but it's very variable. The most obvious signs of teething are lots of dribbling, red cheeks, gumming/chewing their hands/fingers and occasional irritability.

Generally babies can continue to breastfeed while teething without any issues. However, some babies might want to breastfeed more often for comfort and pain relief or may wake more frequently at night. Or teething could cause them to be a bit more fussy when they're feeding. Things that can help include

- 🦷 Giving your baby a teething toy to chew on – the water filled ones that you can cool can be soothing to irritated gums

- 🦷 Make a breastmilk ice pop for your baby to suck on – several brands market *breastmilk popsicle moulds*

- 🦷 Baby teething gel (available in pharmacies)

- 🦷 Wearing a teething necklace for your baby to chew on. These necklaces are made using chunky and colourful BPA-free silicone beads.

– Providing your baby with lots of cuddles and reassurance

Nursing Strike

A *nursing strike* is when a baby who has been breastfeeding well suddenly starts refusing to feed. It is usually temporary – a few days at most. There are a number of reasons why a baby might go on a nursing strike:

- 💧 Your baby is sick and breastfeeding is uncomfortable for them eg, Ear or throat infection

- 💧 Your baby is teething and has sore gums

- 💧 Something is different about your milk – maybe it tastes different due to a medication you've taken or a mastitis infection (it can make milk taste salty)

- 💧 Your milk supply has dropped – this could be caused by a return of your period or pregnancy

- There has been some big change in the family that your baby is finding it difficult to adjust to. For example, a return to work or a bereavement
- You have started using a new perfume or body lotion that your baby doesn't like
- Thrush can make feeding uncomfortable for some babies
- It could be something sensory – sometimes this can happen at around three months. See the section on feeding aversion in Chapter 13.

Try not to panic if your baby suddenly starts refusing to feed. Reassure them that you can still comfort them with your body, without any pressure to feed. Doing skin-to-skin might be helpful. Offer your breast when they are calm or sleepy. They might be willing to feed more during the night. Hand express or pump if you need to. If your baby is not taking any milk at the breast, you may need to offer them milk in a bottle or cup.

If your baby has any symptoms of being sick, bring them to your GP. And make contact with a breastfeeding supporter to talk through the nursing strike. A little bit of reassurance and a listening ear could go a long way to helping you through a difficult few days.

CHAPTER 20

Stopping Breastfeeding

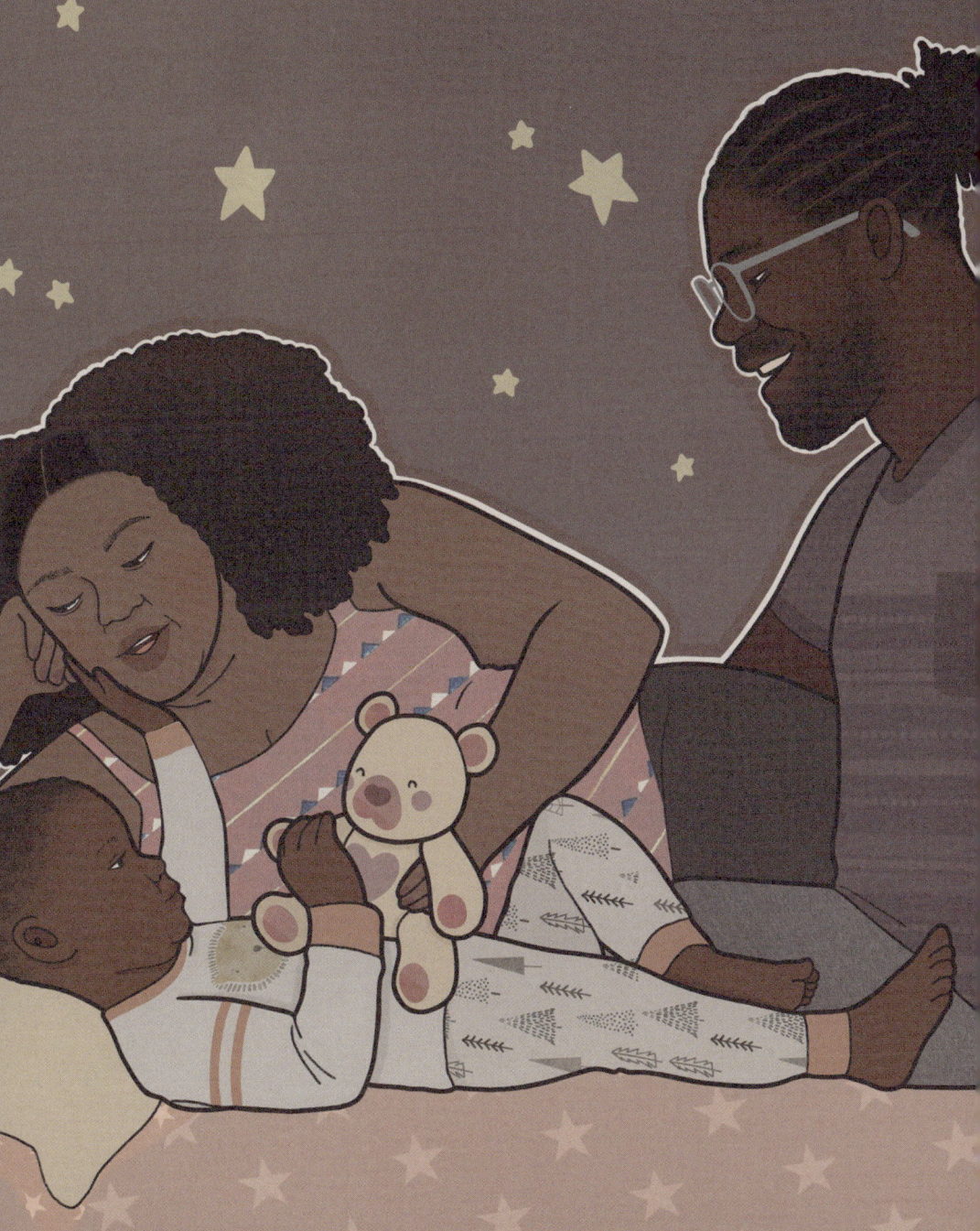

This chapter will help you navigate the practicalities and emotional aspects of ending your breastfeeding journey and hopefully help you feel more confident about making decisions around this process.

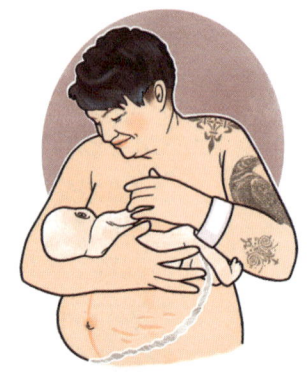

How Long Should You Breastfeed For?

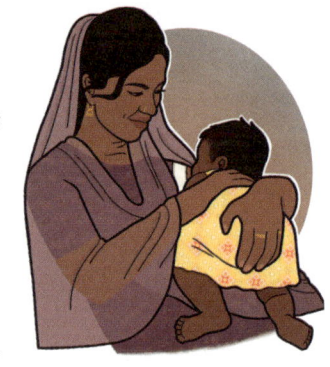

No one can answer this question for you. The World Health Organisation recommends breastfeeding exclusively for six months and then continuing to breastfeed alongside solid foods for up to two years and beyond. You can adhere to these guidelines, but you might choose to breastfeed for a shorter period. As I stated at the beginning of the book, any amount of breastfeeding you do is a good thing – whether it's a week, a month or longer. Everyone is different, has a different set of circumstances, and experiences breastfeeding and new motherhood in varying ways. You may love breastfeeding and want to breastfeed your infant until they start school or you might have more ambivalent feelings about it and be keen to wean after a few weeks or months. Whatever you decide, whatever you feel is the right decision for you, your baby and your family is valid and should be respected. It's OK to feed beyond toddlerhood and it's also okay to make a firm decision to stop breastfeeding, at any point in your breastfeeding journey!

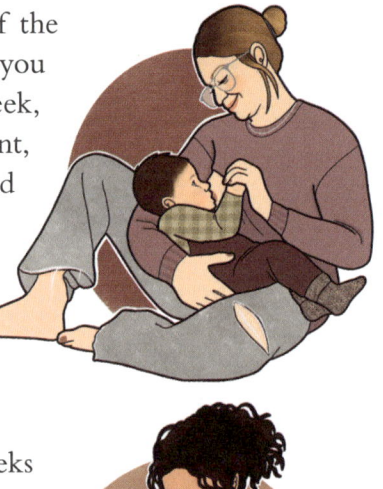

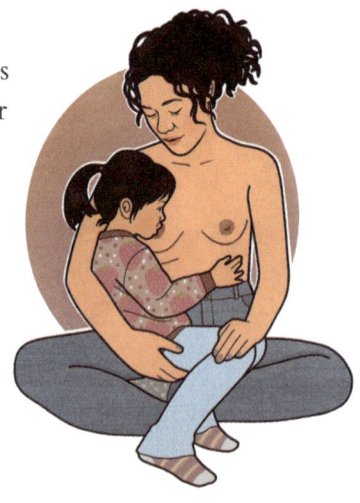

Are You Ready to Stop?

If you are thinking about stopping breastfeeding, give yourself some time to reflect on the reasons why you want to stop. You could talk it through with a friend, your partner or a breastfeeding supporter – sometimes articulating your thoughts and feelings with someone can give you greater clarity. Some people find writing things down or journalling can be a helpful way of gaining insight when they are trying to make a decision. Taking time to reflect might provide confirmation of an instinct that it's time to bring the breastfeeding chapter with your infant to an end, or it could lead to a realisation that you're not ready, or that you're still unsure. Sometimes when parents take time to reflect on stopping breastfeeding, they realise that they may be feeling pressure from family or from societal narratives about when to stop breastfeeding. Are questions from people you know about when you plan to stop breastfeeding undermining your confidence? Are you thinking about stopping because you feel you should or because you really want to? Or are you feeling like you have to? I find a common assumption that mothers make about breastfeeding is that they have to stop when they return to work. Lots of mothers return to work and find a way to continue breastfeeding. There is no one size fits all when it comes to stopping breastfeeding.

The are lots of reasons why you might want to or need to stop – wanting to get your periods back and conceive another baby, overwhelm or exhaustion, concerns about your own health (breastfeeding can be taxing for people with long-term health issues), an upcoming separation from your baby, not enjoying breastfeeding or finding it difficult, or feeling touched out breastfeeding your infant. You don't even have to have a reason. It could be a gut feeling that stopping is the right thing for you.

Give yourself latitude and time to determine when YOU want, feel and/or need to stop. If you're ready, well done on making the right decision for you and your baby. If you're not sure, give yourself more time.

You've Decided to Stop – What Now?

There are a few factors to consider once you've decided to stop breastfeeding:

- **It is a process that can take two-four weeks.**

- **Will you need to give your baby other milk?** If your baby is less than six months old, you'll need to replace breastmilk feeds with stage one infant formula. If your baby is six to twelve months old there is a little more flexibility around what milk you give them in place of breastmilk. You can give them stage one infant formula (as per national health recommendations),

  or you can give full fat cow's milk. If you give your baby cow's milk, it is important that you ensure they get sufficient iron from other food sources. If you are unsure, discuss these options with a healthcare professional.

- **Avoiding blocked ducts and mastitis** When you decide to stop breastfeeding, you need to give your body sufficient time to downregulate milk production. This means gradually doing less breastfeeding or pumping, leaving your breasts a little bit fuller than usual but also ensuring that you don't allow your breasts to become painfully engorged. This could lead to blocked ducts and/or mastitis. When your breasts are fuller for longer periods, the level of FIL (the feedback inhibitor of lactation) rises and milk production starts to slow down.

- **Ensuring your emotional well-being during and after the process** Stopping breastfeeding means a shift in levels of your breastfeeding hormones. This can result in a temporary drop in mood. If you stop breastfeeding or lactating too quickly, the drop in mood can feel quite dramatic and leave you feeling very sad. So, it's important to allow time for your hormones to settle gently and gradually.

- *Your baby* – Stopping breastfeeding will be a change for your baby too. They will adapt and the process will probably be easier on them than on you! But it could be helpful to talk them through what's happening and expect that for a time they might need some extra cuddles and reassurance. If you are stopping breastfeeding an older baby or a toddler, they may protest and struggle to understand why they can't have *boobies* or *milkies* anymore. It's important to factor their needs into your plan to stop breastfeeding and think about how the process can be made as easy as possible for them.

- *Who can support you?* Both the practical and emotional aspects to stopping breastfeeding can be difficult. Some support from your partner, friends or a breastfeeding supporter can help to get you through. For example, your partner might need to become more involved in getting your baby to sleep. And it could be helpful for them to understand how you are feeling about weaning and the potential for a temporary drop in mood.

- *When are you going to stop?* Because of the practical and emotional challenges that stopping breastfeeding can throw up, it's a good idea to pick an appropriate time to start the process. It's best to avoid times that are busy or stressful (for example, the Christmas holidays) and instead pick a time period where you don't have a whole lot going on and don't have other stresses to deal with.

Stopping Breastfeeding Your Baby At Under 6 Months

If your baby is less than six months old, try to take at least a few weeks to phase out breastfeeding and transition to formula feeding. A realistic goal is to drop one feed every few days. Head into the process with an open mind and go at your own pace. Remember, it is important to give your body the time it needs to down-regulate milk production and adjust to less breastfeeding.

Decide which feed you would like to drop first. Some mothers like to give the bottle feeds themselves, while others prefer for a partner to do them. Allow three-four days to fully replace it with a formula feed. This is how I suggest you go about it:

Day 1: Give your baby a 20-30ml formula supplement by bottle followed by a breastfeed. Your breasts might feel a little bit fuller than usual.

Day 2: Give your baby a 30-50ml formula supplement by bottle followed by a breastfeed. Again, your breasts might feel quite full. Hand express a small amount of milk for comfort if you need to.

Day 3: Give your baby a 50-70ml formula supplement followed by a breastfeed. Hand express for comfort if you need to.

Day 4: Give your baby a full replacement formula feed (depending on their age and size, that could be somewhere between 80 and 120ml). Your breasts may feel quite full but only hand express for comfort if you need to.

Once you have fully dropped one breastfeed, you could think about dropping another feed over the course of three-four days. See how you feel. The volumes and times given above are guidelines. You may need to adjust them to suit you.

What kind of bottle should you use?

There are many different brands of feeding bottle available. There is no one-size fits all. Pick one that you think might suit your baby and use an age-appropriate teat. Sometimes parents have to try a couple of different bottles or teats before they find one that they feel works well for their baby.

Try *paced bottle-feeding*. This technique lets your baby control the flow of milk. Hold the bottle relatively level with the floor so that when your baby sucks they get milk, and when they stop, milk stops flowing. Using paced bottle-feeding helps to ensure that your baby doesn't over-feed. Keep the teat in your baby's mouth for the duration of the feed, but tip milk out of the teat if they need a break.

An alternative to the approach outlined above would be to start on day one with a full replacement formula feed and pumping as much milk as you need to feel comfortable. Continue doing this for a few days, gradually pumping less and less each day until it's no longer necessary. Once you have fully replaced the breastfeed with a formula feed, you could decide to replace a second breastfeed and so on until you have completely transitioned to formula feeds.

Stopping Breastfeeding Your Baby Aged 6 Months-Plus

If your baby is between six and twelve months, you can use the approaches outlined above, but you will probably not need to do as much pumping or hand expression. Depending on the age of your baby and how well they are taking to solid foods, they may be able to take stage one infant formula in a sippy cup during the day★. Remember that milk, whether it is breastmilk or infant formula, will continue to be your baby's main source of nutrition up to twelve months. It is also important to bear in mind that your baby may still need some feeds during the night, especially up to nine months. From this point on you might be able to phase out night-time bottle-feeds. A lot depends on your baby.

Enlist the support of a partner of family member. If there are times when the process is feeling hard, it could be helpful to leave the house for a few hours and get them to care for and feed your baby. You may also need their support when it comes to bedtimes or to settling your baby. Consider how you might create new routines around sleep and bedtime, and expect that this process may take some time. During the day, distraction and keeping busy can help to divert your baby's attention from breastfeeding if they are looking for breastfeeds at times when you don't want to breastfeed.

If you are really struggling with getting your baby to sleep and nighttime waking, you could consider enlisting help from an IBCLC or an holistic sleep consultant (some IBCLCs have trained as holistic sleep consultants).

Please Note: Both the NHS and the HSE recommend stage one infant formula up to twelve months for babies who are not breastfeeding. However, the WHO states that babies older than six months can have cow's milk, if stage one formula is not available. Care should be taken to ensure they get sufficient iron from other food sources.

Stopping Breastfeeding Your Toddler

Stopping breastfeeding a toddler can be challenging, especially if your toddler is very head strong and/or has a strong emotional attachment to breastfeeding. These are tips that might help:

Talk to your toddler about your plans to stop breastfeeding. Help them understand what's going on and why for example, "You're a big kid now" or "Mum needs to go back to work" or "Mum's boobs are going to stop making milk".

Do you want to drop daytime or night-time feeds first? If you drop daytime feeds first, do it one at a time, and consider replacing the feed with something to distract your toddler, for example a trip to the playground or a meet-up with other parents and toddlers. If you would like to night-wean first, go to the next section.

Rather than saying an outright "no" when your toddler asks for a breastfeed, tell them they can have a feed "later" or "at bed-time".

Expect that the process will be difficult, and that there may be days when you feel like you are taking one step forward and two steps back. Talk to other mothers who have stopped breastfeeding toddlers and/or chat to a voluntary breastfeeding supporter.

Do something nice for yourself, for example, have a massage or a pedicure or go arrange to go the cinema. Sometimes just a few hours away from your toddler can lessen the sense of overwhelm or exhaustion.

If you have been breastfeeding your toddler to sleep, it will be helpful to change the bedtime routine and get your partner involved. Some mothers find it helps to get out for an hour in the evening while their partner puts their toddler to bed and establishes a new routine, for example, having supper, reading a bedtime story and cuddling to sleep.

It's okay to take a break. Let it go for a while – in the greater scheme of things a few weeks isn't going to make any difference.

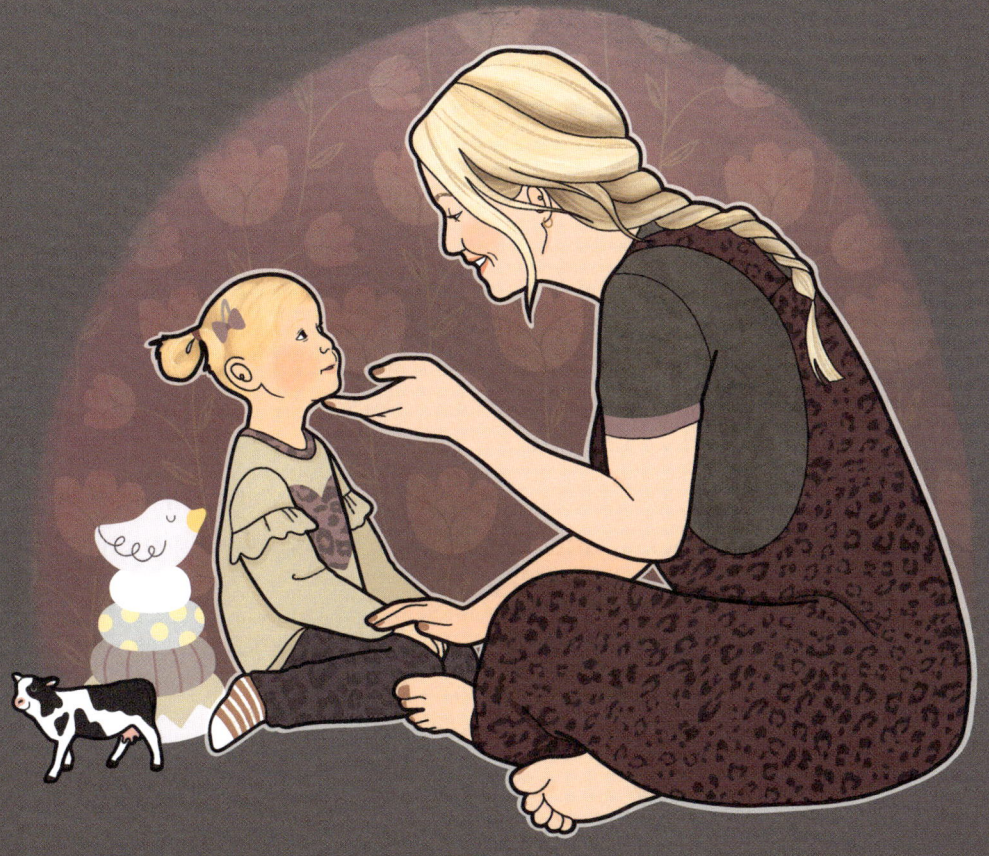

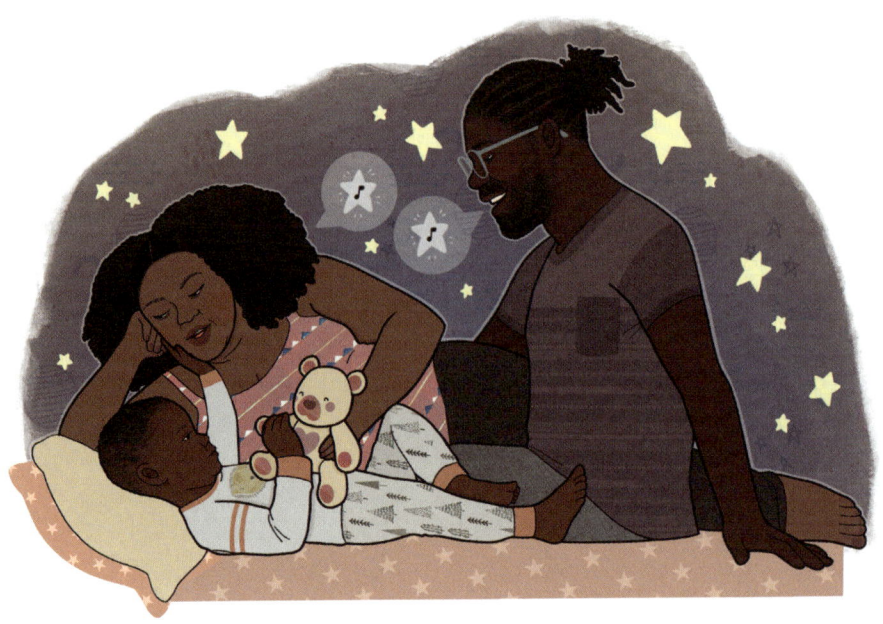

Night Weaning Your Toddler

Some parents choose to stop breastfeeding their toddler at nighttime but continue with feeds during the day. Because of the associations your toddler may have with nighttime breastfeeds – contact and cuddles with you, comfort, feeling safe – this can be a trying process, especially if your toddler is a *boobmonster*! There is no one failsafe way to night wean, but these tips might help:

Expect that it is going to be difficult. Night-time feeds are probably something that your toddler loves and derives comfort from. You're going to be taking that away from them, albeit gradually and gently. That might make them feel upset, confused and angry. These feelings will pass, and you will both find new ways to get through the night together.

Night-time weaning your toddler could mean a few difficult nights, so try and pick a suitable time when there isn't too much else going on for you or the family.

Chat to a voluntary breastfeeding counsellor or an IBCLC. They can give you emotional support and provide you with practical ideas for easing the process.

Explore other ways you can settle your toddler at night – cuddles, a favourite toy, rubbing their back, singing to them. Start introducing these other comfort measures before you start the process of night weaning. When your toddler wakes at night they are looking for reassurance – it's not about food – they need to receive the message that they are loved and they are being responded to.

Talk to your partner about how they can help. They might be able to soothe your toddler during the night.

Could you temporarily change your family's sleeping arrangements? Some parents find that having their toddler sleep in a separate bedroom with their non-nursing parent, or putting their toddler in their own room can help.

You could start by deciding to block off a chunk of time at night during which you are not going to breastfeed – for example, 12am to 4am, and then gradually extend it.

Some parents choose to go away for a couple of nights to help break the night-time feeding habits, but this may not be for everyone. A lot depends on the age of your toddler, how much they breastfeed during the night and how you feel about being apart from them for a night or two.

Some toddlers will continue to wake in the night even after they have stopped breastfeeding.

It is OK to put boundaries in place. Breastfeeding is a relationship, and it has to work for both of you. Don't let yourself guilt-trip about this!

Time for Reflection

Even if you are relieved to have stopped breastfeeding, you might also feel some sadness that this chapter with your infant has come to an end. This is very normal and it will pass. It can be helpful to focus on the positives. No matter how long you breastfed for or how much breastmilk you gave your baby, you have positively impacted

Your baby's health

Your health and well-being

Your relationship with your baby

The environment

Your community and wider society

Be proud of what you have achieved. Think of all the hours that your baby was in contact with you while feeding, and how lucky they are to have had your milk, tailor-made for them, to help them grow and develop optimally.

If you have saved some breast milk you could create a memento of your breastfeeding journey by commissioning a piece of breastmilk jewellery. Or you could frame a nice photo of you breastfeeding your baby. Acknowledge the end of breastfeeding as a milestone and congratulate yourself on every single drop of milk you've provided to your baby.

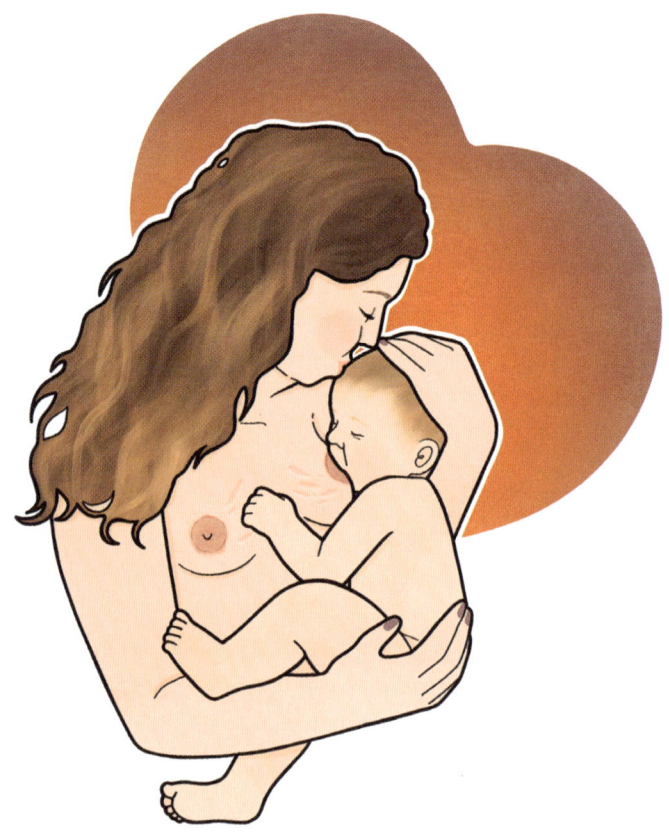

Additional Resources

BOOKS

Sleep:

Let's Talk about your Baby's Sleep, Lyndsey Hookway
Three in a Bed, Deborah Jackson
Sleeping with your Baby, James McKenna

Breastfeeding:

Breastfeeding Take Two: Successful breastfeeding the second time around, Stephanie Casemore
Breastfeeding Twins, Kathryn Stagg
Breastfeeding Without Birthing, Alyssa Schnell
Breastfeeding and Medication, Wendy Jones
Supporting the Transition from Breastfeeding: A Guide to Weaning for Professionals, Supporters and Parents, Emma Pickett
When Breastfeeding Sucks: What you need to know about nursing aversion and agitation, Zainab Yate
Making More Milk, Lisa Marasco and Diana West'
Why Infant Reflux Matters, Carol Smyth
Mother Food: Foods and Herbs that Promote Milk Production and a Mother's Health, Hilary Jacobsen
Your Baby's Bottle-feeding Aversion: Reasons and Solutions, Rowena Bennett
Where's the Mother: Stories from a Transgender Dad, Trevor McDonald

Motherhood Memoirs:

Don't Forget to Scream, Marianne Levy
Milk, Alice Kinsella
Unlatched, Jennifer Grayson
The Baby on the Fire Escape: Creativity, Motherhood, and the Mind-Baby Problem, Julie Phillips
Motherhood: On the choices of being a woman, Pragya Agarwal

Mental Health:

Inferno, Catherine Choo
Pangs: Surviving Motherhood and Mental Illness, Michelle Bradley'
Why Breastfeeding Grief and Trauma Matter, Amy Brown
Why Postnatal Depression Matters, Mia Scotland

Parenting:

What Mothers Do – especially when it looks like nothing, Naomi Stadlen
The Nurture Revolution, Greer Kirschenbaum
Our Babies Ourselves: How Culture and Biology Shape how you Parent, Meredith F. Small

Your Baby is Speaking to You, Dr Kevin Nugent
The Wonder Weeks, Hettie van de Rijt
Baby Led Weaning: The Essential Guide, Tracey Murkett and Gill Rapley

WEBSITES

Breastfeeding Support:

UK

UK National Breastfeeding Helpline
https://www.nationalbreastfeedinghelpline.org.uk
The Association of Breastfeeding Mothers https://abm.me.uk
The Breastfeeding Network https://www.breastfeedingnetwork.org.uk
La Leche League UK https://laleche.org.uk
The National Childbirth Trust UK, antenatal classes and postnatal support
https://www.nct.org.uk
The Twins Trust UK https://twinstrust.org
Lactation Consultants of Great Britain https://lcgb.org

Ireland

Friends of Breastfeeding Ireland https://www.friendsofbreastfeeding.ie/home
La Leche League Ireland https://www.lalecheleagueireland.com
Cuidiu Breastfeeding Support in Ireland https://www.cuidiu.ie
HSE Ireland Breastfeeding Support
https://www2.hse.ie/services/ask-our-breastfeeding-expert
Association of Lactation Consultants of Ireland https://www.alcireland.ie

Breastfeeding Resources:

Global Health Media – excellent videos of hand expression and baby's first
feed www.globalhealthmedia.org
Academy of Breastfeeding Medicine Protocols
https://www.bfmed.org/protocols
First Droplets website with information on hand expression
https://firstdroplets.com
Human Milk Foundation
https://humanmilkfoundation.org/hearts-milk-bank/need-support%20
Breastfeeding Medically Complex Children
https://breastfeedingthebrave.com/
Information on Breastfeeding after Breast Cancer or Breast Surgery (and more)
https://physicianguidetobreastfeeding.org
Unicef UK Breastfeeding Resources https://www.unicef.org.uk/babyfriendly/
baby-friendly-resources/breastfeeding-resources
Protocols for Inducing Lactation https://www.canadianbreastfeeding
foundation.org/induced/medical_conditions.shtml

"Breastfeeding Mums undergoing Fertility Treatment/IVF" support group
www.facebook.com/groups/bfduringivf

For Babies Born Sick or Premature
https://www.bliss.org.uk/parents/about-your-baby/feeding/breastfeeding

Eats on Feets – Community Milk Sharing Information Source:
https://www.eatsonfeets.org

Mental Health:

UK-based Peer Support for Postnatal Depression and other perinatal mental health conditions https://pandasfoundation.org.uk

Support and Advocacy for Families in the UK affected by Postpartum Psychosis https://www.app-network.org

Maternal OCD Charity https://maternalocd.org

Support for Birth Trauma https://www.birthtraumaassociation.org/home

APNI Association for Postnatal Illness https://apni.org

Irish Mental Health Charity Aware https://www.aware.ie

Support for Mothers in Ireland affected by Postnatal Depression
https://www.pnd.ie

Medications and Breastfeeding:

The Breastfeeding Network Drugs in Breastmilk Factsheets
https://www.breastfeedingnetwork.org.uk

The website of UK pharmacist Dr Wendy Jones
https://breastfeeding-and-medication.co.uk

The LactMed Drugs and Breastfeeding database
https://www.ncbi.nlm.nih.gov/books/NBK501922

The e-lactancia website to check the compatibility of drugs with breastfeeding https://www.e-lactancia.org

InfantRisk Information on Medicines and Breastfeeding
https://www.infantrisk.com

Information on medications and exposures during pregnancy and breastfeeding https://mothertobaby.org

Evidence-based information on medications and breastfeeding
www.trashthepumpanddump.org

PODCASTS

Milkshakes Podcast with Nicole Longmire
Makes Milk with Emma Pickett Podcast
Breastfeeding Outside the Box Podcast
The Bad Ass Breastfeeding Podcast
The Boobingit Podcast
Australian Breastfeeding Association Podcast
Breastfeeding Medicine Podcast
All Things Breastfeeding Podcast with Barbara Robertson

Acknowledgements

Before I start thanking the people in my life who've helped me as I was writing this book, I want like to acknowledge all of the people around the world who in various ways are helping mothers and parents meet their breastfeeding goals and are endeavouring to make the world a more breastfeeding-friendly place – voluntary counsellors, peer supporters, lactation consultants, healthcare professionals, researchers, scientists, policy makers, breastfeeding advocates, educators and journalists. Everyone has a role to play, because supporting breastfeeding is everyone's responsibility. There are so many people that I have learned from since I became a parent and started breastfeeding my first baby. I continue to learn from and be inspired by numerous experts in the field of lactation and breastfeeding and the families that I support in my work as an IBCLC. I feel immense gratitude to all of them.

The first person that I would like to say an enormous thank you to is my husband Ronan. He has always given me unconditional love and support, and never once doubted that I could see this project through (even when I didn't believe myself that the book would come to fruition). I also want to thank my children Ruairí, Lorcan and Orlagh. The taught me how to be a mother and how to breastfeed. They also helped me to understand how breastfeeding is about so much more than food – it is love, connection, and comfort.

There are a number of strong women in my life to whom I am indebted. They've given me friendship, love, encouragement and belief in myself, and they continue to do so. First and foremost is my sister Ruth Whelan. I know she is so proud of me and excited to see this book published. My cousin Sinead Andrews has always been there for me and has helped me to realise my worth and to accept myself, just the way I am. My IBCLC colleague Nicola O'Byrne, who wrote Chapter 10 on Pumps and Pumping, has encouraged me while I was writing this book. I am grateful to her for her friendship, her expertise and her wisdom. Another person who helped me through the creative process is my friend Ciara McKeown. She always understood what it meant to me to create this book and her excitement and enthusiasm for the project (discussed at length on Saturday morning walks in Marley Park) gave me so much encouragement and confidence to keep going. I am also grateful to Noelia Molina. She knew I would write a book before I did – I don't know how, but she kept the spark of the idea alight even when writing a book seemed like a pipe dream.

I am very thankful to Doreen Finn, Orla Neligan and Berni Stack for their friendship. They are women that I spend time with every week – walking the dogs, drinking coffee, laughing, crying, bemoaning the challenges of motherhood and menopause, and putting the world to rights. They've helped me to stay sane through the ups and downs of writing this book (in between work, school runs and family life).

When I completed the first draft of the book, I tentatively asked a few of my IBCLC friends to read over some chapters for me. They obliged and offered very useful insights and comments, all of which have helped to make this book better. So Naomi Hurley, Ciara Butler, Sue Jameson and Pauline McLaughlin, thank you from the bottom of my heart. Not just for reading and giving me feedback but for everything over the last number of years. For being there for me, for always being available for chats over the phone and for all you do to help and support breastfeeding families.

In my job as an IBCLC in private practice I have had the privilege of working with hundreds of families. I've learned so much from them – just as much as they have learned from me. I'm immensely grateful to them. I also owe gratitude to the women who took part in my MSc. research. They opened up their hearts to me and helped me come to understand not only the profound meaning that breastfeeding can hold for people, but also, how important it is for us as individuals to find meaning in our life experiences.

I owe a sincere thank you to Martin Hickman at Canbury Press. Within hours of emailing him our book proposal, Martin responded with such positivity and certainty, that we knew he was the publisher that we wanted to work with. I really cannot thank him enough for understanding our vision for the book and for supporting us every step of the way. I'd also like to thank the book designer Megan Sheer at

Sheer Book Design. She understood how important it was to us to create a book that was full of useful information and also beautiful to look at and we couldn't be more pleased with how it has turned out. Last but not least I want to say a heartfelt thank you to the talented illustrator who created the amazing images in this book, Lauren Rebbeck. I'm so grateful to Lauren for agreeing to accompany me on this journey and for always being so wonderful to work with. It has been a joy.

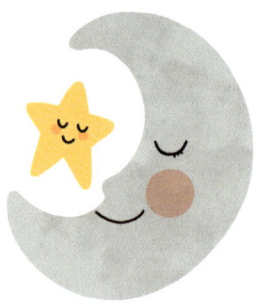